SURVIVING NURSING

SURVIVING NURSING

Emily E. M. Smythe, R.N., M.N.

THE ADDISON-WESLEY PUBLISHING COMPANY, INC.

Nursing Division • Menlo Park, California
Reading, Massachusetts • London
Amsterdam • Don Mills, Ontario • Sydney

Sponsoring editor: *Deborah Collins-Stephens*
Book designer: *Lisa S. Mirski*
Cover designer: *John Edeen*
Illustrations: *Jack Tandy*
Front cover: *Franco Grignani*
  Architetto Designer
  Milan, Italy

Library of Congress Cataloging in Publication Data
Smythe, Emily E. M., 1946.
  Surviving nursing.

  Bibliography: p.
  Includes index.
  1. Nursing—Psychological aspects.   2. Nurses—Job stress.   3. Self-care,
Health.   I.   Title.
RT86.S66 1984   610.73'019   83-22300
ISBN 0-201-16418-3
  BCDEFGHIJ-MA-8987654

Addison-Wesley Publishing Company • Nursing Division
2725 Sand Hill Road • Menlo Park, California 94025

In remembrance of my "Granny,"
BERTHA HENRY MORRISON,
who at eighty-nine years of age
remained physically active, mentally alert,
and always proud of being a nurse.

E.E.M.S.

Contributors

SHEILA K. BYRNE, RN, MN, received her AA from San Bernadino Valley College, her BS from California State University, Los Angeles, and her MN from the University of California, Los Angeles in Psychiatric/Mental Health Nursing. She is Director of the Institute for Continuing Education for Nurses, University of Southern California School of Medicine, Postgraduate Division, and a Mental Health Consultant for the Los Angeles County/USC Medical Center Department of Nursing. She has lectured on Stress Management for Nurses in Hawaii, Europe, and throughout Southern California.

JANET MUFF, RN, MSN, received her diploma in nursing from St. Vincent's College of Nursing, Los Angeles, and her BSN and MSN in Psychiatric/Mental Health Nursing from the School of Nursing, Columbia University, New York. She is currently in private practice as an individual and group psychotherapist in South Pasadena, California and does consultation and education for health-care and business organizations. She is the editor of *Socialization, Sexism, and Stereotyping: Women's Issues in Nursing*, St. Louis: C. V. Mosby Co. 1982.

JESSICA G. SCHAIRER, PhD, earned her doctorate in Clinical Psychology from the City University of New York. She is a member of the Consultation-Liaison Psychiatry Service at Kaiser Permanente's Los Angeles Medical Center where she works with the psychological problems of the medically ill, helps nurses deal with the psychological stresses of the ICU, and teaches courses in relaxation therapy and self-hypnosis. She is in private practice in West Los Angeles and Tarzana, California.

EMILY E. M. SMYTHE, RN, MN, received her AA in Liberal Arts from Colby-Sawyer College, New Hampshire, her BSN from Cornell University, New York, and her MN in Psychiatric Nursing from the University of California, Los Angeles. She is currently a Clinical Nurse Specialist of the Consultation-Liaison Psychiatry Service at Kaiser Permanente's Los Angeles Medical Center and a Mental Health Nursing Instructor at Mount St. Mary's College in Los Angeles. As a part of her private mental health nursing consultation practice, she has lectured on Stress Management for Nurses in Hawaii, Europe, and throughout Southern California.

JEFFREY STOLROW, MS, received a BA in Psychology (Phi Beta Kappa) and a MS in Educational Psychology from the University of Southern California. Currently he is the Director of Stress-Management Services at Kaiser Permanente in Orange County and an Adjunct Professor at the University of Southern California, Department of Counselor Education, teaching Stress Management. Since 1975 he has been conducting research on the clinical application of biofeedback with stress management. He is an APA supervisor and lecturer on stress management and biofeedback.

MICHAEL Z. WINCOR, Pharm D, received his BS in Zoology from the University of Chicago and his Pharm D and Residency Certificate in Psychopharmacy from the University of Southern California. He is currently an Assistant Professor at the University of Southern California School of Pharmacy and a Psychiatric Pharmacist at Kaiser Mental Health Center in Los Angeles. His research interests are in sleep and sleep disorders; he has written a number of book chapters and articles for professional journals. Both governmental and private organizations throughout the United States have called on him as a consultant and lecturer in clinical psychopharmacology.

Preface

This manual was written for every nurse who is having difficulty coping with her or his job. It is the only manual available that offers effective coping strategies specifically aimed at dealing with the many stressors inherent in the nursing profession. It will teach you how stress can be controlled and minimized. This manual will also enable you, the nurse, to recognize stress and to control its manifestations, such as discouragement, disenchantment, anger, depression, stress-related illnesses, and even abandonment of the nursing profession.

This manual speaks directly to you, engaging you in self exploration through the use of numerous exercises, activities, and self-assessment tools. These tools will increase your self-awareness of stressors, personal dynamics, and stress responses. It gives a concise overview of stress-management theory as this theory relates to the nursing profession. It describes, in simple terms, how you can make better use of your clinical skills by reducing your susceptibility to stressors. Stress reduction can also lead to increased active participation in creative problem-solving. The ability to cope with stress can positively influence one's nursing practice, health, and sense of well-being.

The logical place to begin managing stress is within your "self"—that is, as an individual nurse. Your lifetime of experiences colors your perception of events and determines whether or not you perceive a given event as distressing. Stress is a highly personal experience. Therefore, the causes and reactions to stress are individual and must be handled individually. This manual allows you to determine your own weaknesses in stress management and gives you the tools to create your own, personally tailored stress-management program.

Each exercise and activity for learning stress intervention describes the principles and theoretical concepts on which the exercise or activity is based. In-depth coverage (including relevant supporting research) is presented to provide you with the knowledge to understand why the intervention works and how it can be altered to fit your particular needs. Detailed instructions for each intervention activity are given, along with suggestions for applications in typical nursing settings. Ideally, you should practice each approach until you are familiar with it and are able to decide if it has value for you. Then you should incorporate your chosen approaches into a stress-management program.

Because this how-to manual endorses a lifelong stress-management process, an extensive, annotated bibliography and resource section is provided to assist you in your continued growth and self-exploration.

Knowing how to provide patient care is not enough; nurses must be able to manage job stressors in order to do their best. They need to learn how to care for themselves in order to effectively care for their patients. The energy that is squandered on coping with stress can be put to better use. With this newly channeled energy, you can manage stress, improve your life, and also improve the health care system and the profession of nursing.

Acknowledgments

Few books come into being without the efforts of many people who share a belief in the importance of the topic and who are willing to struggle together to create the finished product. There are many unnamed friends and co-workers whom I appreciate for all the encouragement, resources, and personal insights they willingly shared.

All of my contributors, besides being friends, made essential additions to the book. Ann Ludwig, freelance developmental editor, provided invaluable assistance by offering the infinite wisdom of an experienced editor. It is impossible to imagine how any book is written without the help of someone like her. My typists, Cindy Chumley and Jill Fortham, met all their deadlines despite numerous other commitments. The limitless enthusiasm of several people from Addision-Wesley—Tom Eoyang, Editor; Elaine Henderson, Assistant Editor; Pat Waldo, Special Projects Manager; and Deborah Collins-Stephens, Sponsoring Editor—and their watchfulness for pertinent books or articles greatly enhanced the writing process.

Many reviewers provided critical insights that helped with the development of this book, particularly Ann Baldwin, Carolyn Kaiser, and Rosemarie Scully. I would also like to thank Jerrie Allison-Melton, Elizabeth Braun, Phyllis Burton, Karen Lee Fontaine, Marjorie A. Habeeb, Carol Ren Kneisl, and Jo Anne Powell.

My husband, Michael, in addition to coauthoring two chapters, at times was the only person who kept the book alive; he maintained his confidence in me and offered continual encouragement. We shared hours reading each chapter and clarifying ideas.

Most of all, my appreciation and unconditional love go to my daughter, Meghan, who adds immeasurable joy and meaning to my life.

Emily E. M. Smythe

Contents

PART 6   STRESS REDUCTION TECHNIQUES / 260

SURVIVING NURSING

1

The Effect of Stress Upon the Nurse's Sense of Well-being

Nursing takes place in a stressful environment. We have little direct control over many of the stressors that affect our job satisfaction and sense of well-being. We only have real control over ourselves and over how we allow events to affect us. Yet taking control of our lives and caring for our "selves" are acquired skills that we must learn.

If we acknowledge current problems in nursing while accepting personal responsibility for managing our individual stress levels, we will grow through learning how to cope with stress. We may also be able to tackle professional problems and the problems of health care systems that contribute to the stress of nursing.

I hope that the present crisis will provide us with the opportunity to redefine what nursing is. It will if we maintain worthwhile values and services while discarding the useless rituals, positions of subservience, and outmoded functions that have made nursing a less desirable profession.

We may, however, choose to ignore current problems or spend our energy casting blame on others and continue to experience high levels of stress. We may simply go through the motions of a job with which we are dissatisfied and then become early retirees from it. We make personal choices that ultimately determine how we experience our jobs—as opportunities for personal growth and challenge or as sources of distress and dissatisfaction. We need to learn to make stress work for instead of against us.

To gain personal control over our stress, we must understand the general dynamics of stress and the factors in the nursing profession and the health care system that contribute to our job stress. We need to explore how unsuccessful adaptation to stress affects people in order to recognize characteristics of negative response to stress.

This first section examines what stress is and where stress and the negative responses to it originate in nursing.

CHAPTER 1

Stress and the Nurse

MICHAEL Z. WINCOR AND EMILY E. M. SMYTHE

Until recently, there was, unfortunately, a conspiracy of silence regarding stress in nursing. It was almost as if we said, "Ignore it. It'll go away." But the stress remains.

When you discuss problems that you believe contribute to job stress in nursing, some nurses may angrily respond, "Nursing is a worthwhile profession. There is nothing wrong with nursing; the problem is you—your bad attitude and your unwillingness to work." Others may tell you, "It's time to stop talking about the problems in nursing! The real problem is with health care and administrators that produce stress in nursing." Discussing job stress in nursing and its contributing factors should not start a battle with opposing sides attacking and defending the profession, nor should it develop into a struggle to place blame.

INDICATIONS OF STRESS IN NURSING

Statistics show that nursing is a stressful occupation. One study, in which 130 occupations were ranked according to their level of stress, showed that practical and vocational nurses ranked third, nurses aides ranked tenth, and registered nurses ranked seventh—all extremely high (Ivancerich and Matteson, 1980).

Signs of our stress-related problems are everywhere. Recently, some hospitals closed units because of staff shortages. Others had to reduce the nursing care provided to all but essential life-supporting tasks and functions. Some hospitals even had to rely on as much as 60% registry personnel to meet their need for nurses.

Many people believe that simply increasing the number of schools of nursing will solve this apparent nursing shortage. Ironically, however, there are, at present, enough registered nurses to fill all the vacant nursing positions. The real problem is not a lack of qualified nurses; it is a lack of qualified nurses who want to work. Of the 1.4 million registered nurses in the United States, only two-thirds are working. Of the two-thirds, many are part-time or per diem staff (Sullivan, 1981). In other words, at least one out of every three nurses drops out of nursing at some point in her or his career (Hallas, 1980).

Though some have become inactive for various personal reasons unrelated to job stress, these reasons alone do not explain the annual turnover rate of approximately 30% that occurs in some hospitals. Unless the reason for these high drop-out and turnover rates is due to professional restlessness in nursing, many of us seem dissatisfied with our jobs.

Not only are there high drop-out and turnover rates in nursing, but there is also a decline in nursing school enrollments. According to the American Nurses' Association (ANA), nursing student enrollment declined by 30,000 from 1980 to 1981. In the last five years, enrollment has reportedly dropped 1%–2% annually (Green, 1981). Some experts believe the enrollment decline reflects the impact of the women's movement. Since 96% of all nurses are women, the women's movement naturally has had an impact on the nursing profession. Women now have increased opportunities to enter occupations previously restricted to men. Women are now taking a critical look at nursing and many are choosing occupations with better working conditions, greater social status, and more pay.

Nurses are therefore working in a stressful occupation that is not only attracting fewer members into its ranks but is unable to retain those who have received training. "Reality shock" and burnout are problems closely identified with nursing. There is absolutely no question that all of us, in one way or another, are aware of and affected by the stressors within nursing.

What causes qualified nurses to leave nursing? They are leaving not only to become housewives and mothers or to retire, but because the demands of nursing are so great that many of us are simply not able to survive in our chosen occupation. There are a great number of dissatisifed nurses—some who no longer work and others who work but do not enjoy their jobs.

When nurses are asked why they leave nursing or what they find stressful in their jobs, the majority emphasize stressors in the work environment or the nursing profession. For example, in one study of 1,800 ICU nurses (Bailey, 1980), the following situations were identified as particularly stressful:

- Conflict with other health care providers
- Inadequate staffing patterns
- Lack of support in dealing with death and dying
- Inadequate work space and other inadequate factors in the physical work environment
- Unresponsive nursing leadership

A survey conducted by *RN* magazine entitled "Why Nurses Are Giving It Up" identified the following three main problems:

- Inadequate staffing
- Poor communication among staff
- Poor administration

In this survey, dropouts who responded identified their number one reason for leaving as "steadily diminishing patient contact due to an increase in other work demands" (Hallas, 1980).

Participants in stress management workshops I have conducted over the last five years have identified many additional environmental and professional stressors. They cited everything from unappreciative patients, disruptive family members, and inconsiderate, rude, or abusive physicians to inadequate parking, food services, and lounges as stress inducing.

In all of these identified causes of our job stress, we see the sources outside ourselves—as coming from our work environment or the nursing profession in general. Few of us relate the causes of our job stress to personal problems, for example, difficulty being assertive or having unreasonable expectations and quick tempers. More importantly, few of us relate our difficulties to our inability to cope with predictable job stresses, many of which are not unique to nursing.

The truth is that the source of our stress is not simply one or the other—the system or ourselves. The stress each of us experiences comes from an interaction between our "self" and the system within which we work. Stress-producing problems in the health care system and the practice of nursing are complex and diverse. Although many of these problems are beyond our immediate control, we allow them to affect how we feel about our jobs.

Certainly some major changes need to occur in health-care settings, in the health-care system, and in the nursing profession. In some places the work conditions are so poor that the hospital should be forced to post signs saying, "Working here is hazardous to your health." The nursing shortage is so severe in many hospitals that it would be difficult to prove that any nurse could safely practice nursing—many are playing a sort of Russian roulette with their nursing licenses and patients' lives.

Despite the existence of these system- and profession-generated pressures, we nurses must begin to take care of ourselves by learning how to cope with job stress—regardless of its origin; otherwise we will not be effective agents of change. Too many of us are so exhausted from the day-to-day struggle on our jobs that we have no energy left to become involved in making constructive changes. The types of changes that need to occur require energy and commitment. Our first priority should be to learn how to take care of ourselves. Only then can we tackle the problems of the system or the profession. If we are so exhausted we can barely drag our tired bones home after work, I doubt we will be able to do much creative problem solving. Most approaches to systems change that I am familiar with require level-headed problem-solving techniques, but it is next to impossible to think clearly when you are over-stressed.

The issue, therefore, is not how to avoid stressors but how to learn to cope with them and to maintain a reasonable level of job satisfaction. When we accomplish this, stressors become challenges rather that defeats.

WHAT IS STRESS?

Stress is becoming one of the most overused and misused words in America. Every time you pick up a magazine or listen to a talk show, it seems there is a discussion on stress—the stress of parenting, of overeating, of bad economic times, of discrimination—in fact, the stress of everything and anything. We are experiencing a stress epidemic. But what exactly is stress?

Hans Selye, the father of stress research, has defined stress as follows:

> . . . the non-specific response of the body to any demand made upon it. . . . All agents to which we are exposed produce a non-specific increase in the need to perform adaptive functions and thereby to reestablish normalcy. . . . It is immaterial whether the agent or situation we face is pleasant or unpleasant; all that counts is the intensity of the demand for readjustment or adaptation (Selye, 1974).

Part of what is confusing about the word *stress* is that we use it to describe the things that upset us, which are more correctly called *stressors,* and to describe our response to the things that upset us. In the case of using stress to describe stressors, we might say, "There's a lot of stress in my job." In describing stress as a reaction we would say "I'm really stressed because of my job." In correct usage, the term *stress* describes a physiologic response that occurs, regardless of whether the feelings we have are pleasant or unpleasant and irrespective of whether the stressors producing our distress are pleasant or unpleasant.

Fight-or-Flight Response

Let's take a nursing situation to illustrate physiologic stress response. As you walk to your patient's room, he begins to scream at you, "You're the worst nurse in this place. I don't have to take this kind of treatment. I don't plan to either! Get the supervisor." Immediately your body begins to respond to his accusation by going into a state of alarm. Your heart starts pounding faster, your breathing becomes more rapid, your pupils dilate, your mouth becomes dry, your hands become cold, and you begin to sweat; your muscle tone increases and your throat begins to feel tighter. In this example of unpleasant stress, you experience what is called the fight-or-flight response. The idea of picking up the bed tray and clobbering this hostile patient might cross your mind, or you might consider running out of his room and never returning. Because of social decorum and your educational training, you will probably do neither; instead you will begin reasoning out the situation while your body is literally stewing in its own adaptive juices (see Figure 1-1).

Cannon first described this fight-or-flight response in *The Wisdom of the Body* in 1932. He believed this response was part of a homeostatic regulatory mechanism to provide the body with the adaptive energy it needed to deal with situations that threatened the individual's survival (Cannon, 1932). The fight-or-flight response prepared primitive human beings to attack the threat or to flee from it as their only means of survival. This all-out gearing up of the body is anachronistic, since in our society it is no longer acceptable to discharge our adaptive energy by fighting or taking flight. We are thus left with a mechanism that prepares our bodies for action that never occurs—similar to revving up a car engine as high as it can go but keeping the car in neutral.

Interestingly enough, you would experience the same *physical* reactions if, instead of being confronted with an attacking patient, you were given a greatly deserved promotion. Your body would again make the same adaptive response, except that, in this situation, your subjective emotional evaluation would cause you to feel happy and excited instead of angry and excited.

Eustress/Distress

Selye has suggested using the term *eustress* to describe "good" stress that we experience as positive or pleasant, such as being promoted, preparing for competitive sports, or making love. The term distress more accurately describes the unpleasant or "bad" stress we experience, such as when coping with a screaming patient, a cardiac arrest, or with other frustrating situations (Selye, 1978). Any situation or event then can cause us to be stressed if we perceive it as a change that requires us to adapt or adjust.

You can even experience this fight-or-flight response simply by *describing* an upsetting event to another person long after it actually occurred. Or you can experience the stress response when you anticipate doing something you *imagine* will be upsetting to you. In fact, most of the distress experienced in modern times is psychologically induced rather than

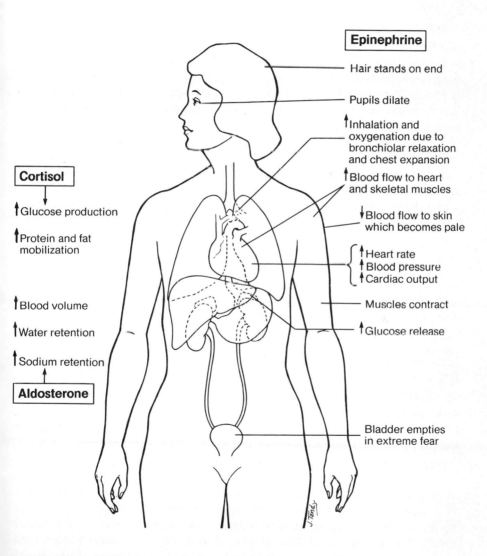

FIGURE 1-1.

Physical manifestations of the fight-or-flight response.

caused by actual physical events. These mental stressors tend to linger long after real stimuli disappear. For example, if someone is angry with you because of something you have done, this will cause you stress. However, by worrying about their reaction, you create additional distress for yourself, which is harder to dissipate. Many real external stressors cannot be avoided, but you can avoid and control the self-induced ones.

Stressors

The stress-producing factors, or stressors, that initiate the stress response can come from many sources. Stressors can be internally or externally generated, positive or negative events, or real or imagined situations. Regardless of their nature, they induce stress by demanding that we adapt to stress. The physiologic response that our body makes is identical to that of our primitive ancestors and also to the response of animals when they are threatened or excited.

Probably the most harmful external stressors are chronic, ongoing conditions that appear to have no direct resolution. When we experience these continual demands, it seems impossible to neutralize our psychophysiologic systems, and we are left in a constant state of "red alert," prepared for action that never comes. The stressors that are specific to the nursing profession are discussed in detail in Chapter 2, "Origins of Stress in Nursing."

NEUROENDOCRINE RESPONSE TO STRESS

What happens in our bodies to cause the characteristic physiologic changes known as the "fight-or-flight" response? The neuroendocrine processes involved are complex. For the purpose of this discussion, we will take the liberty of oversimplifying to some extent. Much of the response is mediated by the hypothalamus—a part of our "primitive brain"—that receives output from the reticular activating system as well as from higher (evolutionarily speaking) brain structures, that is, the limbic system and cerebral cortex.

The adrenal glands are set into motion by the hypothalamus in two ways. The hypothalamus produces a releasing factor that, in turn, increases pituitary secretion of adrenocorticotropic hormone (ACTH). ACTH circulates through the bloodstream to the adrenal cortex—the outer layer of the adrenal gland—where it increases the secretion of corticosteroids (primarily cortisol and aldosterone). The acute effects of increased cortisol include dramatically increasing glucose production for energy needs and mobilizing proteins and fats in the blood. The increased aldosterone causes sodium retention, which increases water retention and blood volume.

The hypothalamus also has direct connections with the adrenal medulla—the central portion of the adrenal gland—via the sympathetic nervous system. Following stimulation of the hypothalamus, nervous impulses along these pathways result in immediate release of epinephrine (also known as adrenalin) from the medulla. Beyond causing an increased heart rate, epinephrine, combined with the aldosterone-induced increase in blood volume, increases blood pressure and cardiac output. In addition, the pupils of the eyes dilate, improving visual sensitivity; muscles contract; the liver releases more glucose to serve as fuel; the volume of inhaled air and available oxygen increases as bronchioles relax; blood is shunted to vital organs, such as the heart and skeletal muscles, and away from less essential areas, such as the skin surface (hence the skin becomes pale). If the skin is broken, blood coagulation occurs more rapidly to prevent severe loss, hair stands on end, and, in extreme cases, the bladder empties. (Hence the expression, "I just about wet my pants.")

These responses, with the exception of the piloerection and bladder emptying, can be of great survival value when one is attacked in the wild or in a dark alley in a big city. However, in more civilized settings such as the professional environment, where you may not have the option to fight or flee, this physiologic turmoil, especially if chronic and not dissipated, may be severely detrimental to your continued existence (see Figure 1-2).

Stress-Related Disorders

Selye described the stress response as a three-stage process called the *general adaptation syndrome* (Selye, 1978). The three stages include (1) the alarm reaction, (2) resistance, and (3) exhaustion. The alarm reaction stage is characterized by the generalized stress arousal described previously. During the resistance stage, the stress response is channeled into the organ system most capable of dealing with it. In the exhaustion phase, the organ system coping with the stress breaks down, the alarm reaction stage appears to repeat itself, and resistance shifts to a stronger system. This process of adaptation, involving as it does different body systems, is what many contend is a major contribution to stress-related disorders.

If muscles are the organ system affected, we may experience headaches, backaches, or generalized "muscle tension." Respiratory disorders (asthma, for example) may be exacerbated. If the gastrointestinal system is involved, we may experience anorexia, nausea, "heartburn," diarrhea, constipation, or even ulcer disease. Chronic stress may contribute to cardiovascular disease— hypertension and related renal problems, vascular headaches, arteriosclerosis, and myocardial infarction. If the immune response is compromised, we may be more vulnerable to infection and perhaps even to cancer. If innate inflammatory processes are affected, we may be at greater risk for rheumatoid arthritis.

There is mounting evidence that chronic, undissipated stress can be at least a contributing factor to each of the just mentioned disorders. Each of these disorders most likely is a product of complex interactions involving environment (for example, external events, social interactions, and stim-

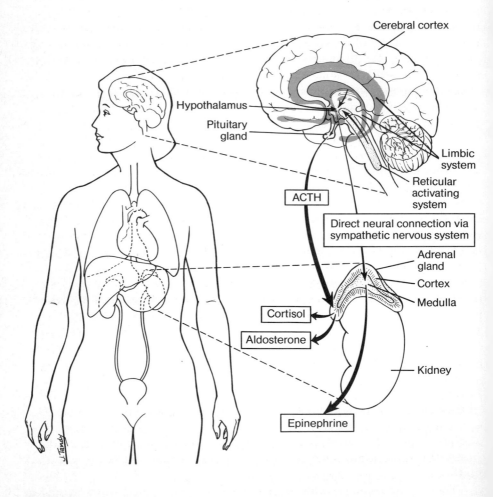

FIGURE 1-2.

Neuroendocrinologic scheme of the fight-or-flight response.

uli), internal perceptions that may be a product of personality style as well as genetic determinants, and the interaction of primitive brain structures with more advanced, civilized brain functions. We should not be too surprised if, in the not too distant future, we receive a warning from the surgeon general that it "has been determined that stress may be dangerous to your health."

CONCLUSION

Stress is not something that can be totally avoided. The only time you are really free from stress is when you are dead! What we can avoid is the negative response to stress—distress. The process of adapting to demands—pleasant or unpleasant—occurs constantly. Stress becomes a problem when the demands are so intense and so prolonged that we are unable to meet them.

Few events are inherently stressful. We largely create stress in situations by the way we evaluate and interpret events. Each person's response depends on his or her personality make-up and personal conditioning factors. Whether or not a stressor is experienced as distress depends on our perception of that stressor. If we interpret a stressor as desirable or pleasant, then the good stress we experience passes quickly, and our bodies quickly return to the balanced state of equilibrium.

We can also block our perception of an event so that there is little, if any, physical arousal (Lazarus, 1976). The reverse is also true: our minds can create a disaster out of a small event. For example, the stress-prone individual can interpret a supervisor's frown as an attack. We are all familiar with people who "create mountains out of molehills." Some individuals seem to be supersensitive to any change or demand that occurs to them, whereas other individuals appear to handle overwhelmingly stressful situations masterfully without even becoming upset or aroused. Though the stress response is universal, what we perceive as stressful and whether it becomes destructive to us are largely individual matters that can be altered by each of us for better or worse. We can learn to avoid stressors that needlessly tax us and enhance our relaxation response to avoid the pitfalls of overreacting to stressors.

Stress is not destructive in and of itself. It is what we do with it that can be destructive and unpleasant. Stress is a normal by-product of growth and progress. Part of living is a constant struggle to improve the quality of life and undo the multitude of wrongs that seem to occur on a daily basis. From the beginning of time, each generation has confronted its own stresses and disasters. Stress is an inescapable and accepted part of the human condition. If there were no stress, there would be no need or motivation to grow. Too little stress leads to boredom and disinterest. The

"Thinking Your Way Out of Distress" and "Stress Reduction Techniques" sections of this book explore further the conditioning factors that influence our stress response.

Stress also has a positive side to it. Selye has referred to stress as the spice of life—too little and your life is tasteless and bland; too much and you are overwhelmed.

Selye also uses the analogy of a "race horse and a turtle" to demonstrate the importance of recognizing your level of stress tolerance. There are race horses who thrive on stress and are only happy with a vigorous, fast-paced life style and turtles, who, in order to be happy, require peace, quiet, and a generally tranquil environment, which would frustrate and bore most race horse types (Selye, 1978). Which are you?

We need the adaptive energy of stress to stimulate the personal growth that will enable us to meet the unending demands of our society and environment. Stress cannot be totally avoided—nor would you want to totally avoid it. Just because stress is a part of living, you do not need to live with every stressor that confronts you. If there are stressors you can avoid, by all means do not subject yourself to them. "An ounce of prevention is worth a pound of cure." Although stress is a part of life, distress does not have to be. Stress and change are inescapable events in all our lives. We need to make stress work for us rather than against us.

REFERENCES

Bailey, J. T., Steffen, S. M., and Grant, J. W. 1980. Stress audit of 1,800 ICU nurses. *J. Nurse Ed.* June 19(6):25.

Cannon, W. B. 1932. *The wisdom of the body*. New York: W. W. Norton.

Green, L. 1981. Nurse recruitment at fever pitch. *Los Angeles Times*, 17 May, p. 5.

Hallas, G. 1980. Why nurses are giving it up. *RN* 43:17–21.

Ivancerich, J. M., and Matteson, M. T. 1980. Nurse and stress: time to examine the potential problems. *Superv. Nurse* 11:17–20.

Lazarus, R. 1976. *Patterns of adjustment*. New York: McGraw-Hill.

Selye, H. 1974. *Stress without distress*. Philadelphia: J. B. Lippincott.

Selye, H. 1978. On the real benefits of eustress (interview by Laurence Cherry). *Psychol. Today* 11(10):60–70.

Selye, H. 1978. *The stress of life*. New York: McGraw-Hill.

Sullivan, R. 1981. Nurse scarcity forces cut in care in New York municipal hospitals. *New York Times*, 6 August, p. B-6.

CHAPTER 2

Origins of Stress in Nursing

JANET MUFF

"How can you work with kids who have cancer?"
"How can you work 12-hour shifts?
You must get exhausted!"
"How can you stand there so calmly
while Dr. Smith is yelling his head off?"
"How can you get up and talk in front of
200 people?"

There is much evidence to indicate that nurses, individually and collectively, perceive nursing as stressful. Newspaper headlines proclaim the nursing "shortage"; vacancy rates for nursing positions soar (Mullner et al., 1982); statistics indicate that nearly one-third of all registered nurses are not working (Hallas, 1980); and among working nurses, only a small percentage are "very satisfied" with their jobs.* Nursing is indeed stressful, but what is stressful for one person may not be stressful for another. In fact, one nurse's stress may be another's challenge. Perception, or how the nurse sees a situation and her or his role, is the key (Claus, 1980; Seliger, 1982). Stress and one's response to it are individual phenomena. External factors may create an environment conducive to stress, but it is the individual with his or her unique personal history and personality structure who experiences certain events as stressful.

Nurses often attribute stress to the nature of the job, to organizational factors, and to interpersonal conflict. They discuss these things among themselves, they write about them—in short, they understand them. But what is less easily recognized and understood is that a nurse's perception of these factors as stressful is based on her or his frame of reference. What *is* a nurse's frame of reference? That she is (most likely) a woman, that she is a nurse, and that she has a role in whatever setting she works. These concepts of self and role come from socialization, both individual and professional.

Ninety-six percent of nurses are women and, as such, they experience stresses common to all women in our society. In addition to these, nurses experience stressors related to the fact that nursing is traditionally a "woman's job" in a traditionally "man's world." This chapter, then, concerns the contextual stressors in nursing (nature of the job, organizational factors, and interpersonal conflict) but also gives considerable weight to their antecedents—individual (female) socialization and professional socialization—the learning processes that determine a nurse's perception that such factors are stressful.

CONTEXTUAL STRESSES

Most nurses describe stress as coming from the nature of the job, organizational issues, and interpersonal conflicts. Whereas socialization and

---

*A study of vacancy rates (nursing vacancies per 100 beds) in 4,022 community hospitals nationwide indicated that 37.4% of hospitals had a vacancy rate of 10.0 or higher and 35% had a vacancy rate of 0.1–9.9 (Mullner et al., 1982).

Increased demands placed on nurses and decreased contact with patients were cited as major stressors for practicing nurses (67%) and dropouts (33%) in a survey of Florida nurses (Hallas, 1980).

A survey of 1,051 nurses across the country found that 10.8% of nurses were "very" satisfied, 54% were "fairly" satisfied, and 35.1% were "somewhat" and "not" satisfied.

identity issues produce stress in subtle ways over time, the stresses of understaffing or poor working environments are immediately apparent.

The Nature of the Job

Because of the kind of work they do, nurses have been identified as a population at risk for high stress and burnout (Anderson, et al., 1981; Garfield, 1980; Patrick, 1979; Storlie, 1979). Chronic exposure to pain, suffering, death, and hopelessness increases nurses' vulnerability. Even in areas where patients may not be critically ill, the work is fast paced. Nurses have many decisions to make and daily crises to handle. The environment itself, whether noisy, drafty, hot, cold, or poorly laid out, may contribute to nursing stress.

In addition to patient and environmental factors, workload is described by nurses as a major source of stress (workload meaning not only the amount but the degree of job difficulty). Included in this catchall phrase are the following:

- 24-hour patient care responsibility
- 24-hour nursing coverage responsibility
- Chronic short staffing or high patient-nurse ratios
- Necessity for floating to other than regularly assigned units
- Necessity for rotating shifts
- Perceived barriers to efficiency (unnecessary rules and regulations, unnecessary paperwork and other work, more and longer meetings, inefficient systems for processing patients, resources, and/or information)
- Absence of sanctioned "time-outs"

In a study of burnout among nurses, Pines and Kanner (1982) examined the presence of negative conditions and the absence of positive conditions. They found nurses usually expected negative conditions—daily confrontation with death, large patient loads, and time pressures—and could handle them. The absence of positive factors—challenge, variety, appreciation, sense of significance, and good interpersonal relations—was more distressing. In short, nurses experience disappointment, frustration, and stress not so much from the nature of the job as from the lack of personal growth and satisfaction.

Organizational Issues

Nurses (and departments of nursing) do not exist in a vacuum. System needs and values often determine the nature of the job, which in turn reflects system problems. Nursing is stressful because nurses often have little control over nursing, patient management, the environment, or the system (Daley, 1979; Pines and Maslach, 1978). Historically, as we have seen, the origins of nurses' lack of control have been their dependent relationships in the hospital and medical hierarchies, a result of socialized and institutionalized paternalism. Consider, for a moment, the status (or lack of status) of nursing reflected in the following examples:

- Among the hospital triumvirate—administration, medicine, and nursing—only nursing does not report directly to hospital boards of directors in most institutions.
- The medical staff bylaws determine many hospital- and patient-related policies and procedures. The work is done in medical staff committees from which nurses are often excluded entirely, and certainly as voting members.
- Nursing care is not valued as highly as other services. It is not reflected in the patient's bill but is generally subsumed under room rate charges.

How can nurses have forgotten the lethality of "legislation without representation?" Having representation and being heard are important, but having a vote is more important. Suffrage is essential to self-determination. How can nurses have ignored the importance in today's business world of the "bottom line"—money? For nursing departments to have political clout, they must first have financial clout. To have financial clout, they must generate revenue. To generate revenue, they must charge for their services. Consider the clout of high-revenue-producing departments such as pharmacy, laboratory, and radiology. Given the increasing fiscal constraints upon hospitals, those who contribute to the wealth will have greatest say in its distribution.

Nursing's lack of control over practice, then, stems from lack of formal representation and failure to demonstrate revenue generated. Such antecedents, however, seem of little importance to the staff nurse faced with a shortage of trained personnel. To her or him, lack of control means lack of control over the immediately stressful situation—the patient, the workload, and/or the environment. On a somewhat broader scale, nurses at all levels experience stress when they are given responsibility without authority, resources, or commensurate rewards, when they cannot manage their own time but must conform to the schedules of others, and when they are expected to perform non-nursing functions routinely or to assume the work of others who are absent (Veninga, 1979). When describing stressors, nurses cite workload, environment, and other factors, but it is not these things in themselves that are stressful—it is the nurse's perceived inability to control or alter them.

Interpersonal Issues

Although the nature of the job and organizational factors are the most frequently cited sources of stress in nursing, interpersonal difficulties are often more personal and painful. Interpersonal issues, as I define them, are broad (the way the system views individuals) and narrow (the way two individuals interact). Broadly interpreted, then, any philosophy, spoken or unspoken, of the organization may contribute to stress. For example, an organization that values homogeneity rather than heterogeneity and that curbs creativity and independent thinking may be stressful for certain individuals. Another organization that values physicians more than other workers creates stress in those who are valued less, simply *because* they are less valued and also because they are not supported in conflicts with physicians. Yet another, rarely admitted, philosophy is adherence to crisis management rather than long-range planning. Again, individuals in such a system succumb to the capricious whims of the system and have little control over their work. These individuals often experience stress.

The rules, spoken and unspoken, that affect interdepartmental relations can also generate conflict and stress. For example, the shortage of nurses has led to intensified recruitment efforts in many hospitals. Other departments then perceive nurses as "getting all the goodies" and become jealous. Siblinglike rivalry develops, and non-nursing personnel thwart nursing goals in numerous indirect and covert ways. The process is often unconscious. Nurses are oblivious to the power others perceive them to have and experience only an inability to get the job done—supplies arrive via the "slow boat," vital information gets lost in transition, other departments do not cooperate. The simplest task assumes insurmountable proportions, and the nurse feels stress. On the other hand, nurses may view other fair-haired (read revenue-producing) departments as getting all the goodies; the jealousy thus engendered is stressful.

Much has been written about conflicts between physicians and nurses. Such conflicts are related to historical antecedents, power and status inequities between medicine and nursing, mutual lack of knowledge and respect, and individual personality differences. Despite the many analyses of the problem, however, conflict with physicians continues to be a major source of stress for some nurses.

Less well documented, but equally destructive, are conflicts among nurses. At the organizational level, conflict among nurses can be seen in vertical and horizontal dimensions. Vertical conflicts, for example, occur between staff nurses and supervisors. Some may be related to personality differences, others to the staff nurse's limited view of the situation (she sees that she is short-staffed and does not see the hospital as a whole). Other conflicts may result from a supervisor's loss of nursing identity and his or her identification with the aggressor. This is a defense mechanism used by people who perceive themselves as powerless. Identifying with someone in power reduces the threat from that individual and at the same time gives power by association. Vertical conflicts not only reflect lack of mutual understanding and reciprocity but are further complicated by the individual's personal conflicts over dependence/independence and authority.

Horizontal conflicts among nurses occur between shifts, between units, and between individuals. Often, they are conscious, but more often they go unrecognized. They are seen in not-so-humorous put-downs and, more subtly, in unconscious omissions, as when a med-surg nurse requests a physician consultation for her patient rather than consulting with her nursing colleagues on the psychiatric unit. Sibling rivalry exists within nursing as well as between nursing and other departments, and the goals of such rivalry are parental approval and goodies. Paternalism and maternalism encourage these conflicts. Dependency and powerlessness, for example, enhance nurses' susceptibility to divide and conquer tactics such as flattery. How sweet it is to hear, "you're special, you're not like all those other nurses." And how nurses swallow the bait, hook, line, and sinker, failing to perceive that increased divisiveness in nursing in turn makes nurses more dependent and powerless.

Conflict also occurs between patients and nurses. For example, nurses often complain:

- "Mr. Jones keeps ringing his bell. He only wants attention."
- "I told Sherri she couldn't have her medication now and she called the doctor. He said to go ahead and give it. He always takes the patient's side!"
- "I'm not going to let that patient manipulate me!"

No one asks "What's wrong with wanting attention? That's only human." No one wonders how it is that nurses and patients wind up on opposite sides with doctors as arbiters. No one points out that we all manipulate people and situations daily to achieve our goals. It is as if the battle lines are drawn with nurses and patients as adversaries. This is not matter-of-fact limit setting for the patient's benefit; this is a personal, emotionally charged battle of wills.

Interpersonal conflicts, although not necessarily destructive, are often stressful. Few people manage conflict easily and objectively. Too often, earlier developmental conflicts are reactivated, coloring the current situation, and when identity, role, values, and worth are at stake, the personal (narcissistic) investment is high. The self is on the line, utilizing energy for offensive and defensive maneuvers, and the cost to the individual is great. This is stress.

How have these stressors in nursing evolved? Because they are widespread, they cannot be seen as the problems of certain nurses or certain institutions. For example, a nurse who is unhappy at one hospital will rarely find that "the grass is greener" at another. She or he will often be trading one set of problems for another. The universal problem of nursing—the contextual stressors—have evolved because nursing has traditionally been a woman's profession.

FEMALE SEX ROLE SOCIALIZATION

Little girls, from the moment they are born, are treated differently than little boys. They are wrapped in pink blankets, handled more gently, and given the kind of toys that are "appropriate" for little girls. They grow up

learning that being feminine means being quiet, soft, nurturing, dependent, passive, submissive, and pretty. They learn that female roles most
often involve putting others (men and children) first and themselves last.
Not only do women envy "masculine" roles, which are active and instrumental, but they learn that society values and rewards those roles more
than "feminine" ones.

Women's jobs, derivatives of women's roles, emphasize nurturing, caretaking, and housewifery. Times are changing, but traditionally woman's
place has been in the home, and if of necessity (never from choice) a
woman has worked, her jobs have been nursing, teaching, waitressing, or
taking dictation, all extensions of her natural maternal, wifely functions.
Because of the way they have been socialized, females have rarely aspired
to nontraditional kinds of work. Typically, they have not been taught the
kinds of skills necessary for success in male-dominated professions, such
as mathematics, sciences, and the manual arts. Neither have they developed the personality characteristics, such as independence and assertiveness, so vital to management and leadership positions in the professions.
Understanding financial data, thinking in business terms, having political
savvy, doing research, and keeping written records have traditionally been
"masculine" prerogatives. Women have not thought in terms of lifelong
careers but have seen jobs as stopgaps for marriage.

Sexism and Stereotyping

Throughout history, philosophy, religion, and other social institutions
have perpetuated the myths of woman as evil, woman as inferior, and
woman as servant (Ashley, 1980). These negative images of women reflect
both men's longing for and fear of women, who they cannot fully understand and whose powerful natural function, childbearing, they can never
hope to acquire. By viewing women as sex objects, men have projected
their own aggressive and sexual impulses onto women (and have seen
them as coming *from* women), a mechanism that absolves men of responsibility for their actions ("She's asking for it"). By viewing women as objects of ridicule—dolls, sissies, gossips, nags, and battle-axes (with huge
syringes and enema cans)—men can laugh at and thus diffuse women's
awesome power (Muff, 1982).

A less obvious, but equally destructive, form of sexism has been men's
idealization of women. To be placed on a pedestal may at first seem ap-
pealing, but women soon realize the idealization has three negative effects: it imposes unrealistic expectations on the idealized woman and thus
assures her downfall; it denies her humanness, her sexuality, her anger,
her "negative" attributes; and it creates a relationship based on a false image, which is no relationship at all (Muff, 1982).

Women have long been the focus of media propaganda intended to
keep them in their rightful place—barefoot and pregnant. *Beautysell* and
babysell have been coined to describe the glut of advertising that exhorts

women to pluck, deodorize, make up, diet, and dress themselves into society's arbitrary definition of beauty that glorifies childbearing and child-rearing. Women have heard and accepted two potent media messages: "Beauty wins, and beauty keeps (a man)" and "A woman's main aim in life is to get a man and have his children."

Woman's place, then, has been in the home, and women who work outside the home from choice have been suspect. Their femininity has been questioned. They have been accused of neglecting or depriving their children. [It is interesting that when social exigencies such as war have necessitated the entry of women into the work force, the propaganda and the sanctions have changed. Nurses during World War II, for example, were exhorted to work. "Duty" to patients and country, together with images of mom and apple pie, were bound together in one patriotic, emotionally charged packaged deal. Women were told that nursing was an eminently suitable occupation for them because it might help them snare a man, preferably a doctor, and because it prepared them for marriage and motherhood (Hughes, 1982).]

Myths about women and work flourish. They tell us that women's work is an extension of maternal and housekeeping functions, women are unreliable, transient workers, and women work for "pin money."

Certainly these myths have evolved from fact. First, society has segregated occupations according to sex and has discriminated against women through socialization, education, and institutional barriers, thus preventing their attaining or even aspiring toward certain careers. Second, women have been made responsible for housekeeping and childrearing roles, which has meant that jobs outside the home have taken second place to domestic responsibilities. If, for example, a couple's child is sick, it is generally the mother, not the father, who stays home from work, and it is *her* employment record that suffers. Finally, society fails to recognize that, increasingly, women are becoming heads of households, single parents, and breadwinners. The economic climate is such that even in families with two incomes, the wife's paycheck is as necessary as her husband's.

It is no wonder, then, that women's jobs have been valued less than men's jobs. Domestic labor, for example, is not seen as work (Greenleaf, 1980) but as an extension of natural feminine functions. Female occupations, therefore, are not thought to require specialized education or remuneration. Having one's work viewed in this light is stressful, because it is stressful to be devalued and idealized; to be limited in one's choices; to have one's self, one's intelligence, and one's work go unrecognized; and to be underpaid.

Female Stress—The Conflicts of Traditional and Changing Roles

The purpose of this discussion is not to denigrate traditional feminine attributes or roles but to suggest that restricting women to these attributes and roles limits the development of their human potential and creates conflict and stress. The issue is choice. Socialization, sexism, and stereotyping limit women's choices to certain socially "acceptable" behaviors, roles, and careers. On the other hand, feminism encourages women (and men) to be whatever they choose—traditional, avant garde, or a little of both. Choosing to be different also creates stress but of a different kind. Nurses who are women share these stresses with all other females in our society.

Stresses of Traditional Roles Women have been socialized to believe that *female* or *feminine* means second best and that their role is to be subservient. Male identity and masculine values or characteristics are the norm (Menikheim, 1979). Men retain their names after marriage, but women change theirs. Our language is rife with examples of sexism: the use of masculine pronouns when implying both sexes and the use of terms such as brotherhood, chairman, and mankind. All "men," women soon learn, are *not* created equal.

How do females integrate the devaluation of women into their personalities and self concepts? With difficulty and conflict (Muff, 1982). Society's low opinion of females becomes a part of each woman's opinion of herself. Studies have repeatedly demonstrated that women have more depression and lower self-esteem than men (Lasky, 1982) and that they achieve less in terms of careers, power, prestige, and money—society's indices of success. As women become aware of status and power in their personal and business relationships, they experience conflict that is reflected in their thoughts and behaviors.

Women learn self-hate and hatred of their own kind because society devalues them. Minorities share these attitudes, and although women are not in the numerical minority, they experience the same sort of discrimination. Behaviors associated with subservience and second-class status include obsequiousness, coyness, slyness, cunning, and denial of membership in one's own group. Women learn to achieve their goals by deferring to authority figures, using feminine wiles, playing the male-female game, and "identifying with the aggressor" (aligning themselves with those in power)—often to the detriment of other women (Muff, 1982).

Women's life options are restricted to the homemaker role or to female professions. Although housework, child-rearing, and female jobs have been advertised as glamorous, they are in fact often frustrating and unrewarding. These roles are unstructured, invisible, and have unclear expectations. Achievements are difficult to define. Many women have only one source of gratification, their housewife-mother role, whereas men often have two roles, domestic and business. When the female role is frustrating or disappointing, women cannot turn to an alternate role for satisfaction and self-esteem (Muff, in press). Although women who work therefore have a potential advantage, most kinds of women's work, including nursing, reenact familiar domestic roles.

Women have a higher incidence of mental illness. However, statistics fail to reflect that women have been socialized into mentally "unhealthy" behaviors—subservience, dependence, and passivity, for example. In addition, women are seen as mentally unhealthy whether or not they accept the traditional role: We are told that "women who *act out* the female role are depressed, incompetent, frigid, and anxious; women who *reject* the female role are aggressive, castrating, and "promiscuous" (Muff, in press).

One might imagine that strict adherence to the traditional role for which women are socialized would leave a woman conflict-free, but this is not the case. No one is completely or perfectly socialized. No woman is fully dependent, or fully subservient, or fully passive. Women, even traditional women, experience conflict and stress over marital and parental roles, particularly when they perceive themselves as lacking autonomy, achievement, or control over life situations.

Stresses of Nontraditional Roles   Changing gender concepts and identifications, women's demands for equal rights, changing marital roles and family styles have given rise to stresses for both sexes. For some women, a decision not to marry or not to have children causes stress. Other women experience conflict in making a career choice when feelings about aggression, competition, and role behaviors are activated. Guilt over assuming "masculine" traits, acquiring power, and abandoning "feminine" traits is common (Steck, 1981). For others, discrimination in the workplace, exclusion from "old boy" networks, and the expectation that women must do more than men in similar positions to *prove* themselves are additional burdens.

Nurses, then, most of whom are women, share with all women the conflicts and stresses of being female. Nursing, as a predominantly female profession in a male-dominated health care system, is prey to the same discrimination, paternalism, and power inequities as individual male-female relationships. Having looked at stresses related to the "feminine" role, we can move on to the unique stresses of nursing—those engendered by the professional socialization process, identity and role issues, and the nature of the job.

NURSING AS WOMEN'S WORK

Female nurses are twice socialized into subservience and traditionalism: first as women and second as workers in a work setting that mimics social roles. Those who choose to remain traditionalists must develop coping mechanisms for dealing with subordination and lack of autonomy; those who choose nontraditional nursing roles or who behave assertively or independently face personal and professional risks. Both choices involve stress.

Professional Socialization Issues

In their roles as caretakers, women have been healers of sorts. The history of modern nursing conventionally begins with Florence Nightingale, whose objective it was to rid nursing of its promiscuous, sinister, and lower-class images. "Ironically," says Helen Cohen (1981), "Nightingale established and promulgated an educational system that does not produce professionals like herself: staunchly independent women who discard the female stereotypes and refuse to accept the convention of traditional health care." How and why has this happened? Because nurses have not recognized the issues of all women as *their* issues? Because paternalism in nursing has meant that nurses (women) have traditionally been dominated by physicians and hospital administrators (men)? Because the nursing education process itself has failed in some way?

Nursing as an Outgrowth of Women's Role   "The development of nursing and the status of women have been parallel," say Glass and Brand (1979); however, "There is evidence that the women-nursing relationship is diverging . . . women are taking an increasingly active role in shaping the attitudes, norms, and values of society . . . nursing is not in this shaping position; by nature it responds to the trends taking place in society and is thus shaped by it." Some nurses react vehemently against any connection with feminism; others perceive the connection but choose to remain uninvolved (Lieb, 1978). How has this happened when nursing as a female-dominated profession reflects the status of women in society?

- Is not the stress of a nursing administrator who is responsible for, but does not control, her budget similar to that of a housewife whose husband doles out the weekly household allowance?
- Is not the stress of a staff nurse who not only cares for her patient but cleans beds when housekeepers are not available, assumes secretarial duties when the ward secretary is absent, runs to the pharmacy because the delivery system is broken, and catches hell from a physician and hospital administrator for not being at the desk to greet that physician similar to the stress of a supermom who cares for the house, cares for the kids, cares for her husband, cleans, chauffeurs, juggles, and manages, and who catches hell for forgetting to pick up the drycleaning?
- Is not the stress of a nurse who is addressed by physicians as "honey" or "Susie" yet who calls them "Doctor" similar to that of countless secretaries, waitresses, and airline stewardesses who respond to the males in their lives as "Mister," "Sir," or "Captain?"
- Is not the stress of a critical care nurse who can't say "no" and is pressured into working a double shift because "we can't get anyone else and you can't abandon patients" similar to that of any woman who has ever said "yes" when she meant "no," who has ever been coerced in the name of selflessness or duty into doing more or giving more than she is able?

We know the stresses are similar, but the commitments and attitudes of nurses and feminists appear to be diverging. Once nurses were leaders in women and women's health issues. They are now followers. Where are the Florence Nightingales, Margaret Sangers, and countless marching nurse suffragettes of today?

Propaganda and Paternalism   The myth that nursing is a natural female function gives rise to the following misconceptions:

- Because nursing is not an intellectual process, it need not take place in institutions of higher learning. Nursing skills are best acquired through apprenticeship.
- Because nursing requires no specialized skills, anyone (any female) can do it.
- Because nursing consists of caretaking and domestic functions, it provides ideal training for marriage and motherhood. It is not a lifelong career but a stopgap.
- Because nursing comes so naturally, women can return to nursing and perform competently after many years hiatus.

Historically, how has this propaganda affected the nursing profession? It has led to masculine domination of this "feminine" profession in educational and clinical settings. The system of apprenticeship learning, fostered by hospital schools, insured that nurses were seen as cheap labor, had little life away from the hospital, learned only what was deemed necessary by physicians, remained subservient to physicians, allied themselves with physicians rather than other nurses, and had little time to develop independent theory and practice. "The role of women (nurses)," says JoAnn Ashley, "was very early conceived as that of caring for the hospital family" (Ashley, 1976). Traditionally, nurses have reenacted the "feminine" domestic roles of housekeeper, wife (to hospital husbands—doctors), and mother (to hospital children—patients). In addition, they have been dutiful daughters (to hospital fathers—doctors and administrators).

Nurses themselves have often accepted the lower-class status of nursing and have consistently denied the need for formal education, research, and theory development. For example, it is nurses who are most impassioned over the technical-professional split between baccalaureate and nonbaccalaureate practitioners. It is nurses who argue that they should not be required to take the same science courses as premedical and other professional students but should be given courses specially designed (and less difficult) for nurses. It is nurses who deny the value of written care plans, failing to see that it is reliance on oral history rather than written documentation that has equated nursing theory with folklore rather than fact.

Nursing as a profession has suffered the consequences of inequality and deference to medical authority: low status, low pay, and lack of autonomy (Passav-Buck, 1982), which are added burdens for the individual nurse.

Authoritarianism, Perfectionism, and Isolationism in Nursing Education The problems and stressors in nursing education can be viewed from faculty and student viewpoints. For example, paternalistic constraints upon faculty are not restricted to diploma schools but are equally prevalent in university-based programs where nursing departments remain under the control of medical schools and where nurse educators encounter sex biases in obtaining promotions and tenure. The stress is severe. Economic and political factors also impinge upon nursing education. The notion that nursing is natural and does not require formal education, together with budgetary cutbacks, threaten the survival of baccalaureate programs.

How *do* faculty survive? By adapting—by adopting many of the values of the paternalistic system within which they work. In this way the stress is transmitted to students.

Aspirants to nursing historically have been young high school graduates. In contrast to medical and law students, few have had college educations or extensive work experience. Most have been female because traditional images of nursing as a feminine profession have lacked appeal for potential male recruits. *And young women have traditionally required guidance and protection!* This has led to authoritarianism in nursing education and practice. Remember the strict curfews and dormitory regulations of school days. Bring to mind a teacher or supervisor who was convinced there was only one way of doing things—the right way—her way. Recall the stereotype of the "battle-ax" nurse. These practices and stereotypes are not past history. They are experienced by many nurses practicing today. Authoritarianism is alive and well in nursing.

Often nursing faculty continue to be critics and evaluators rather than role models and demonstrators (Raabe, 1980). Despite assertions by educators that they value creativity and independent thinking, they reward obedience (Cohen, 1980; Flanagan, 1982). Nursing faculty, themselves in powerless situations, perpetuate powerlessness and subservience in their students. They foster dependency. Think, for a moment, of the difference between the clinical experiences of a medical student and a nursing student. The former has considerable independence of action; the latter cannot give a bed bath, much less a medication, without the watchful, ever-present nursing instructor. It is noteworthy, too, that the medical student's experience is guided by interns and residents, fledgling practitioners, clinically oriented members of the profession, whereas the nursing student often is solely responsible to and learns from the nursing instructor. Two issues are involved: trust in the student (and the intern or resident) and belief in the educational process.

This brings us to the issue of perfectionism in nursing education. Not only must the nursing instructor observe her student's first injection, but often the student must practice giving injections (and bed baths) to her peers beforehand in the nursing laboratory. Imagine the consternation of a diploma nurse who, after working in an intensive care unit (ICU) for seven years, returned to the university to obtain her BSN and was duly required to demonstrate giving bed baths and injections in both laboratory and clinical settings before being "turned loose." The messages are clear: tasks and details are most important, and they must be practiced until perfect; the student is incapable of executing even minor tasks without supervision; the instructor's presence will assure perfection and "proper" learning of technique. Are there not ways of teaching nursing that value independence while teaching skills?

Along with perfectionism comes exaggeration. The smallest detail is imbued with undue significance. Is a bed bath really an undertaking that warrants practice and observation? Are most medications so lethal that their administration must be fraught with anxiety? Of course, medications must be carefully administered, but that in no way accounts for overvaluing certain tasks and magnifying negative outcomes. Few situations in nursing are life and death and rarely is a nurse's license on the line, yet nurses fervently believe the contrary to be true. Not only is this approach grandiose, but it is undoubtedly (and unnecessarily) stressful. In addition, adherence to the "there's only one right way to do things" school of thinking destroys creativity, problem-solving potential, and the ability to translate learning from one situation to another.

Another problem of nursing education has been isolationism. Traditionally, hospital schools have been isolated from the mainstream of professional education. Students of these programs have suffered in several important aspects: their education has been restricted by the prejudices and concerns of the hospitals with which their schools are aligned; their curricula have often narrowly focused on medical sciences, technical skills, and sometimes on "professional" issues but have not conveyed the broader picture so necessary in developing their full human potential; their isolation from the campus setting has denied them a sense of collegiality with other nursing and non-nursing professionals.

Traditionally nursing did and does value skills over concepts. In practice, both are necessary. Again consider the medical student whose basic education is grounded primarily in the sciences and who learns techniques secondarily in clinical and advanced education settings. How different is the nursing student, by comparison, who values the skill first? (This is not an advocacy of medical education, which is often appallingly deficient in interpersonal and interprofessional considerations, but is an illustration of differing viewpoints.)

Even in collegiate settings, nursing students often prefer special, less complex science courses (Cohen, 1981; Lowery-Palmer, 1982). How can nurses begin to think of themselves as professionals, equal with other professionals, without expecting equally rigorous educational and practice requirements? To illustrate isolationism in a less controversial way than by comparisons with medicine, consider a nursing colleague who was writing a book pertinent, not just to nurses, but to all health professionals. She was told by her publisher to restrict the book to nursing because nurses would buy only books specifically aimed at them.

The pendulum, however, may now be swinging the other way to the extent that nursing education may isolate itself from the concerns of nursing service. For example, the new theoretical models of nursing taught in schools are often unpractical in work situations. The effort to "professionalize" nursing, and set it apart from other health professions, has led to a surfeit of nursing theories and even language. Although demonstrating nursing's uniqueness and preserving its identity are laudable goals, many nurses in clinical settings abandon unwieldy ivory tower tenets. It is stressful enough to collaborate with other professionals without adding a language barrier to further isolate oneself.

The combined effects of these three influences—authoritarianism, perfectionism, and isolationism in nursing education—produce graduates who often are unprepared to meet the sophisticated demands of patient care and unit management situations. Many have not learned to think critically and mistrust their own judgment. Those who cannot quite accept all they have learned frequently react passively rather than rebelliously. They are surprised and experience stress when faced with bureaucratic and role conflicts. Often they feel isolated and do not see themselves as part of a larger group of professionals.

Nursing Image and Identity Issues

Nurses, we hear, are having an "identity crisis." They are "at the crossroads." Well, they have *been* in crisis at the crossroads for as long as anyone can remember. The indecision, bickering, and struggle over identity, role, and professionalism contribute to the conscious stresses experienced by nurses. Harmful stereotypes, myths, and unreasonable expectations, together with individual narcissism, take their toll.

The Impact of Stereotypes Stereotypes are initially pigeonholes, or mental boxes, that categorize people in an attempt to speed up information processing. Eventually, however, the expeditious pigeonholes become prisons. They are no longer facilitators; they are no longer optional. Rather than simple ways to sort preliminary information about people, they become rigid *expectations of* people and, as such, *all* stereotypes are limiting and potentially harmful.

The most common stereotype of a nurse is that she is a woman. After that she is an *angel of mercy,* a *handmaiden* to the physician, a *woman in white,* a *battle-ax,* a *sexpot,* or a *torturer* (Muff, 1982) or any combination of these. Such stereotypes reflect myths, fears, and fantasies about women. They represent an idealization of how a nurse ought to be or a depreciation of how nurses are. What is missing from these formulations is the notion that nurses are real people and that nursing requires intelligence.

Naturally, there is some truth in stereotypes or they would not persist, and naturally, nurses themselves defend "good" aspects of each. For example, the angel of mercy image is not without appeal. Most nurses become nurses to "help" people and few would deny the need for caring and compassionate traits in nurses. Many nurses, however, become defensive when traditional stereotypes are examined. My suggestion is not that we abandon valuable traits, but that we question all stereotypes and their relationships to nursing stress.

The angel of mercy, for all its value and appeal, creates stress when self-lessness as an ideal and caring for others mean that nurses forget or are told to forget themselves. In addition, angels are superhuman creatures—they are not limited by human considerations, neither do they experience human emotions such as anger, frustration, and physical desire. The angel of mercy stereotype creates an impossible ideal and denies nurses important aspects of their humanness.

The handmaiden stereotype also combines desirable and undesirable qualities. Following physicians' orders is certainly part of nursing, but following them unquestioningly or following them exclusively is not. Yet many people (mainly the public and physicians themselves) view nursing practice in this narrow, confining way.

The woman in white stereotype, derived from the traditional nursing uniform, conjures up mental associations of cleanliness, purity, and virginity. Uniforms are linked to professionalism and are often mandatory, even when they are not indicated clinically. Again, the humanness of nurses is denied and personal choice is restricted, in this case by narrow definitions of "appropriate" dress.

The battle-ax, the epitome of a controlling, stiff-necked old maid, is both feared and scorned. She may give or demand excellent patient care and run a tight ship—both priorities and positive characteristics of the battle-ax—but these characteristics are outweighed by the negative image of this stereotype—that of frigid, unyielding womanhood.

The sexpot stereotype twists something of value, such as scientific anatomic knowledge, into something degrading—sexual promiscuity. ("You're very familiar with the human body aren't you, honey?") The image is not that of a healthy sexual human being, but of an immoral, unintelligent sex object.

The torturer image, so prevalent in comedy and get-well cards, is typified by the nurse wielding an enema or syringe. In reality, it *is* often the nurse who is an agent of pain or discomfort as she implements doctors' orders, but she does not do so with the relish and glee evidenced in this stereotype.

Whether angel or sexpot, nurturer or torturer, handmaiden or battle-ax, stereotypes are limiting. They restrict nurses to certain narrowly defined roles and rules of conduct. They cause nurses to repudiate parts of themselves: their need to be cared for, their sexuality, their frustration and anger. They cause nurses to have unrealistic expectations for themselves. The stresses, then, arise whether one complies with or defies the stereotypes (the system and society). The first means giving up oneself; the second means being oneself, but at great cost.

Myths and Unreasonable Expectations A lot of what people believe is based on fantasy rather than fact. We see things as we think they ought to be, or as we expect them to be, rather than as they are. At its simplest, this means that when you proofread something you have just written, you can easily miss typographical errors because you read words as you expect to see them, not as they are. At its most complex, this means you tend to measure yourself against unreasonable expectations.

Myths about nurses, as we know, come from stereotypes. They also come from society's, nursing educators', and nurses' *wishes* for what nurses *should* be. Here are some examples:

Myth. *A "good" nurse cares for all patients equally and is concerned about people all of the time.* This is an expectation. The "should" is implicit. A good nurse *should* care. Yet nurses, even good nurses, soon realize that it is impossible to care for all people equally, and it is also impossible to care for people adequately, given today's workload and system constraints. It is impossible for a nurse to care all the time, yet the expectation persists, not only externally but internally, and many nurses who do not or cannot care enough feel guilty, stressed, or burned out.

Myth. *A nurse's worth, whether or not she does a "good" job, is related to patient compliance, patient outcome, patient improvement, and patient happiness.* There is, in fact, no direct cause-and-effect relationship between the nurse's activities and the patient's improvement. Administering a certain medication may raise or lower a patient's blood pressure, but in the overall context of patient improvement or deterioration, few things are so easily measurable. Of course, actions have consequences, but to disregard the multitude of factors impinging on the patient and to negate the patient's own conscious and unconscious contributions is unnecessarily burdensome. Yet this myth persists and is institutionalized by laws, for example, that mandate outcome criteria for quality assurance audits.

Myth. *Total patient care means solving all the problems of a patient's whole life: finding him a job, putting a roof over her head, providing food for the table, curing his pain, making her life meaningful, saving their relationships, and so on.* How unrealistic! And yet many nurses have difficulty defining the limits of their role and setting priorities. They feel guilty because somehow, someway, if they were "good" enough or organized enough, or if the system were perfect enough, they would or should do all these things.

Myth. *Patients can make us mad, happy, guilty, irritated, and so on.* If there is any single "truth" in life, it is that we *make* ourselves. Not that genes, parents, environment, and circumstances do not play a large part in each individual's development, but each individual as an adult must assume responsibility for her or his personality, its strengths and weaknesses, irrespective of origin. Often, nurses will say "Dr. Smith *made* me so mad," or "The head nurse *makes* me feel guilty." Just semantics? Maybe partly, but if we admit that words reflect our thoughts and wishes, then we must also admit that the idea that people *make* us feel implies that we are not responsible for or in control of ourselves. By blaming others, by refusing to accept responsibility, nurses perpetuate their victimization and stress. (Choosing to be responsible entails stress, too, but of a different kind.)

Myth. *Being a role model means offering oneself as an example of normalcy; being an expert means judging what is right and wrong.* Being a nurse role model means exemplifying a "right" way of doing things. However, there is no *one* right way to do anything. What makes one nurse good does not make another good. "Goodness" and "rightness" are individual values, not the arbitrary standards of any school or person. A good nurse is someone who acts in accordance with his or her own values and who respects those who do the same, whether or not they agree. Perfectionism, as we have said, is stressful, as is trying to bring others around to our truths.

Just as there is no *one* right way for nurses, there is no one right way for patients; yet nurses in the role of expert often judge patients or give patients permission to do something, behaviors that imply moral or professional superiority. Even simply saying "It's OK to cry" involves judgment (of what's OK or not OK) and permission.

Myth. *Patients and supervisors and co-workers should appreciate us and our work.* Most people like to be appreciated. Being thanked makes the day seem brighter, diminishes frustrations, and balances the hurts. However, nurses who expect thanks and measure the value of their work by whether others appreciate it are doomed to disappointment. The value of the work is the work itself. A psychiatric nurse, for example, may work very hard with a substance-abusing patient who may tell the nurse he hates her or may improve only to return again to drugs or, even worse, may commit suicide. Through words or actions, the patient may be saying that he does *not* appreciate or agree with the treatment plan. Does this mean that the nurse failed to do a good job? Many patients do not appreciate what nurses do for them. Some reject the help outright. Does that mean that the nurse's work is valueless, that the nurse did not do enough, did not do the "right" thing, or missed the key thing that would have altered the patient's outcome? Think about it.

Myths such as these create unrealistic expectations and link the nurse's personal worth to outcomes beyond her or his control. Such myths are detrimental to real self-esteem and patient-centered care. They keep the nurse feeling frustrated, disappointed, and stressed.

Victim versus Narcissist: Apparent Contradictions in the Nursing Personality
Nurses are dependent and see themselves as victims. At the same

time, they are egocentric and narcissistic. Nurses' (and women's) dependency has long been acknowledged and is being examined, not so much as a character flaw, but in the light of the symbiosis into which they have been socialized. Women are dependent, not because there is something innately wrong with them, but because they are taught to be that way. Although dependency has been recognized and addressed, narcissism has not (except in sexist psychologic theory that fails to see that narcissism is as much a function of socialization as enforced dependency). Female narcissism has been stereotyped as overconcern with beauty, appearance, make-up, and clothes. The real issues of narcissism—developmental arrest, identity conflicts, and interpersonal difficulties—are not nearly so frivolous and lie at the heart of many nursing stresses. For this reason, they will be examined in depth.

Most nurses, as women, have been socialized to be dependent, to be mirrors, to exist primarily as reflections of the needs of others. Most women have been defined, and have defined themselves, as someone's wife, or someone's mother, or someone's appendage. Women's self-identity and self-esteem, then, traditionally have been derived from their relationships with others rather than from a real sense of self.

Women who are nurses react similarly. It is as if they hold up the mirror of themselves to reflect what other people wish to see. For example, consider the response of some nurses whose head nurse said, "I know you've been feeling overwhelmed, so let's talk about how your day went and try to do some problem-solving." This was an innocent enough statement, yet most nurses felt that the head nurse was telling them they were not doing a good job. When they met with her, nearly all gave her responses they *thought* she wanted to hear rather than discussing their day's problems. They left the meeting upset and full of fantasies as to what the head nurse was "really" getting at. Instead of voicing their confusion or discomfort, they tried to second-guess her. The session was disastrous.

Why does this happen? Is there a nursing personality that would explain it? Some studies of nurses describe them as highly dependent, nonassertive traditionalists who often believe and do what they are told. My own experience, while partially validating this, has shown me that there is more: nurses go through the motions, mirror what others wish to see, act compliantly, appear to be victims. But, on some deeper level, they actually reject what is happening. The rejection is rarely overt but is passive and indirect. Mirroring and this type of passive resistance are well-known behaviors in seemingly powerless people; they occur because of the sanctions against open rebellion.

Victims are, in fact, powerful. Passive resistance uses power negatively. For example, consider a poor, browbeaten OR nurse whose passivity, inability to make decisions, and lack of "authority" to release certain equipment can effectively slow down the flow of cases, and make the physicians crazy and bring them to their knees.

If dependence and seeming victimization are one aspect of the nursing personality, narcissism is the other. Two authors have recently addressed narcissism (without labeling it) in relation to stress and burn-out. Freudenberger (1975) suggests that recruits to nursing are commonly seeking self-fulfillment, self-aggrandizement, and self-sacrifice and that they deny personal problems. Veninga (1979) describes scripts used by nurses that include "I trust only myself," "Everybody should see the world as I see it," and "I'm going to succeed even if it kills me." Sound familiar? These statements reflect narcissism or overevaluation of self.

Nursing education teaches nurses to trust only themselves. When teaching students about medications, fundamentals instructors inevitably say *"Never trust anyone but yourself!"* Many nurses have extrapolated this to all areas of their practice. They never trust anyone else. They believe that there is only one right way to do things—their way. They engage in power struggles with patients, doctors, and co-workers. Statements like "Then the doctor took the patient's side" invariably reflect a power struggle. Fulfilling one's own needs for love and approval through patients, trusting only oneself, and engaging in power struggles create stress *and* indicate narcissistic overinvolvement.

What is the relationship, then, between victim and narcissist? How do we resolve the apparent discrepancy between nurses whose behaviors are alternately passive-dependent and narcissistic-egocentric. How can these two extremes coexist in one person? We can reconcile the apparent dichotomy by looking at psychologic development.

Think for a moment of an infant who wants to be cared for yet is greedy and wants to control. Not very different from this is the nurse who relies on a physician to handle a touchy patient problem (thus being dependent and nonassertive) yet who criticizes the same physician for failing to manage the situation as she would have liked (thus being narcissistic). Think of the idea of "having your cake and eating it too." Impossible? Ambivalent? It is all of these things. It symbolizes internal conflict similar to that of early childhood. One cannot be taken care of and be in charge or refuse responsibility yet demand control. Having one's cake and eating it too (in nursing) creates conflict and stress.

For example, nurses are quick to point out their victimization, especially when the subject of "floating" comes up. "Can't they see I'm an ICU nurse, not a med-surg nurse?" "How can they expect us to work where we've never been oriented?" "We're specialists now, not generalists. There's been such a proliferation of technology and theory that we can't possibly know everything!" So the story goes. What are we hearing? That all nurses cannot do the same job. "A nurse is *not* a nurse is *not* a nurse." But flip the coin and see how these same nurses describe float and temporary help who come to their units. "You should have seen the nurse they sent us. She couldn't even do a dressing." "She's from the psych unit and you'd think she never went to nursing school." Scorn and sarcasm punctuate these comments. Suddenly, all nurses should be able to do the same job. The tune has changed from "a nurse is *not* a nurse is *not* a nurse" to "a good nurse *is* a good nurse *is* a good nurse," and a good nurse is someone like me. Narcissism.

On the one hand, nurses are asking how "they" ever got the idea that a "good" nurse can work anywhere. On the other hand, nurses themselves secretly believe that there is such a thing as a "good" nurse and that he or she *should* be able to work anywhere. We may never know where "they" got the idea originally, but we can begin to understand why it persists. It is the old chicken-or-the-egg story; which came first, social expectations that nurses be supernurses or nurses' own expectations? Are nurses victims of society or victims of their own narcissism?

The confusion and anger over "entry into practice" reflects the same problem. Again, the inconsistencies are striking. On the one hand, nurses perpetuate the conflict actively or passively, stressful as that confusion and rivalry is. They feel victimized. On the other hand, these same nurses adhere to a simplistic concept that there is only one definition of what a "good" nurse is. People with and without degrees battle on, each firmly believing that their way is the *right* way. Again, we find victimization and narcissism, opposite sides of the same coin, at the root of the conflict. Again, we find the fantasies of *one* real truth and "my truth is the *real* truth" at work.

The real problem exists in the conflict between nurses' *expressed* belief that each nurse is unique (a nurse is *not* a nurse is *not* a nurse) and the *unconscious,* narcissistic belief that a "good nurse is what I believe her or him to be" (a nurse *is* a nurse *is* a nurse). Each narcissist, by definition, makes victims of others, and nurses play both roles. By viewing "my way" as the right way, each nurse perceives other ways as lesser, wrong, whatever. Unflattering comparisons, infighting, and sibling rivalry are the natural consequences for a group of people, each of whom thinks that her or his way is right. When people take "sides," think in terms of "winning" and "losing," become moralistic and judgmental, there is no easy solution. No one gives up or gives in. The struggle (and the stress) continues.

Identity, self-esteem, and one's perception of personal power reflect one's degree of separateness and independence. Nurses, symbiotically attached to paternalistic physicians and maternalistic supervisors, experience a reactivation of primitive conflicts over the issues of narcissism and dependence and independence. One step in growing up and becoming separate, for individuals and professionals, is recognizing one's dependency needs and one's narcissism. Women's (nurses') dependency is widely documented and many steps are being taken by women (and nurses) to overcome their socialized passivity.

Narcissism, as I have said, is less well recognized and perhaps harder to swallow than dependency. Most people, not just women or nurses, fight such revelations about themselves or their professions because they think of egoism or narcissism as bad or unflattering or "undesirable" when, in fact, they are natural personality characteristics. Sometimes these traits help, sometimes they hinder. In any case, they cannot be ignored. Narcissism is not the same as independence. Independence means valuing the separateness and independence of oneself *and* others; narcissism means wanting others to be like oneself and do what one wants. A second step, then, in growing up and becoming separate means giving up the fantasy that "my truth is the real truth" and, to some extent, giving up one's narcissism. As if that were not painful enough, a third step means giving up the fantasy that there is any such thing as *one* real truth.

CONCLUSION

Stress in nursing often leads to burn-out, the three major causes of which are (1) a mismatch between efforts and results (Chance, 1981), leading to disappointment and frustration, (2) a mismatch between nurse and environment (Bailey, 1980), leading to role ambiguity and conflict, and (3) a mismatch between people (Pines and Maslach, 1978), leading to interpersonal conflict. The issue in all three is control or, more specifically, the discrepancy between the nurse's need to control events, environment, and people and his or her inability to do so. Storlie (1979) says disillusionment and burn-out follow "confrontation with reality in which the human spirit is pitted against circumstances intractable to change."

The reality for many nurses is that they feel powerless to change their circumstances. This is partly due to the fact that, as women, most nurses have been socialized to traditional, dependent behaviors. In addition, their professional socialization, with its often skill-oriented focus, has failed to educate them in the ways of the business world. They learn neither fiscal and managerial strategies nor political savvy, both of which are necessary for business effectiveness. This contributes to their sense of powerlessness. Finally, contextual stressors and interpersonal conflicts, not to mention actual discrimination in work situations, are the proverbial straws that break the camel's back. But, the reality is that nurses are *not* powerless. Their expertise gives them power. Their numbers (1 out of every 44 women voters is a nurse) give them power. The long-range goal, then, is to alter their *perceptions* of themselves and their situation; the short-range goal is to assist them in coping with stress in the meantime.

REFERENCES

Anderson, C. A., and Basteyns, M. 1981. Stress and the critical care nurse reaffirmed. *J. Nurs. Admin.* Jan:31.

Ashley, J. 1976. *Hospitals, paternalism, and the role of the nurse.* New York: Teachers College Press.

Ashley, J. 1980. Power in structured misogyny: implications for the politics of care. *Advan. Nurs. Sci.* 2(3):3.

Bailey, J. T. 1980. Job stress and other stress-related problems. In *Living with stress and promoting well-being*, editors K. E. Claus and J. T. Bailey. St. Louis: The C. V. Mosby Co.

Bush, M. A., and Kjervik, D. K. 1979. The nurse's self-image. In *Women in stress: a nursing perspective*, editors D. K. Kjervik and I. M. Martinson. New York: Appleton-Century-Crofts.

Chance, P. 1981. That drained-out, used up feeling. *Psychol. Today* Jan:88.

Claus, K. E. 1980. The nature of stress. In *Living with stress and promoting well-being*, editors K. E. Claus and J. T. Bailey. St. Louis: The C. V. Mosby Co.

Cohen, H. 1980. Authoritarianism and dependency: problems in nursing socialization. In *Current perspectives in nursing: social issues and trends*, editors B. C. Flynn and M. H. Miller. St. Louis: The C. V. Mosby Co.

Cohen, H. 1981. *The nurse's quest for a professional identity.* Menlo Park, Calif.: Addison-Wesley.

Daley, M. R. 1979. Preventing worker burnout in child welfare. *Child Welfare* 58(7):443-450.

Donovan, L. 1980. What nurses want (and what they're getting). *RN* Apr:22.

Eisenstein, H. 1982. On the psychosocial barriers to professions for women: Atlanta's apples, 'women's work,' and the struggle for social change. In *Socialization, sexism, and stereotyping: women's issues in nursing*, editor J. Muff. St. Louis· The C. V. Mosby Co.

Flanagan, M. K. 1982. An analysis of nursing as a career choice. In *Socialization, sexism, and stereotyping: women's issues in nursing*, editor J. Muff. St. Louis: The C. V. Mosby Co.

Freudenberger, H. J. 1975. The staff burn-out syndrome in alternative institutions. *Psychotherapy: Theory, Research, and Practice* Spring, Vol. 12.

Garfield, C. A. 1980. Coping with burn-out. *Hosp. Forum* Jan–Feb:15.

Glass, L., and Brand, K. 1979. The progress of women and nursing: parallel or divergent? In *Women in stress: a nursing perspective*, editors D. K. Kjervik and I. M. Martinson. New York: Appleton-Century-Crofts.

Greenleaf, N. P. 1980. Sex-segregated occupations: relevance for nursing. *Advan. Nurs. Sci.* 2(3):23.

Hallas, G. G. 1980. Why nurses are giving it up. *RN* 43:17-21.

Henley, M., and Freeman, J. 1979. The sexual politics of interpersonal behavior. In *Women: a feminist perspective*, editor J. Freeman. Palo Alto, Calif.: Mayfield.

Horner, M. 1972. Toward an understanding of achievement-related conflicts in women. *J. Social Issues* 68:158.

Hughes, L. 1982. Little girls grow up to be wives and mommies: nursing as a stopgap to marriage. In *Socialization, sexism, and stereotyping: women's issues in nursing,* editor J. Muff. St. Louis: The C. V. Mosby Co.

Kjervik, D. K. 1979. The stress of sexism on the mental health of women. In *Women in stress: a nursing perspective,* editors D. K. Kjervik and I. M. Martinson. New York: Appleton-Century-Crofts.

Kramer, M. 1974. *Reality shock: why nurses leave nursing.* St. Louis: The C. V. Mosby Co.

Lasky, E. 1982. Self-esteem, achievement, and the female experience. In *Socialization, sexism and stereotyping: women's issues in nursing,* editor J. Muff. St. Louis: The C. V. Mosby Co.

Lieb, R. 1978. Power, powerlessness, and potential—nurse's role within the health care delivery system. *Image* 10(3):75.

Lowery-Palmer, A. 1982. The cultural basis of political behavior in two groups: nurses and political activists. In *Socialization, sexism, and stereotyping: women's issues in nursing,* editor J. Muff. St. Louis: The C. V. Mosby Co.

Menikheim, M. L. 1979. Communications patterns of women and nurses. In *Women in stress: a nursing perspective,* editors D. K. Kjervik and I. M. Martinson. New York: Appleton-Century-Crofts.

Muff, J. 1982. Handmaiden, battle-ax, whore: an exploration into the fantasies, myths, and stereotypes about nurses. In *Socialization, sexism, and stereotyping: women's issues in nursing,* editor J. Muff. St. Louis: The C. V. Mosby Co.

Muff, J. 1982. Why doesn't a smart girl like you go to medical school? The women's movement takes a slap at nursing. In *Socialization, sexism, and stereotyping: women's issues in nursing,* editor J. Muff. St. Louis: The C. V. Mosby Co.

Muff, J. (In Press). Women's issues in psychiatric nursing. in *Lippincott manual of psychiatric nursing,* editor S. Lego. Philadelphia: J. B. Lippincott.

Mulligan, J. E. 1980. Together we go, separate we stay: women's studies and nurses' studies. In *Current perspectives in nursing: social issues and trends,* editors B. C. Flynn and M. H. Miller. St. Louis: The C. V. Mosby Co.

Mullner, R., et al. 1982. Hospital vacancies. *Am. J. Nurs.* 82:592–4.

Passau-Buck, S. 1982. Caring vs. curing—The politics of health care. In *Socialization, sexism, and stereotyping: women's issues in nursing,* editor J. Muff. St. Louis: The C. V. Mosby Co.

Patrick, P. K. S. 1979. Burnout: job hazard for health workers. *Hospitals* 16:53(22):87–8, 90.

Pines, A. M., and Kanner, A. D. 1982. Burnout: lack of positive conditions and presence of negative conditions as two independent sources of stress. *Psychiatric Nurs. Ment. Health Serv.* 20(8):30.

Pines, A., and Maslach, C. 1978. Characteristics of staff burnout in mental health settings. *Hospital and Community Psychiatry* 29(4):233.

Raabe, M. S. 1980. Diploma school socialization: survival and defense. In *Current perspectives in nursing: social issues and trends*, editors B. C. Flynn and M. H. Miller. St. Louis: The C. V. Mosby Co.

Seliger, S. 1982. Stress can be good for you. *New York* 2 August, p. 20.

Steck, A. L. 1981. The nursing shortage: an optimistic view. *Nursing Outlook* May:302.

Storlie, F. J. 1979. Burnout: the elaboration of a concept. *Am. J. N.* Dec:2108.

Styles, M. 1980. Change and challenge in nursing—the road ahead. In *Living with stress and promoting well-being*, editors K. E. Claus and J. T. Bailey. St. Louis: The C. V. Mosby Co.

Veninga, R. 1979. Administrative burnout—causes and cures. *Hospital Progress* Feb:45.

CHAPTER 3

Negative Responses to Stress

JANET MUFF

Because of the many stressors in our profession, it is not surprising that nurses often experience their practice, their environment, and their interpersonal relationships as stressful. With their expectations unmet, they often see themselves as trapped in disappointing and frustrating situations. Faced with seemingly unrelenting stressors, many nurses develop symptoms of *dis*tress.

When chronic, these symptoms lead to burn-out. Physical symptoms were discussed in Chapter 1. We will concentrate here on mental and emotional symptoms and their consequences (Figure 3-1).

Not everyone who experiences frustration and disappointment will manifest the same set of symptoms. How you respond to stress, positively or negatively, depends on numerous factors: your character, your perception of a situation, the context of the situation (what else is happening in your life), and the presence or absence of support systems, to name just a few.

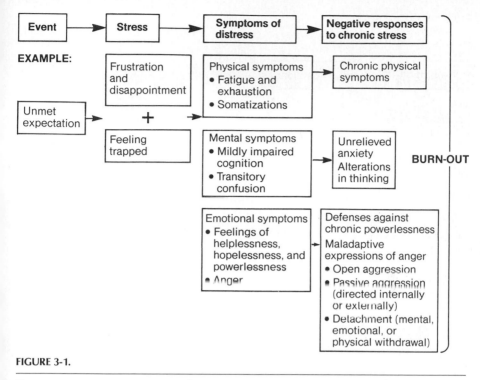

FIGURE 3-1.

Event—stress—symptoms of stress—negative responses to chronic stress.

SYMPTOMS OF DISTRESS

Perception, Cognition, and Emotion

Recall, for a moment, the relationship of cognition and emotion to our perception of the environment. From birth, human beings experience the world through events, interactions, and objects. We integrate the incoming perceptions *mentally* by developing a cognitive framework, mental pigeonholes and processes, and then respond to them *emotionally*. Each experience adds to and alters the cognitive framework and emotions that, in turn, alter how future events are perceived and handled (Figure 3-2).

There is a growing controversy over which comes first, the mental state or the emotional state. Traditional psychology holds that emotions determine thought. That is, if you feel down, you'll begin to think negative or depressed thoughts. There is a growing body of research by Beck (1967, 1976) and others, however, indicating that one's cognition (mental state) determines one's emotional responses. Perhaps it is the individual who determines (probably unconsciously) whether mental or emotional symptoms come first. In any case, the controversy concerns our perception of

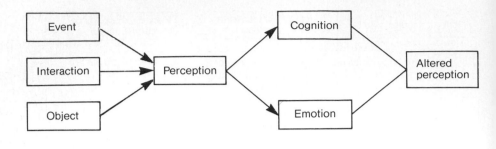

FIGURE 3-2.

Perception alters cognition and emotion, which in turn alter perception.

certain events as stressful and the resulting interrelated mental, emotional, and physical symptoms.

Mental Symptoms

Stress may impair thinking, both the process of thinking and the actual content of one's thought. The nurse who is being shouted at by a physician may, for example, become confused, begin to doubt her perceptions of the situation and herself. She may then feel stupid. Another nurse, faced with the stress of an examination, may forget what he knows. Yet another nurse, floated to an unfamiliar unit or confronted with several problems simultaneously, may be unable to think straight or may forget routine activities in the stress of the moment. If the stress is alleviated, these mental symptoms disappear.

Emotional Symptoms

Helplessness and *anger* are two predominant emotional responses to feeling trapped in a frustrating and stressful situation. Helplessness is a sense of impotence in the face of overwhelming odds. The nurse who is trapped in a job because it is the only Monday through Friday position available may indeed *be* helpless and unable to change her environment or the people with whom she works. Other nurses, faced with unresponsive physicians or administrations, lose sight of their options, begin to feel trapped, and become helpless and hopeless. Sometimes they experience anger; more often they feel powerless. Again, if the situation changes or if the nurse sees herself as having choices, the helplessness and anger dissipate.

NEGATIVE RESPONSES TO CHRONIC STRESS

When transitory stress becomes chronic, distress often becomes a chronic negative response. Unrelieved stress, namely chronic feelings of frustration and disappointment in a situation where a person also feels trapped, leads to chronic negative responses. The symptoms of distress, whether physical, mental, or emotional, are no longer transitory and variable, but become fixed, automatic, and often complex patterns of behavior. The nurse whose stomach churns when she feels pressured may develop an ulcer if that pressure is unremitting. Similarly, the nurse who becomes controlling and dictatorial when things get hectic may become increasingly so in a work situation that is unpredictable and chaotic.

Unrelieved Anxiety and Alterations in Thinking

Someone who responds to transitory stress with mental symptoms will respond to chronic stress the same way. The nurse who begins to feel disorganized, who feels she can't cope, who makes several mistakes or errors in judgment often becomes anxious. She knows she is not coping. These failures in coping activate unconscious conflicts about self-worth, self-image, acceptable behavior, expectations, success and failure, and competence. The nurse experiences *anxiety,* a psychophysiologic response to danger—external danger or the danger of internal conflict and loss of control.

Prolonged exposure to stress and unrelieved anxiety alter one's thinking by changing one's sense of reality of the world and of the self. Confusion, impaired cognition, altered self-image, suspicion, and false omnipotence result.

Confusion is the inability to distinguish reality from unreality. A person who is confused has trouble being objective and loses perspective. When, for example, a nurse is asked to handle a problem that rightfully and realistically belongs to someone else, she may become involved, then resentful, then overcome with helplessness and, ultimately, hopelessness. Her sense of personal boundaries may be lost and her judgment impaired. She may have difficulty determining priorities and setting limits on what she can do, reasonably and safely, when overwhelmed by conflicting demands of patients, physicians, co-workers, and supervisors. This sense of being overwhelmed plays a key role in the nurse's ability to assess the task and decide on the best course of action. In short, the ability to delineate a role and react rationally may be lost.

Impaired cognition is the inability to plan and deliver nursing care or to perform managerial and administrative functions in a logical and efficient manner. This is often due to fatigue and a general sense of disorganization, though in some cases it results from the use of drugs or alcohol. The nurse may be unable to plan her work in a logical sequence. She may have difficulty delegating tasks or may delegate inappropriately. She may overlook things or become forgetful. She may make mistakes.

Altered self-image is a change in self and role concepts. There is much in today's health care settings to challenge the identity and self-worth of even the hardiest nurse. Realizing that nurses are often unable to make changes and must yield to others who are more powerful than they are is undoubtedly painful. Nurses often react to such frustrations by questioning themselves, their competency and values. Gradually, their self-image as effective, compassionate caregivers erodes.

As it relates to stress, *suspicion* is the notion that others are unappreciative of our efforts. Cause-and-effect thinking decrees that if things go wrong, someone must be at fault. So we arbitrarily blame others—doctors, hospital administrators, supervisors, and peers. Placing blame is the first step toward paranoia. If we can blame others, they can blame us. Paranoia is the belief that others are deliberately out to get you. The head nurse, for example, who forgets to delete a sick nurse from the day's schedule, is blamed by her staff. A suspicious nurse may even believe that the head nurse intentionally short-staffed the unit. If we become suspicious, we question others' motives and perceive threats where none exist.

Omnipotence refers to a false sense of being uniquely capable and solely responsible, and it signifies a distorted perception of reality, of others, and of oneself. It may result from a need to maintain control in a situation that is perceived as overwhelmingly out of control. Often it contributes to nurses overburdening themselves. The thinking goes, I'd better do it myself if I want it done right.

Defenses Against Chronic Powerlessness

Nurses who feel powerless become defensive. They often stop taking risks and play it safe. They exert control in whatever areas they can: by adhering to policies and procedures, going by the book, or ordering and regulating the environment or patients. They see change as threatening and fear it will disrupt the routine. Their behavior becomes characterized by rigidity, inflexibility, and resistance to change.

Nurses respond to those they perceive as powerful in characteristic ways. Often, they outwardly accept their dependency and engage in a kind of game-playing common among minorities and others who are powerless. This game involves feigned stupidity, obsequiousness, and deferential behavior. For example, women, often powerless in relation to men, play the game in which they chase a man until *he* catches *them*. Nurses, seemingly powerless in relation to physicians, play the game by offering suggestions in such a way that the doctor thinks he came up with the idea.

The game, then, is as old as civilization, existing whenever there have been power inequities between men and women, whites and blacks, bosses and secretaries, doctors and nurses. And, as in any game, both sides have objectives: for the powerless, to get what is needed (resources, services, control, security, recognition, love) without threatening the powerful other; for the powerful, to get what is needed (the work done) without losing face. The game works but at great cost in terms of wasted energy and dishonesty in human relations.

Generally, we see that continual frustration leads not only to powerlessness, but to anger as well, the expression of which depends on each person's character and on perceptions of whether it is safe to express feelings in a given situation.

Maladaptive Expressions of Anger

It is not easy to express anger productively in the face of powerlessness. Anger that is bottled up or feared comes out in a rage, directly or indirectly, or is turned inward. Often, chronic anger may become so painful that it necessitates withdrawal from a situation, if not physically, at least mentally and emotionally.

Open aggression is anger that is directed outwardly toward the perceived source of frustration. It is often nonproductive in that it emerges in a punitive, blaming, attacking manner. Prolonged stress makes people irritable and impatient. When exhaustion and frustration erode the normal defenses, a nurse's anger spills out, perhaps in fleeting sarcasm or rageful outbursts. Rather than focusing on meeting their own needs, nurses blame others. Such interactions often escalate emotions and are nonproductive.

Another form of open aggression occurs when a nurse, perceiving herself as at the bottom of the pecking order, in turn relegates the patient to a step even further down. Occasionally, when this happens, nurses are openly hostile to patients. More often they engage in devaluating ("Oh, she just wants attention."), labeling ("the hysterectomy in Room 307" or "the crock in bed 6"), judging ("He's being manipulative." or "His pain's not real, it's psychosomatic."), and/or stereotyping ("Hispanics are emotional.") behaviors.

Passive aggression, on the other hand, is hidden anger. It may be expressed outwardly or inwardly but is not acknowledged for what it really is. Aggression that is directed outwardly in a passive way can be seen in forgetting, work slow-down, or losing a vacation request. Something or someone is obstructed. Other examples of passive aggression include negativism and cynicism, attitudes that also obstruct, hamper, delay, and undermine. Griping and bitching fall in this category as do comments like "We tried that last year and it didn't work." Passive aggression is seen in the help-rejecting complainer who details all his troubles for his colleagues then methodically negates the value of each suggestion they propose. His sentences are prefaced with "Yes, but . . . ."

Internally directed aggression is experienced as boredom or depression. These emotions are similar in that they are unpleasant feeling states, they imply the existence of frustrated needs to be taken care of, and they immobilize the individual and obstruct activity. Take the nurse, for example, who cannot assert herself with a physician. She knows she is right, yet she questions herself. She feels hopeless about the situation. She goes home depressed. Another nurse, confronted with daily unit frustrations, loses his sense of instrumentality and becomes bored. Frustrated anger, or anger that cannot be expressed, or that is impotent, may be internalized and experienced as boredom or depression. It may also be expressed in physical symptoms.

Detachment is mental or physical withdrawal used as a defense against painful emotions. When the pain of caring, of trying and failing, of hitting one's head against a brick wall becomes too much, the nurse may defend herself by mentally pulling away. Apathy is a state characterized by absence of feelings in which a nurse says, "Who cares? It's not worth it!" This signifies avoiding painful reality through emotional detachment. Other isolating strategies include defenses such as intellectualization (the use of science, rationality, objectivity, professionalism, and other mental processes to avoid experiencing feelings) and compartmentalization (the separation of various aspects of life—home from job—into discrete entities). These mental processes separate painful realities from nonpainful ones so that the pain may be removed from conscious awareness.

Physical detachment as a reaction to anger and helplessness can be seen in a nurse's diminished contact with patients. As stress increases, the nurse's energy is channeled inward to support coping mechanisms and defenses. Her capacity for concern for others is reduced by the need to focus on internal control. There is less energy available for other aspects of work. Nonsanctioned time-outs are taken in the form of extended breaks, absent days, and sick time. The ultimate forms of physical detachment, of course, are resigning the job and dropping out of nursing.

CONCLUSION

What do these chronic negative responses to stress have in common? First, that nurses perceive themselves as trapped in painful situations over which they have little control. Second, that nurses generally perceive the cause of their stress as external (rather than as an internal problem of perception or coping.) Third, that negative, maladaptive responses are rarely efficient, do not improve conditions, and are often deleterious to self and situation.

Physical, mental, and emotional symptoms begin as self-defense mechanisms against stress. They become negative when they consume large amounts of energy, fail to provide relief, and when they further diminish the nurse's capacity to think and work. Structuring one's environment, for example, can be healthy and efficient. It is destructive, however, when structure leads to rigidity, the need to make others conform, and the inability to evaluate individual needs. Controlling one's emotions can be healthy and politically wise, for instance, when one is engaged in delicate negotiations or when one must handle volatile situations. On the other hand, controlling one's emotions can be unhealthy if it results in migraine headaches, or can be politically disastrous if one's extreme reticence means being unable to assert one's views in a committee meeting.

What we, as nurses, need to realize is that strong emotions—frustration, helplessness, and anger—may be altered, limited, controlled, diminished, or masked, but they do not vanish. Their external appearance may be changed, but they remain within us, draining energy from productive work into defensive maneuvers and affecting our relationships with others, albeit subtly.

What we need to do is avoid frustration by altering our expectations and perceptions and by acknowledging and expressing our feelings. If, instead, we attempt to disguise or control painful emotions, or if we try to change others or pit ourselves against impossible odds, then we engage in an endless, painful struggle that leads to burn-out.

REFERENCES

Beck, A. 1967. *Depression: causes and treatment.* Philadelphia: University of Pennsylvania Press.

Beck, A. 1976. *Cognitive therapy and the emotional disorders.* New York: International Universities Press.

Freudenberger, H. J. 1975. Burn-out syndrome in alternative institutions. *Psychother.: Theory Res. Practice* 12(1):73.

Freudenberger, H. J. (with Richardson, G.) 1980. *Burn-out—the high cost of high achievement.* Garden City, N.Y.: Anchor Press.

Gunderson, K., et. al. 1977. How to control professional frustration. *Am. J. Nurs.* 77:1180.

Kleinke, C. L. 1978. *Self perception: the psychology of personal awareness.* San Francisco: W. H. Freeman and Co.

Maslach, C. 1976. Burned-out. *Human Behavior* Sept:16.

Mendel, W. M. 1979. Staff burn-out: diagnosis, treatment, and prevention. *New Direc. Men. Health Serv.* 2:75.

Patrick, P. S. 1979. Burnout: job hazard for health workers. *Hospitals* Nov:87.

Pines, A., and Maslach, C. 1978. Characteristics of staff burn-out in mental health settings. *Hosp. Commun. Psychiatr.* 29(4):233.

Veninga, R. 1979. Administrator burnout—causes and cures. *Hosp. Prog.* 60(2):45–52.

CHAPTER 4

Burn-out: From Caring to Apathy

EMILY E. M. SMYTHE

THE ROAD TO BURN-OUT

What happens to make us feel unable to cope with our chosen profession of nursing? How does the eager, enthusiastic nursing student become a cynic who has nothing to offer but criticism? Why do some idealistic new graduates begin to doubt their ability to offer anything meaningful to their patients or profession? What happens that we go from caring to apathy?

In Chapter 2, we discussed sources of stress in the nursing profession that can provide a climate of unresolved conflict and job strain. Many of these stressors are interpersonal or systems issues that strongly affect us but that usually are beyond our control. These stressors and their subsequent conflicts can initiate a variety of responses in us—among them the fight-or-flight reaction of the general adaptation syndrome (discussed in Chapter 1). Frequently, our responses to the stresses we perceive as beyond our control are destructive, rather than creative, problem-solving solutions (see Chapter 7: Focusing on the Possible: A Problem-Solving Approach).

If, over a period of time, our responses to continual stressors do not decrease the stress and concomitant physiologic reactions, we become physically and emotionally exhausted. When the unresolved stresses are caused by the job, this stage of exhaustion is called burn-out. We don't become burned out from a stressful day or a bad week. Many people describe themselves as being burned out when, in fact, they are overstressed, bored, or frustrated. Burn-out is much more than this; it is the *terminal phase* of failure to resolve work stress. We can, however, become burned out if, over a long period of time, we are unable to cope with the day-to-day job stresses.

Burn-out is a syndrome characterized by the presence of negative job attitude, negative self-concept, and the loss of concern and feeling for patients (Pine, 1981). The dictionary defines burn-out in another way: "worn-out by excessive or improper use; exhausted" (*Webster's New Collegiate Dictionary*, 1977).

The progression from caring to apathy goes something like this: overwhelmed with a sense of failure in your chosen profession, you slowly disengage from a commitment to provide care and concern for your patients. You simply become a robot, following the prescribed treatment regimen, "putting in time" for your salary—feeling emotionally vacant. What's missing is the caring in your nursing care. You just go through the motions, waiting for the work day to end so that you can escape. Clearly, you feel nothing can be done to correct what is perceived as a destructive work situation. The only avenue left open is withdrawal; withdraw your involvement, enthusiasm, or even your physical self by retreating to paper work, calling in sick, or job-hopping.

Being concerned for patients and watching them suffer or die while not getting optimal help is more than you can tolerate. Working short-staffed with inadequate supplies or equipment frequently means just barely surviving. You start to feel as if you are single-handedly supposed to manage all the patients' problems and make up for the deficits in the work environment—a herculean (and impossible) task. After functioning in this way for a long period of time, you may decide that there is only one way to protect yourself from a sense of inadequacy. You decide not to put yourself out—to avoid interacting with the patients and seeing or hearing their concerns. You begin to feel there isn't anything *you* can do about them!

There are numerous ways you can protect yourself from becoming emotionally involved or concerned with patients. Patients can become diagnoses, labels, or derogatory terms instead of human beings. For example, you might find yourself referring to your patients as "the 22-year-old drugger," "the quad in ICU," "the quack," or the "GI bleeder in room 47." When patients are referred to by labels, they can easily become objects or things. No longer are they real, live, suffering human beings with families, jobs to return to, and personal reactions to their illnesses and/or hospitalization. They are now flat, one-dimensional problems. We have abbreviated their lives into nonemotional and safe terms. When we think of patients only as their diagnoses, we stop seeing the complexity and richness of their lives; instead, we now have "a problem" (a diagnosis or label) that has a prescribed treatment. For example, every nurse knows how to handle a GI bleeder, but not all of us feel emotionally able to care for a frightened, depressed man who is begging us to help him talk with his family.

By the time you become burned out, you've already cared so much and felt so inadequate to relieve your patients' suffering that this impersonal way of viewing patients is a relief. There is now an invisible barrier between you and the patient, so no real contact ever has to occur.

As a consultant, whenever I watch burned out nurses care for patients in this dehumanizing fashion, I feel pain and, frequently, anger. I create fantasies for myself to relieve the stress I feel and to give me a humorous perspective that then allows me to help the burned out nurse and her or his patients. One of my fantasies is that the patient suddenly vanishes but the nurse doesn't even know that he's gone, because he simply never "existed" for the nurse. Or another fantasy is that two patients with the same diagnosis switch beds and continue to receive the same medical treatment as before the switch. The burned out nurse would never even know the difference because she or he clearly didn't *know* the patients.

This type of humor relieves the horror I feel witnessing burned out nurses attempting to handle their work responsibilities. Once I'm no longer furious with the nurse, I can start to look more clearly at the situation; I can begin to get a sense of the nurse's struggle to avoid hopeless despair by depersonalizing patients. (See Chapter 18, "Creative Imagination.")

Another way you may start to behave when you feel powerless to deal constructively with job stressors is to become the house griper. All your energy is spent complaining about the numerous problems on the ward. Whenever you gripe about a problem, it helps to decrease sense of responsibility for the problem. It's as if you say, "Hey, don't look at me. I only work here. I'm not responsible for this place and all that's wrong with it! Don't expect me to do anything about it. I'm just telling you what's wrong!"

There's nothing wrong with blowing off steam by complaining occasionally, but, with burn-out, this may become a major part of your style or your only way of responding to the stressors you perceive. After a while, this continual griping no longer helps blow off steam; it just becomes one more reminder of the endless, hopeless abyss of your job. It also depletes your energy and spreads dissatisfaction and resignation to co-workers. (See Chapter 14: Controlling Contagion: Disturbing the Stagnant Quo.)

If the job pressures continue and the discomfort is sufficient, you may feel the need to withdraw—not only from patients but also from co-workers, friends, or family. Avoidance becomes your main coping strategy. You feel used up as if you have nothing to offer anyone; furthermore, they too might want something from you—to listen to their problems, to spend time and nonexistent energy doing things, or even to have an answer to their question, What's the matter with you lately? Because your energy is overspent, you start to see any request, no matter how small or reasonable, as an overwhelming demand. Just getting up in the morning and struggling through the workday is more than you can handle. Exhausted and tired, you no longer have interest in hobbies, sports, or going out. It's all just too much of an undertaking!

At this point you may experience any type of change as an impossible strain, even if the change could potentially alleviate some problems. After all, change requires adaptive energy, and in your stage of exhaustion, energy is the one thing you don't have. You might even find that rigidly and blindly adhering to policies or protocols provides some sense of stability and order to your chaotic work situation.

If the symptoms of tension and anxiety become unbearable, alcohol and drugs may seem the only way to relieve the discomfort. After work you may try to escape conflicting feelings about your job by numbing your brain with alcohol or drugs. You find that you can no longer get to sleep without a pill, even though you're exhausted! Thoughts keep running through your head about how to find the answer to your problem. "There's just got to be some solution for my suffering." You keep going over and over the same work problems in an attempt to find the answer; you become more and more fatigued. The more tired you become, the more irritable and sensitive you are to any job hassles.

When all else fails and you still feel burned out, you might give up. Giving up can take many forms. One form is job-hopping (working a few months in one hospital and then going to the next to find a better job, only to repeat the same cycle—a multiple reenactment of the "grass is always greener" syndrome in which the personal dynamics of the problem are ignored). Another form is working for a nursing registry to avoid getting caught up in hospital politics and getting attached to patients. This is not to imply that working for registries is a bad idea; in some situations, it may be an adaptive decision. Another form is moving up the ladder to an administrative job, away from direct patient problems. Usually, you discover that the burn-out process continues, but this time in the form of staff problems. Yet another form of giving up is going back to the books; back to school as a way up and out. The hope is that you will be able to return to a position with more power and control over your professional life. Or you may become an educator, teaching how things ought to be so you don't have to face how awful they actually are. Burn-out can occur in the educational system and in administrative/management positions as well as in the "front lines" of clinical practice. Also, these changes may be adaptive decisions if you've learned from previous mistakes. If you've learned how to cope and are now directing your energies into productive channels that allow for job satisfaction, these changes represent a positive job-related decision.

This has been an overview of what can happen to you if you are unable to cope with the stresses inherent in nursing today. You burn out from improper use. No longer able to find solutions to job problems, you slowly withdraw into a disengaged state of apathy.

YOU KNOW YOU'RE BURNED OUT WHEN . . .

You know you're burned out when you can identify in yourself many of the signs and symptoms listed on the self-assessment exercise that follows. The signs and symptoms of burn-out can be divided into four basic categories: physical stress symptoms, emotional detachment, dissatisfaction with work accompanied by decreased job performance, and negative self-concept.

Physical stress responses are the first symptoms to occur and are also the easiest to recognize. These symptoms are not unique to burn-out and are the same ones that occur during the fight-or-flight response of the general adaptation syndrome. When they occur in conjunction with symptoms in the three other areas, you're looking at burn-out.

As discussed previously, emotional detachment is actually a protective response; it comes into play when you feel unable to handle job stressors in a more direct, constructive fashion.

With increasing job dissatisfaction, your work performance decreases— sometimes to the point of functioning well below a satisfactory or safe level. When you are under intolerable stress, you are unable to function at your best. You rely on instincts and impulses rather than good, critical judgment.

Since a major part of your self-concept comes from your job performance, it is difficult to sustain positive self-regard in the face of repeated failures. Negative self-concept and accompanying low self-esteem are usually the most difficult problems to correct. If you remain burned out for an extended period, you will doubt yourself so much that all aspects of your life can be damaged. You begin to distrust your judgment and competence in all areas—relationships, parenting, and finances, for example. And if the blow to your self-concept is sufficiently severe, the damage will last long after you've left your job and, in some cases, become a permanent scar that severely impairs your ability to trust yourself.

At this point you're probably wondering just how bad off you actually are. Are you burned out? Take a few moments to complete the assessment exercise on burn-out on pages 51 and 52..

When completing the self-assessment exercise, you need to realize that burn-out occurs in degrees or stages. You may not be burned out at all but still may find this tool valuable to provide an early warning system. You may be just beginning to become disillusioned with nursing, or you may be at the advanced, terminal stage of burn-out where every item on the scale seems to fit (Edelwich and Brodsky, 1980). The more items on the

YOU KNOW YOU'RE BURNED OUT WHEN: SELF-ASSESSMENT FOR SIGNS AND SYMPTOMS OF "BURN-OUT"

Directions

1. Place a check (✓) next to each sign/symptom of burn-out that you are presently experiencing at least once a week.
2. Place a check and a plus (✓ +) next to each sign/symptom you have frequently (more than twice a week) or to such a degree that it significantly interferes with your job functioning or personal life.
3. Your score will not determine whether or not you are burned out. The assessment tool should increase your personal awareness and alert you to potential danger signs/symptoms of burn-out. The more check-pluses (✓ +) you have, the more likely you are to be burned out.

Physical Stress-Related Symptoms

1. _____ Chronic fatigue, exhaustion
2. _____ Insomnia or frequent nightmares
3. _____ Marked weight loss or gain
4. _____ Increased anxiety or nervousness
5. _____ Muscular tension (headaches, back pain, teeth clenching or grinding)
6. _____ Increased use of alcohol/medication
7. _____ Menstrual changes
8. _____ Gastrointestinal disturbances (nausea, vomiting, diarrhea, constipation)
9. _____ Frequent body aches and pain
10. _____ Decreased sexual interest

Emotional Detachment

1. _____ Disliking or feeling annoyed with patients
2. _____ Avoiding co-workers
3. _____ Calling clients names or referring to them by diagnoses
4. _____ Feeling apathetic, lacking interest
5. _____ Feeling like "just putting in time and going through the motions"
6. _____ Frequent sick calls
7. _____ Focusing attention on paper work, non-client-related tasks

YOU KNOW YOU'RE BURNED OUT WHEN: SELF-ASSESSMENT FOR SIGNS AND SYMPTOMS OF "BURN-OUT" (Continued)

8. _____ Wanting to be left alone/not bothered by anyone at work
9. _____ Having marital or interpersonal discord
10. _____ Avoiding talking with your patients or their families

Dissatisfaction with Work and Decreased Job Performance

1. _____ Feeling work is meaningless
2. _____ Reduced productivity
3. _____ Negative about everything at work
4. _____ Procrastination or forgetfulness
5. _____ Disillusioned with profession
6. _____ Hate job
7. _____ Generalized irritability
8. _____ Increased opposition to any change
9. _____ Job accidents or frequent mistakes, omissions
10. _____ Low frustration tolerance
11. _____ Unduly critical of co-workers, organization
12. _____ Working below your potential
13. _____ Inability to concentrate or solve problems
14. _____ Feeling as if your job is destroying your personal life

Negative Self-Concept

1. _____ Questioning your own competence as a health professional
2. _____ Feeling depressed (hopeless, helpless, sad)
3. _____ Being unduly self-critical
4. _____ Feeling overwhelmed (too much to do)
5. _____ Feeling as if you have nothing to offer
6. _____ Feeling responsible for your client not benefiting from care
7. _____ Feeling worthless, incompetent, or stupid
8. _____ Being less creative
9. _____ Experiencing isolation or alienation from others
10. _____ Feeling of lowered self-esteem

assessment tool you endorse, the greater your degree of burn-out, especially if they are check-pluses ($\checkmark +$).

Most people who use an assessment tool for evaluating themselves want a definite answer to whether or not they are experiencing a problem. In general, however, many evaluation tools used in health care systems are best applied to inform you of the signs and symptoms of a given problem; they attempt to identify a pattern of responses and evaluate the severity or duration of the symptoms. For example, your only physical symptom may be migraine headaches that keep you out of work whenever they occur; they may require an ever-increasing amount of analgesics to control the pain. This one symptom clearly warrants attention as a severe problem, regardless of whether or not you have any other physical symptoms.

Another function of the assessment tool is to alert you to potential danger signals. This is particularly important with burn-out since prevention of the terminal exhaustion phase can occur more easily if you are sensitive to your less severe stress responses. The goal of burn-out prevention is early recognition of the developing problem; in other words, catch it while you are under stress, but are still able to cope with and be involved in your job.

Many of the signs and symptoms of burn-out occur in normal day-to-day living and are not unique to burn-out. What you are attempting to evaluate in yourself is a *pattern* of responses. For example, we all occasionally get headaches, dislike a patient with whom we're working, don't want to come to work, or feel down on ourselves. That doesn't necessarily mean that we're burned out. On the other hand, if you have these experiences frequently or to the point that they characterize your behavior, then clearly you are burned out.

Furthermore, using an assessment exercise for burn-out may allow you to label the discomfort you were feeling but didn't know how to describe. Many times in workshops I give on stress management, participants will say something like, I felt awful . . . like something was definitely wrong with me, but I didn't know what it was. I'd been feeling like I was going crazy or was different from everyone else! Now I know what the problem is—I'm burned out. Now I can start to do something about it.

If you discovered that you are burned out, don't be alarmed; above all, don't become self-deprecatory. *A word of caution and consolation:* to become burned out, you had to have been "on fire." You would never become burned out if you weren't a caring, sensitive nurse who was once enthusiastic about your job and who once had high aspirations for your chosen profession. In fact, the degree of disappointment you feel is probably directly related to the degree of expectations you have about your job (that is, the more unreasonable your expectations, the greater your sense of disappointment). Nurses who are insensitive, don't care what happens to their patients, or see their job as simply a nine-to-five money-making situation don't risk becoming burned out. So if you identified yourself as being burned out, remember that under your charred exterior is a warm, responsive person who once again can become a contributing member of the nursing profession and who can once again experience satisfaction from providing nursing care!

BURN-OUT TOLL

Burn-out is an expensive and devastating problem that not only affects you, the individual nurse, but also affects every aspect of the health care system—the patient, hospital management and administration, and the nursing profession in general. Once many nurses in a system become burned out, the problem becomes more than an individual problem; the destructive, vicious cycle it develops makes it a system problem. See Figure 4-1 for a graphic presentation of the disequilibrium of burn-out toll.

Although the primary focus of this book is on you, the individual nurse, it is helpful to look at how you, as one burned out nurse, can ultimately have a negative influence upon the total health care system in which you work. After all, you don't practice our profession in a vacuum. Your behavior can have a profound effect upon others with whom you have daily contact. Of course, the idea of having a powerful influence on others—even a negative force—usually seems surprising given the powerlessness and helplessness a burned-out person feels! In fact, one reason you may have become burned out is that you feel unable to change the destructive work

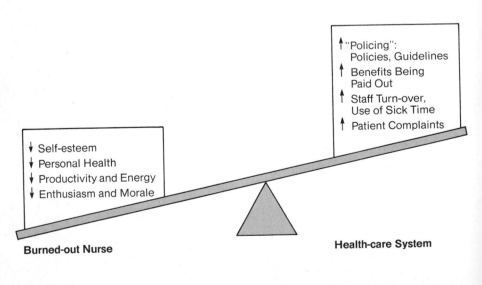

FIGURE 4-1.

Burn-out toll: disequilibrium in the health care system created by a vicious cycle.

situation that influences not only your job satisfaction but also the progress and care of your patients.

I see the vicious cycle of burn-out as a tragedy, a play that is reenacted daily on an unconscious level. The play goes something like this.

Characters:

- Burned-out nurse
- Rigid hospital administrator
- Struggling, unsure head nurse
- Frightened patient
- Angry physician

Stage Directions:

Each character speaks only to himself or herself, and all characters speak at once with forceful conviction. It is imperative that no character recognize the presence of the other characters or hear the other characters' concerns. If these directions are not strictly followed and an open dialogue should occur, it will diffuse the increasing tension and make it difficult for each character to continue in his or her role, thereby ruining the vicious cycle. Furthermore, each character must appear to be unaware of his or her own part in the vicious cycle. The monologues appear to have lives of their own, and the characters only provide a vehicle for the presentation of each archtypical position.

Burned-out Nurse: I can't stand this job. It's ruining my whole life; all I think about is work. . . . I can barely get myself out of bed in the morning. I've started making mistakes, but what can they expect! I can't even think clearly with all the commotion going on. There's never enough staff, and there are so many patients that need me. Half these crocks are just complainers anyway. And for all the education and training I've had, I get paid much less than the plumber or even the grocery store check-out clerk! Why in the world did I ever want to become a nurse? That new head nurse is always coming around spying on us. Now they cut the staff even more because of budget problems. They're always making decisions about how to improve patient care, but no one asks me what I think and, after all, I'm one of the ones who's here 24 hours a day. I'm also sick of these doctors. They're never here when you need them, but they sure expect you to jump at their beck and call!

Rigid Hospital Administrator: It's a disgrace. All those nurses do is complain. Used to be it took one nurse to do what three of them can barely manage. No matter how I try to meet their demands they just ask for more. They said they needed a ward clerk to take doctors' orders; I got one for them. Now they want pharmacy to deliver stat drugs, respiratory therapists for the ICU, phlebotomists, in-service educators; what will they think of next? We've got to cut hospital costs; all this extra help is a waste of money. The more free time they have to sit around and gripe, the more demands they come up with. And that new head nurse—she doesn't keep them in line! She needs to be firmer with them. We ought to fire some of these nurses who aren't functioning. The patients have too many complaints about their care. The next thing I know we'll be having a big law suit. . . .

Struggling, Unsure Head Nurse: Well what do they expect from me? Hospital administration is all over me about those nurses' job performance. The last time I had a counseling session with one of them, she just said, "I've had enough; this is the best I can do. It's a miracle I even come to work anymore! Feel free to fire me!" Of course she knows we're already critically short of staff; how could I fire her? I'll just have to make my expectations clearer, revise a few of the nursing protocols, and spend more time on the unit observing. She even complained about that too, saying I was "policing her." With all the mistakes being made, I've got to supervise more. And their negative attitude! If they just were more positive, everything would work out better.

Angry Physician: The nursing staff in this hospital is incompetent! The nurses make so many mistakes it's amazing any of my patients get well. I'm going to talk with the hospital administrator about the poor patient care here; if he can't shape it up, I'll just admit my patients somewhere else. . . . The nurses here are rude, too—always irritable—maybe they're just castrating women who have miserable home lives!

Burned-out Nurse: Not only do I have the usual job pressures that got me into this state, but now I've got the pressure of constant surveillance, and I have to justify every action. I really resent being treated like a child rather than a professional. They act like the poor patient care is my fault instead of the hospital's.

The Frightened Patient: I don't understand it. The nurses here aren't interested in me. They're not at all like the friendly nurses I see on TV. Why, yesterday the day nurse almost gave me my roommate's pills! I'm getting scared. They don't even care when I put on the call light. I'll have to speak to my doctor about this. I'm paying good money for my health care, and I'm not getting what I'm paying for. I'll just have to be more demanding and insist on my rights!

Ending:

The play ends with each character running through his or her script over and over, day after day. No changes occur. Each character seems locked into a self-deprecating pattern that allows the vicious cycle to continue.

CONCLUSION

Of course there are *many* other possible endings to this play. In fact, I believe for most burned-out nurses the endings are happy or certainly could be happy ones. Their experiences with burn-out can set the stage for personal and professional growth that will, we hope, alter many of the negative stressors in the health care system and enhance their sense of professional competence. Nurses who are in the early stages of burn-out, or nurses who are not burned out, can use their knowledge of the signs and symptoms of burn-out and its causes to prevent the development and spread of the burn-out syndrome. Although burn-out is a serious problem in nursing, it can be prevented and cured.

REFERENCES

Edelwich, J., and Brodsky, A. 1980. *Burnout: stages of disillusionment in the helping profession.* New York: Human Sciences.

Pine, A., and Aronson, E. 1981. *Burnout: from tedium to personal growth.* New York: Free Press.

Webster's New Collegiate Dictionary. 1977. Springfield, Mass.: G. and C. Merriam Co.

2

Philosophy of Self-Care: A Process for Coping with Job Stress in Nursing

After reading the previous section, which focuses on the stresses of nursing, you might believe that because job stressors are so prevalent in nursing you are doomed to feel distress as long as you remain in the profession. Take heart, there is another option. You don't have to become burned out or suffer from stress-related illness because of the stressors in nursing. Many nurses suffer no ill effects from their jobs—in fact they thrive on their work.

The first thing you will have to accept if you hope to control your job stress is that you are ultimately responsible for your own well-being. True, there are stressors everywhere in nursing, as there are in any job. Perhaps nursing has more than its share of stressors. Who is to say? But whether you respond to these stressors by experiencing distress and defeat or challenge and satisfaction is up to you. Sure the health-care system needs some major changes, and nursing is a demanding profession; but you don't have to become overstressed and dissatisfied with your job.

Learning to cope with stress is not an end point by which someday you will have handled all your stress and thus become stress free. Managing stress is an ongoing process that enables you to learn how to handle varying quantities and types of potential stressors—many of which are unavoidable. The first step in learning the stress-management process is to develop a self-care philosophy.

This section presents the essential ingredients of the stress-management philosophy of self-care: (1) self-awareness, (2) personal responsibility, (3) positive self-regard, and (4) a healthy life-style. It explores positive responses to stress that form the basis for developing your own self-enhancement philosophy.

Stress management is presented as a holistic approach to living rather than simply a collection of techniques and coping strategies. Without adopting a self-care philosophy, it is unlikely you will significantly alter your job stress or continue to practice the techniques you learn in more than a haphazard fashion. From a holistic perspective, stress management is not simply learning how to cope with stress; it is a process for promoting an optimal sense of well-being.

Learning to cope with job stress is a process. It is a way of traveling through life, not a final destination. *Bon voyage.*

CHAPTER 5

Self-Awareness: A Means of Taking Charge of Yourself

EMILY E. M. SMYTHE

AWARENESS AND SELF-RESPONSIBILITY

Stress management is a process of self-care that develops logically out of being aware of and responsive to your internal needs and external demands. You cannot adequately manage job stress unless you know how you are feeling emotionally and physically and are able to accept personal responsibility for these feelings. The issue is not learning how to avoid job stressors but learning how to cope with them so that stressors become challenges rather than defeats.

The only person who can manage your stress is you. As long as you consider yourself a helpless victim of job stressors, you will feel hopelessly defeated. Whenever you place blame for your behavior or emotional response on someone or something else, you have automatically given up your ability to control yourself—you have placed your sense of well-being in someone else's care. You may avoid taking responsibility for your self-care because of the negative connotations associated with the concept of responsibility. *Responsibility* is a term often used when the words *blame* and *obligation* would be more appropriate. When someone says to you,

"Who's responsible for this problem?" it probably seems as if she is saying, "Who's to blame for this mess?" Or when someone says, "You are responsible for doing something about this," he is more likely implying, "You are obligated to solve this problem." Blame and obligation beget resentment and resistance. Blaming is a way of avoiding responsibility.

Responsibility more accurately means respond-able, or having the ability to react based upon your sense of awareness. The dictionary definition of responsible is "involving personal ability to act without superior authority." This definition implies a self-directed selected position that can emerge only from a sense of personal awareness.

A word of caution: becoming aware of yourself and personal responsibility for your stress management does not mean becoming self-critical or digging up personal inadequacies with which to beat yourself. It does mean listening to yourself by paying attention to your needs and perceptions. Awareness also comes from acknowledging your limitations, not as failures but as reasonable boundaries. Knowing yourself implies appreciating your uniqueness—a form of self-respect. Self-awareness is not the same as self-evaluation. When you are aware, you suspend your evaluative, critical self and awaken your senses. When you are fully aware, you allow yourself to recognize your internal needs and the external stimuli as they emerge and are experienced by your senses. Once aware, you are able to choose to respond only to those stimuli that are interesting and important to you and need not get trapped by automatic responses that cause you to forfeit your sense of control. When you are fully aware, you will experience a sense of vitality that can come only from being tuned in to yourself and the world around you.

Rather than using our senses to become aware, most of us settle for being critical observers who evaluate our experiences against unrealistic standards of what we should be like. This self-criticism can become a defeating process that will eventually erode our self-support and self-confidence and lead to a sense of inadequacy and helplessness. Negative self-evaluation is self-perpetuating. When you imagine defeat before you undertake a task, chances are good you will fail. The converse of this is equally true—if you feel confident in your ability to manage stressors, you will greatly increase your chances of success. Lazarus (1966) demonstrated that feeling helpless and unable to control your environment significantly contributes to the experience of distress. The more self-support and control you feel in a given situation, the less severe your stress response will be (Lazarus, 1966).

The more out of touch we are with ourselves, the less able we are to be in control of ourselves. If your life is governed by many "shoulds," "oughts," or "musts," you are not operating from your personal value system or current needs; you are responding to someone else's frame of reference—parents or teachers, for instance. Whenever you live your life according to other peoples' expectations of what you should be like instead of how you actually are, you lose touch with your senses and self-support systems by becoming controlled by external demands. You live your life acting out a role much as a small child imitating adults playing at life, not living life. Rotter et al., (1976) has used the term "externals" to describe people who believe their lives are governed by external events. Their sense of well-being is at the mercy of other people's evaluations of them. Because of their lack of self-awareness and self-control, externals experience normal, everyday occurrences as stressful. "Internals," who are governed by their senses and beliefs in their ability to control their lives, are able to handle stress better and are generally happier because they take active control over their lives. Given the same daily stresses, internals do not feel as stressed and upset as "externals" (Rotter et al., 1976). The critical variable in experiencing distress is our self-awareness and sense of control over stressful life events, not the inherent danger of the stressor.

APPROACHES TO STRESS RESISTANCE AND ENHANCEMENT OF WELL-BEING

We can gather a lot of useful information about a philosophy of self-care by examining people who respond positively to stress. Unfortunately, there is no simple or single way to deal with stress. Every religion and philosophy has different "answers." It is possible, however, to study the common traits of people who thrive despite stress and to select the ingredients that best suit your personality and life-style. From other people's collective wisdom, you can weave your own self-care philosophy.

Why do some nurses feel positive and enthusiastic about their jobs despite the numerous stressors in nursing? What wisdom do they possess that can benefit the rest of us? An embittered nurse once said to me, "The only way anyone can enjoy nursing is if she is naive or blind to the problems." Blind, naive optimism, however, quickly wears out in the light of constant day-to-day job hassles in nursing. Interestingly enough, most satisfied nurses did not achieve success by ignoring or avoiding problems but by possessing an accurate awareness of their job stress and taking care of themselves. Instead of seeing problems as obstacles to their job satisfaction, they see them as challenges. They do not waste energy attempting to avoid stress but accept the fact that stress is a normal part of any job. They are able to recognize which problems are worth fighting for and which are better left alone.

Since you can't avoid stress entirely, you need to come to terms with how you are going to allow it to affect you. You have to choose how you will respond to stress. You can spend your energy lamenting that this is not the best of all possible worlds, or you can accept stress and change as a part of life and decide to use your energy to make the best of it. Acceptance is the opposite of hopeless resignation. Accepting stress as part of living involves shifting into a position of self-control—of taking charge of your sense of well-being rather than simply reacting.

The difference between feeling distressed and frustrated on one hand or satisfied and challenged on the other is not caused by environmental or interpersonal conditions of the job alone. Our job perception and responses, positive or negative, are created by the interaction between our inner selves and the systems in which we work. As Kashoff (1976) says,

> Stress is an inside job. We do not have it until it resides inside us. It is not just out there somewhere. It is how we hook up and relate to what is out there that determines whether or not it will be stressful to us. And, finally, once we experience the discomfort of stress, the crucial question is not where or how we got it, but what do we choose to do about it.

When studying "stress-resistant" people, we find the following attitudes toward living: be open to change, be aware of having control over events, and be committed to what you are doing. People who possess these attitudes remain healthier than other people despite exposure to certain stressful life events that are associated with the development of illness (Kobasa et al., 1979). When people believe that they are doing something important and of personal value, they are encouraged to put themselves into their jobs wholeheartedly rather than taking the attitude that they are putting in time for a paycheck. Selye points out that work is a biologic necessity. The aim of work is to find an occupation that is enjoyable. Thus it becomes enhancing rather than defeating or exhausting.

> Labor is doing what we must;
> Leisure is doing what we like.
> George Bernard Shaw

It is not work itself that wears us down but the frustration and failure we experience in our jobs that becomes devastating (Selye, 1975).

Part of what determines a personal sense of failure and frustration is where we place our emphasis. There is a substantial difference between being inclined to influence certain outcomes and having preferences for these outcomes. When you become addicted to certain goals, you feel your life is governed by strong emotional demands that must be met to survive. If you are addicted to being right, knowing all the facts, being loved by everyone, or any other outcome, you will be unable to exercise control over yourself and will continually feel overstressed (Keyes, 1975). Disagreements become life-and-death struggles. Your goal becomes a necessity rather than a personal preference. Getting stuck on one goal and one approach to achieving it also narrows your awareness of other equally valid approaches. Perhaps, for example, you cannot save a patient's life, but you can provide comfort, which is also important. You can miss this opportunity if you are close-minded and addicted to demanding one result. There are many paths leading to the top of the mountain; the trick is not to feel defeated if your efforts are blocked. Whenever events and interactions are emotionally charged, you become locked into defensive reactions—life feels like a frantic struggle for survival. But the only goal worth being addicted to is maintaining your optimal wellness through active self-care.

Traits of Self-Actualized People

Maslow (1968) examined successful people from all walks of life to identify what traits recur in self-actualized individuals. His interest was in determining not only how people successfully cope with life demands but also how they are able to flourish and realize their maximum potential. Self-actualization cannot exist as a goal in its own right; it is a by-product of the active utilization of external resources, such as the pursuit of human rights, promotion of health, and religious beliefs. Maslow identified some of the following traits in these self-actualized people:

- Adequate perception of reality and acceptance of it
- High degree of acceptance of themselves and others, including an unhostile sense of humor and feeling of brotherly love
- High level of autonomy based upon an ethical values system that governs behavior and the ability to hold onto these values despite cultural pressures
- High level of creativity and inventiveness; they search for new solutions to old problems and the positive potential in problems
- Usage of problem-centered approach; they focus attention on tasks or missions instead of on themselves
- Spontaneity in thinking, behavior, and emotions
- Renewed appreciation of basic pleasures—nature, children, friends

Jourard (1974) proposes that people's self-images and beliefs significantly influence their growth toward a healthy personality.

> Descriptions of man do not merely describe, they *prescribe*. A person acts in the world as being with the limits, strengths and weaknesses he believes are his "nature." . . . A person will persevere in a difficult project so long as he has hope, and *believes* he has the capacity to succeed. As soon as he begins to doubt that it is within his capacity, he gives up, and "natural sequences" take over. . . . A man's views of his capacities to cope, to survive, to grow are decisive influences upon the course of his life.

Positive Attitudes

Part of what determines our perceptions of our potentials and limitations is our attitude toward life in general. Attitudes can be changed. Looking for the positive in yourself and others as well as in every situation gives you the ability to deflect many potential stressors. Successful people focus on what can be learned from mistakes and do not let one failure become a personal defeat. They are able to learn from enemies and competitors as well as mentors. Disagreements provide better opportunities to define beliefs more clearly and to learn about the self than do agreements. If you become upset during an interaction, use the opportunity to learn about the vulnerable, sensitive parts of your character. If the other person were not touching a "weak spot" within you, you would be able to brush off the comments as irrelevant or unfounded. Stress survivors are able to let go of stress; they learn to roll with the punches and come up fighting. Selye (1975) wrote the following words of advice on maintaining a healthy attitude:

> Try to keep your mind constantly on the pleasant aspects of life and on actions which can improve your situation. Try to forget everything that is irrevocably ugly or painful. This is perhaps the most efficient way of minimizing stress by what I have called voluntary mental diversion. As a wise German proverb says, "Imitate the sun dials' ways; count only the pleasant days."

Perls (1969), the father of gestalt therapy, said that people do not realize their full potential because they are afraid of living in the here and now. Instead, they live in the past, through obsessive remembering, or in the future, by creating catastrophic expectations and fantasies. Healthy persons trust their own ability and potential for self-regulation and growth through becoming more aware. They trust the wisdom of their bodies to mobilize their innate capacity for self-healing. The Chinese use the term *chi* for this healing force of nature. They believe that a strengthened body can rid itself of disease. As we become more aware of our senses and the world around us, we are more able to respond spontaneously from a position of self-support—to let ourselves go with the flow instead of struggling against the inevitable. Forcing ourselves and others to act differently than we feel causes needless distress. "Maturation is the development from environmental support to self-support" (Perls, 1969). People who achieve peak performances, athletes or musicians for instance, do so by losing themselves in their experience. They do not become self-conscious. They do not think about or attempt to force the experience. Once they stop to become an observer of their performance, they are no longer able to be involved.

CARING FOR YOURSELF IN ORDER TO CARE FOR OTHERS

In nursing we have been taught that client needs come first, and that we must ignore our own needs to better the client's situation. Unfortunately, this way of thinking is entirely wrong! Unless we first learn how to care for ourselves, we will not have much to offer our patients. You cannot give something that you do not have. Stress interferes with our ability to "be there" for the patient and to provide the best care we are capable of giving. Nurses attempting to function when in distress are as impaired as nurses who have a physical illness.

> When job stress in a human service setting is chronic the helper's motivation, involvement and positive regard for the work and for clients may suffer. . . . In fact there is research and theory suggesting that the enthusiasm, idealism, and hope of the helper are critical ingredients in . . . health care. . . . When the helper loses enthusiasm, effectiveness declines (Cherniss, 1980).

Selye (1978) formulated the concept of *altruistic egoism*—"looking out for ourself by being necessary to others and thus earning their goodwill." Putting other people's well-being before our own self-care is against the basic laws of nature and exhausting at the very least. Many nurses have neglected self-care to the point that their own need for support prevents them from giving to their patients (Michaels, 1971). How can we teach health maintenance if we are unable to live by these principles of well-being? Health, from a holistic perspective, is a positive state of being, not just the absence of illness.

Kashoff (1976) uses the term *enlightened self-interest* to describe the concept of self-care in relation to patient care.

> I care a lot about you—so much so, in fact, that I will have a great deal more to offer you by taking good care of myself, saying "no" on occasion to preserve my energy, and making sure that I too get my turn now and then. In this way, I will not be harboring resentment but rather feel far happier to share myself and extend myself to other people.

Do you know what it is like to receive care given by an overstressed, emotionally unaware nurse? Try to remember a difficult time in your life when you went to someone you trusted for help but found the person so preoccupied and inattentive he or she couldn't be there for you. We've all had that kind of experience. When we don't give ourselves care as nurses, we become unable to be fully present for others, including our patients.

If we really want to be in a position to utilize our nursing knowledge and skill, we must first value ourselves enough to practice self-care: martyrs are crucified; they don't survive to help the next person. "If I am not for myself, who will be for me? And if I am only for myself, what am I?" (Hillel, a Hebrew philosopher).

Are you your own best friend or worst enemy? Imagine for a moment that you are required to tell a colleague three positive characteristics about yourself. You are not allowed to attach disclaimers or trailers. ("I'm attractive—except I'm a little overweight.") Pay attention to your feelings as you imagine praising yourself to this other person. Now imagine you have to tell this same person three faults or weaknesses you have. How do you feel about this?

Did you notice any difference between praising and criticizing yourself? Most people find it uncomfortable to imagine praising themselves. We are taught not to brag or be conceited. Unfortunately, many of us have learned to neutralize our "positives" by ignoring or minimizing them. Even when other people give us praise, we generally deflect it. ("Oh, it was nothing.

You would have done the same thing.") On the other hand, we usually personalize our mistakes. For example, not having an answer to every question seems to be a sign of our basic stupidity. Obviously, after years of this selective inattention to our good points and preoccupation with our shortcomings, we find it difficult to maintain self-confidence.

No one can support you as well as you can support yourself. Learn to be self-nurturing. We all need to build up our own self-esteem and confidence to tackle stress without becoming stress-related casualties. We need to become as familiar and comfortable with our strengths as we are with our limitations. Force yourself to write down what you've accomplished each day rather than focusing on the day's mistakes. Whenever you catch yourself chiseling away at your own self esteem **stop immediately.** Give yourself support by telling yourself, "Yes, I could have done that better, but this is an entirely new experience. I can't expect to be a pro the first time. . . . I've come a long way. I'm really proud of myself!"

A philosophy of self-care involves holding yourself in high esteem. So what if you're not perfect! After all, no one is. See your life instead of as a failure as in the process of becoming a success. If you encounter a limitation, accept it as a part of yourself and look elsewhere for your strengths.

> The effects of chronic self-hate and low self-esteem are insidious and pervasive even though they may not be immediately obvious. Generalized feelings of worthlessness and inadequacy invariably lead to a disastrous total life-style. . . . Compassion is the only antidote to self-hate. . . . Compassion is, ultimately, a state of mind in which benevolence reigns supreme. . . . Being responsible for ourselves without guilt or other forms of self-hate take precedence over all other activities (Rubin, 1975).

OWNING YOUR "I"

One way to increase your awareness and sense of control is through the gestalt therapy technique of "owning the I." Owning involves acknowledging yourself by what you say. For example, the statement, "I can't . . ." helps you avoid responsibility. Saying "I won't . . ." or "I'm not willing to . . ." indicates personal control. Using the word *try* is a way of disowning ability and intention. Trying does not accomplish much except to help you avoid commitment and to give an excuse if (when) you fail. Forcing yourself to take a clear stand by saying either "I will do . . ." or "I won't do . . ." makes you aware of your choices and gives you a sense of power. Not owning your I is another way of decreasing your awareness. Unfortunately, most nurses are notorious for not taking a personal position on issues. How often do you make statements like, "We think you ought to . . ." or "It would be good if . . . ?" When you avoid making I statements, you discount all that you think, feel, believe, and want. Disowning only decreases your awareness and sense of control. These may seem like semantic gimmicks, but I have found that by acknowledging myself—owning my I—I have a greater sense of personal power over my life and more awareness of my choices.

PERSONAL AWARENESS AND SELF-RESPONSIBILITY ASSESSMENT

It is easy to lose touch with yourself as you frantically attempt to meet work demands as well as juggle personal concerns. Part 3 provides self-assessment tools designed to increase your awareness of stress-related symptoms and of how you respond to stress. The following questions are to help you explore your attitude towards your self-care:

1. Do you think your needs and wants are as important as those of other people?
2. Do you actively make choices that influence your job and personal life?
3. Do you pay attention to your body's messages *before* you experience illness or pain?
4. When you have an emotional reaction such as sadness or anger, do you consider it valid, or do you rationalize that you shouldn't feel the way you do?
5. Do you have clear personal goals for your life, or do you seem to be drifting from day to day?
6. Do you generally feel self-confident in your abilities to handle daily stress and change?
7. Are you able to identify your strengths as well as your weaknesses?
8. Are you able to let go of angry, resentful feelings, or do you spend a lot of energy ruminating about conflicts?
9. Are you in control of your sense of well-being, or do you tend to blame others for the way you feel?
10. Do you generally respond positively (feel enthusiastic and excited) or negatively (feel overwhelmed and uncomfortable) to stress?

CONCLUSION

Anyone in a healing profession must become acquainted with his emotional nature, his personality conflicts, his strengths and weaknesses, and generally be willing to engage in a process of self-exploration (Pelletier, 1978).

Ultimately, you are the person responsible for your sense of well-being. The more aware you are of yourself, the more able you are to manage your distress and contribute to your optimal level of well-being.

REFERENCES

Cherniss, C. 1980. *Staff burnout: job stress in the human services.* Beverly Hills, Calif.: Sage Publications.

Jourard, S. M. 1974. *Healthy personality: an approach from the viewpoint of humanistic psychology.* New York: Macmillan.

Kashoff, S. 1976. Nursing your stress. *J. Emerg. Nurs.* 2(2):12–20.

Keyes, K. 1975. *The handbook of higher consciousness.* Berkeley, Calif.: Living Loving Center.

Kobasa, S. C. 1979. Stressful life events, personality, and health: an inquiry into hardiness. *J. Pers. Soc. Psychol.* 37(1): 1–11.

Lazarus, R. S. 1966. *Psychological stress and coping process.* New York: McGraw-Hill.

Maslow, A. A. 1968. *Toward a psychology of being,* 2nd ed. New York: Van Nostrand Reinhold.

Michaels, D. R. 1971. Too much in need of support to give any? *Am. J. Nurs.* 71:1932.

Pelletier, K. 1978. *Toward a science of consciousness.* New York: Dell Publishing Co.

Perls, F. 1969. *Gestalt therapy verbatim.* New York: Bantam Books.

Rotter, J. B., Chance, J. E., and Phares, E. J. 1976. *Applications of a social learning theory of personality.* New York: Holt, Rinehart and Winston.

Rubin, T. I. 1975. *Compassion and self-hate.* New York: Ballantine Books.

Selye, H. 1978. On the real benefits of eustress. *Psychol. Today* 11(10):60–70.

Selye, H. 1975. *Stress without distress.* New York: Signet Books.

CHAPTER 6

Balance: A Way of Developing a Healthy Life-Style

EMILY E. M. SMYTHE

> Those who flow as life flows
> Feel no wear, feel no tear
> Need no mending, no repair (Lao Tse 1973)

There is a tendency in all organisms to correct any imbalance by self-regulating processes that reestablish homeostasis, or balance. In discussing the body's balance, Goldway (1979) points out that balance occurs naturally without our striving to achieve it.

> Disease is merely a series of adaptations (otherwise called signs and symptoms) mobilized by a fantastically complex system that keeps adjusting itself in order to try to preserve its survival (by maintaining equilibrium/balance).

Maintaining this equilibrium is a continual, active process. Because each action causes a reaction, which in turn causes another action, and so on, there really is no true cause-and-effect, linear relationship in living organisms. Instead, what occurs is a cyclical life process.

In Western thinking we have tended to break down the life processes into linear equations to logically understand complex systems. We have also isolated or reduced aspects of the whole system in an attempt to understand their function—sometimes to the extent that our comprehension of the living system is distorted. When those of us in the health profession make a mind-body-environment split and fail to see the interaction and interrelationship among these arbitrary divisions, we lose sight of their interdependence. For example, people who become physically ill have changes in their moods, thinking, and perceptions. They also respond to and interact with their environment in an altered fashion. For that matter, to truly understand the function of each organ or body system, heart, lung, kidneys, or brain, you must understand the body as a whole, the person who inhabits the body, and the individual's environmental context. For instance, the heart of an overweight and highly anxious person with renal damage functions very differently from the heart of a healthy young athlete. A heart is *not* just a heart. It needs to be understood in context, as must all living systems and their components.

We in the Western world also have a tendency to classify natural events as good or bad. Warm weather is good, cold is bad (unless you're a snow-skier); light is good, darkness is bad. . . . Of course we don't all agree on what is good or bad, but we all seem to classify things in this way. Stress is usually seen as bad, which as indicated in previous chapters is not really the case. Whenever we experience stress, whether distress (bad stress) or eustress (good stress), we experience a state of imbalance or disequilibrium that can eventually lead to exhaustion and cellular breakdown. Of course, for undetermined reasons, eustress doesn't produce the same degree of wear and tear on the body as distress. However, being in a constant state of positive excitement or "high" also can be exhausting. No one can sustain the keyed-up excitement of sexual orgasm or competitive readiness for long. Our bodies need to rebalance.

In stress management the approaches used are designed to return the body to a state of equilibrium by enhancing the body's own self-regulatory mechanisms. With minor stresses our bodies readily readjust to a state of balance. However, when stress is prolonged or the compensatory adaptive resources depleted, balance is not restored automatically. Various stress reduction techniques and coping strategies discussed in Parts 3 and 5 are designed to assist us in returning the body to a balanced state.

Ideally, however, we should be able to prevent the prolonged states of disequilibrium that contribute to distress and illness by practicing a healthy life-style. A healthy life-style's primary focus is the enhancement of an optimal sense of well-being. Its basic elements are good nutrition, physical fitness, a vibrant spirit, stress management, and relaxation. All these elements can be achieved through a healthy life-style based on the principle of balance, that is, maintaining equilibrium by enhancing the body's self-regulatory, homeostatic mechanisms. These components are interrelated and combine to maintain balance in the individual life-style and in the individual's relation to the universe.

You can consciously adopt a healthy life-style by assuming personal responsibility for reinforcing the natural healing capacities of the body, avoiding unnecessary stress, and maintaining system balance as an approach to developing high-level wellness. Unfortunately, as Selye (1979) points out,

> We have been so overwhelmed with the abnormalities of modern living that we have come to believe that the abnormal is normal. We overlook the fact that natural harmony, balance, and homeostasis are the norm.

Certainly when all we see is misery, suffering, and irrational acts of cruelty or violence, it is easy to get a jaded view of life. We lose our sense of balance. There is, however, another perspective to life. There are also acts of true generosity and love, miraculous feats of overcoming hopeless odds, and collective striving to better the lot of humanity. The evening news doesn't present the world accurately—it certainly does not report all the news. The *good news* is usually missing and thus the "news" doesn't present a balanced picture of our times.

We have also lost our sense of balance and appreciation for nature. We cut through mountains to build highways and pollute the streams, the air, and the earth with noxious wastes and fumes; we denude forests and irrigate the deserts with little thought for the fact that our resources are finite and that this earth is the only place we have to live. We act as if whatever goes wrong can be fixed by technology. "If we squander all our natural resources, we'll just create new ones" seems to be a common, distorted philosophy. Many of us also apply this erroneous logic to our bodies. Oh, I can always go on a diet tomorrow. What does it matter that I "pig-out" today? We eat the wrong thing, fail to exercise, we smoke, drink excessively, and push ourselves without resting. In general, we grossly neglect ourselves as if the way we live will have no ill effects on our health or well-being. Many of us believe that modern medical technology will be able to save us from our life-styles—there's always surgery or pills. We look for instant answers to lifelong problems. Many of us give better care to our cars than we do to our bodies.

There simply isn't any easy, quick, magical answer to achieving high-level wellness. What we do, or neglect to do, on a daily basis, has an accumulative effect on our health and sense of well-being. Developing a healthy life-style involves daily living practices that assist the body in maintaining its balance and thus its health. A healthy life-style is based on a philosophy of self-care that includes the ingredients of self-respect, self-awareness, self-control, and self-responsibility discussed in the previous chapter. If you misuse your car by racing it around, never changing the oil or getting a tune-up, eventually it will die on you. Simply adding gas or replacing the tires won't keep it going. Every operating part of your car is necessary; failure to care for each part will ultimately lead to breakdown. Sure you can get an engine overhaul when your car breaks down, but when it comes to your body, what is an "engine overhaul"? A heart transplant? Kidney dialysis? A face-lift? When your car falls apart, you can always replace it with a newer model. Unfortunately, we only get one body. We are totally dependent on our bodies; if we destroy them, we destroy ourselves. "Your body is beautiful just as nature designed it—please don't do anything to void the warranty" (Ardell, 1979).

What I propose, and what most holistic health care practitioners advocate, is the same basic healthy life practices your parents probably preached to you years ago, even if they didn't live by them. Here are seven basic rules for good health practices that have been demonstrated to decrease incidence of illness and promote a sense of well-being (Breslow and Belloc, 1972).

1. Get regular physical activity.
2. Obtain seven to eight hours of sleep each day.
3. Don't smoke.
4. Use alcohol moderately or not at all.
5. Maintain proper body weight.
6. Eat three well-balanced meals (especially breakfast).
7. Don't snack between meals.

As you attempt to switch over to a more healthy life-style, be realistic about your immediate goals and be appreciative of your current life-style. For you, developing a healthier life-style may only require adding a few coping strategies or new stress-reduction techniques. However, if you have not been taking responsibility for your health by not exercising, eating too much junk food, and letting work take over your life, remember that "the journey of 2000 miles begins with one step." Pace yourself, and attempt to accept your starting position as a part of who you are at this time—someone evolving. Avoid comparing yourself with others who have been living optimal life-styles. Their life-styles consist of comfortable habits that by now require little energy. For you, in the beginning, becoming healthier may be a foreign experience that requires much energy and attention. One of the reasons the best-laid plans fail is an all-or-nothing attitude. If you swear, "I'll never eat junk food again," or, "I'll go jogging absolutely every evening," one slip will make you feel like a total failure. The easiest way to avoid this attitude is to be realistic with yourself by not making absolute, unreasonable rules. Instead, acknowledge that you might slip up once in a while, but *use* the slip-up as an opportunity to learn more about what conditions led to your defeat or when you are most vulnerable. The most common cause of these relapses is our tendency to cope with negative emotional states by using old habits (Goleman, 1982). We get upset and decide to be good to ourselves by eating candy or not pushing ourselves to run—in a way we spite ourselves much as little children try to spite their parents by refusing to eat dinner or to go play when their feelings have been hurt.

Switching to a healthy life-style demands accepting a lifelong commitment to your own well-being. Try to keep the advantages of this life-style in mind; don't view it as a sacrifice or as drudgery but as a form of self-care and self-respect, a gift to yourself. "I'm abstaining from these sweets, not to deprive myself, but because I love myself."

Adopting a new life-style can only be done gradually. None of us learned to walk in one day. Learning to live a well-balanced life will also require time, patience, and repeated effort. Chapter 7, "Focusing on the Possible: A Problem-Solving Approach," focuses on ways to develop personal contracts and prioritize self-help goals in your development of a healthy life-style.

When I started toward a healthier life-style six years ago, I was drinking two pots of coffee and smoking two packs of cigarettes each day. I frequently got headaches, felt pressured, hated my job, and was one big grouch. A lot has changed since then, but I still have self-improvement goals to achieve. Remember, a philosophy of self-care is a lifelong process—a way of traveling. We never reach perfection. We are, hopefully, constantly striving to become self-actualized and to fulfill our potential.

This chapter is not designed to teach you all you need to know about the elements of a healthy life style. As nurses we have all had nutrition, physiology, and anatomy courses that focus on the physiologic needs and capabilities of the human body. This chapter concerns the consequences of neglecting self-care and some possible approaches to improving our life-styles. It should merely suggest a beginning for your further growth.

SPIRITUAL AWARENESS

What particular spiritual beliefs an individual holds—humanitarian, Catholic, Buddhist, existential—are not so important. What matters is the existence in each of us of a belief or beliefs that provide meaning, direction, or purpose to our lives. This spiritual dimension can stem from religious, humanitarian, or philosophic values. The beliefs that emerge from our spiritual sense give hope in times of crisis, provide a perspective for the day-to-day struggles of living, and offer guidance to our lives. Our beliefs contribute to our perception of stress and our notion of what can be done to handle distress.

We have long neglected the moral/ethical issues of health-care. All nurses will have to confront views of humankind, death, and life at some time in their practice. At times, nurses must also determine what is *reasonable* intervention as opposed to intervention that oversteps the limitations of our knowledge and ability to provide a quality life. In my job as a consultation-liaison psychiatric nurse, I am frequently asked to intervene with patients who have decided to refuse recommended treatment or who wish to be left alone to die. The physician feels the patient needs psychiatric intervention. Often what is occurring is a conflict in values that is enacted as a power struggle between patient and physician.

In nursing, we also face the suffering and pain of humanity on a daily basis. We all need some inner strength and direction to help us respond to the dilemmas this causes us. There are no magical right answers; the answers for each of us come from our spiritual sense. There are simply no understandable explanations of why a child should suffer from severe burns, a teenager become paralyzed from an accident, a young mother die of cancer, or a father die or become crippled from coronary disease. Nor can we give adequate *scientific* explanations of why some people who sustain severe physical injuries from accidents recover completely to live full lives, why some with incurable illnesses are cured, or why some in their time of dying or suffering have a true sense of acceptance and peace.

As nurses, we see the worst and the best of people. Our beliefs, from whatever origin, influence our understanding of the suffering we encounter and our ability to cope with it. I believe that none of us can deny the existence of something holy, mystical, or unexplainable that occurs in the healing or dying process. At best, as health professionals, we are facilitating a process of restoring a natural balance in the universe or perhaps of a God-given gift of health.

Albert Schweitzer's wisdom was that a temple and a healer exist within each of us. Even if we have lost touch with it, within each of us there is an imprint or memory of a sense of faith—hopefully a nurturing and sustaining belief.

There is ample evidence that our beliefs can produce changes in our body chemistry. Our healing systems and our belief systems are closely related. For example, a strong will to live combined with faith and hope can influence our fight against disease (Cousins, 1976). Probably the best example of how effective beliefs are in producing physiologic responses is the placebo effect. For some unknown reason, 30% of the population will show demonstrable clinical improvement when given a placebo. Their faith and belief that the placebo has power to help them produce improvement (Cousins, 1977).

Attitudes that stem from a spiritual wellspring, regardless of the faith held, are love, hope, forgiveness and acceptance, and joy in and appreciation of life. We know, as nurses, that these positive attitudes enhance the recovery process and the patient's sense of well-being. The same attitudes can also diminish our own sense of distress. If we have them, we can allow life's problems and hassles to pass without demanding that things "ought to be different," because "life's not fair." If we are able to let events "flow like a leaf on a mountain stream," or, from a Christian perspective, to accept "not as I will, but as thou wilt" (Matthew 26:39), we avoid creating unnecessary stress or holding onto distress. This does not mean developing a deterministic, helpless position. It does, however, encourage us to acknowledge natural forces and to appreciate our responsibility for our lives within the parameters of nature.

Personal Sharings for Spiritual Awareness

Some of my ways of getting in touch with my inner spirit when I feel overstressed, pessimistic, or lost might be of use to you.

- *Meditation,* as described in Chapter 17, "Relaxation: An Active Process," allows me to quiet the daily noise and chatter of superficial concerns and helps me get in touch with my inner beliefs. Prayer can be equally as effective. In many ways, prayer and meditation share the same process of putting daily events into a larger perspective or value system.
- An effective way for me to get in touch with my beliefs during interpersonal conflict is to force myself to see "the God" in my enemy. All people are of the same species, and although we have tremendous differences, we also share a few basic commonalities. No matter how evil or misguided another person may seem, there is still potential for goodness and caring. Consciously forcing myself to see that potential for goodness helps me to see conflicts as differences of opinion or personality rather than as struggles between good (my beliefs) versus evil (their beliefs).
- When I feel off balance and overstressed, I go where natural balance is more easily seen and felt to renew a sense of personal calm and direction. In my case, being near the water or in the wilderness puts me in touch with the rhythm and balance of the universe. Seeing the stars and the moon come out each night, no matter what absurdities and stress the day has brought, gives me hope and a sense of perspective.
- Remembering moments of unspeakable joy and beauty can bring a reappreciation of the miracles in life—of a spirit beyond my mere understanding. For me, my daughter's birth is the joyous miracle that reminds me of the hope and beauty in life that coexists with the sorrow and pain.

Value Clarification

It takes a lot of energy and conscious focusing to hold onto the good and natural in daily living. However, unless we exert these efforts, living can feel like a pointless struggle of no consequence. Value clarification is an approach to increasing your awareness of the beliefs you hold and the directions you wish to follow. Acknowledging your values does not mean that you can immediately fulfill your desires or become self-actualized. However, being aware of personal values can help put external and inter-

CLARIFYING VALUES EXERCISE

Answer the following questions about your beliefs:

1. What do I feel are the most important values I hold? (For example, love, power, happiness, security, others.) Which value (or values) is most important to me?
2. Who are the people I admire most (living or deceased)? What are the values these people live by or represent?
3. Imagine that someone is describing you to another person. What things would you like this person to say about you and what you stand for?
4. What do you feel would be worth dying for? What would you strongly endorse even if people you respect ridiculed you for it? What would you support with your time and/or money? What would you vote for in a secret ballot?
5. What are the beliefs and values you want to pass on to your children or future generations?
6. What do you believe is your greatest personal achievement? Your greatest failure?
7. Are there things you presently do that compromise your beliefs or values? Are there things you don't do that could further support your values or beliefs?
8. What are some personal goals you would like to reach over the next year, five years, or ten years?
9. When was the last time you endorsed your beliefs or values by taking specific action. (For example, if you believe in preserving the environment, do you turn out lights, walk to work, or vote for someone who supports environmental issues?)
10. At this time, are you willing to make a contract to change or support something in your life that you believe is important and that requires some action on your part? (For example, if you are opposed to nuclear arms, do you donate money to antinuclear groups, wear a blue ribbon to symbolize your position for nuclear disarmament, talk to your children, friends, or colleagues about this belief?)

nal demands and needs into perspective while providing a thread of consistency and stability in your life.

Our behavior, both verbal expression and nonverbal actions, represents our values. Many of us have values that are inconsistent with the way we live; it is how we spend our time that proclaims our beliefs. Many of us maintain conflicting values that produce a sense of confusion and tension in our lives.

Value clarification focuses upon the process of valuing rather than the development of any specific value or belief. It involves "choosing, prizing, and acting" on our values (Rath, 1966). How we function as nurses is based upon our spiritual or philosophical beliefs. The more we are aware of our beliefs, the more consistent we can be in our activities, and the clearer we can be about taking control of our lives and basing them upon these values. And, as we have seen, taking control of our lives decreases personal distress.

PHYSICAL FITNESS

The human body was created to be active and must move to function properly. Our bodies fall apart from disuse or improper use.

> Habitual inactivity is thought to contribute to hypertension, chronic fatigue, and resulting physical inefficiency, premature aging, poor musculature and lack of flexibility, which are the major cause of lower back pain and injury, mental tension, coronary heart disease and obesity (HEW, 1976).

Just reading this quote may make you feel like getting up and moving immediately before these disasters befall you. Besides preventing problems, various types of exercises are also credited with increasing lung capacity, decreasing excess fat, facilitating digestion and elimination, strengthening blood vessel and heart efficiency, relieving common complaints of pregnancy, decreasing depression, improving self-image, eliminating anxiety and muscular tension, and increasing a generalized sense of well-being—and this is only a partial list of the positive, health-enhancing benefits of regular exercise (Ardell, 1981).

The type of exercise you select is not as important as doing something to get yourself moving to maintain physical fitness. Certainly you will hear people say jogging, aerobic exercises, or swimming are the best exercises—if not the *only* good exercises. But what is most important is that you select forms of exercise you prefer and feel you can stick with. You may select several activities and vary them throughout the week. Try to include physical exertion in your normal pattern of living by walking up stairs instead of taking the elevator or walking to the store rather than driving.

Often, when we feel exhausted or overstressed, the mere idea of physical activity seems as if it will kill us. "I just can't drag my tired bones to the gym tonight," we say. Physical exercise actually can rejuvenate you—give you a surge of extra energy. It can also decrease your muscular tension and promote relaxation. The rhythmical diversion of physical exercise can also allow you to suspend your mental haranguing and quiet your worrying. Exercise is one of the safest tranquilizers. It has been found that one way to relax after a particularly mentally stressful day is to become involved with some type of physical activity (Selye, 1975).

Unfortunately, some of us associate physical fitness and exercise with our earlier experiences with gym classes in school. The emphasis was usually on boring drills and routine exercises or on competitive sports and the expectation of winning. Given these previous experiences, the idea of exercise may not sound exciting or may even be intimidating. However, you can find an active sport or exercise that interests and rewards you. Whatever you decide to do, don't be afraid to use your body!

RELAXATION

Although specific relaxation techniques and coping strategies are discussed in Part 6, "Stress Reduction Techniques," it might be helpful in this chapter to introduce a key idea. Many of us are *afraid* to relax. That may sound strange. Of course everyone wants to relax, to let go of stress, you may think. In fact, many of us feel guilty relaxing—we may think of it as loafing and wasting time. Our society operates upon the Puritan work ethic: work makes you pure; idle hands are the devil's workshop; you'll never get ahead if you don't work harder than the next guy. Certainly there is nothing wrong with hard work—as long as it is also balanced by relaxation.

Some of us view being calm and able to relax as something to scorn: How can she be so cool in the middle of all this craziness? What's the matter with her? I'll bet she doesn't work very hard! She always looks so mellow.

There's an advertisement for a brokerage firm that seems to typify this notion. In the ad, you see various scenes where people are relaxing at lunch or breakfast. Then the ad tells you that while other brokerage houses employ people who *waste time,* these brokers are always working, getting that competitive edge—at lunch, at the crack of dawn, and into the early hours of the morning. When I see this ad, I always think to myself, "Thank God they're not managing my money! I'd hate to think what kind of decisions are made by such overstressed, exhausted people." But that is the American image of a successful person. We reward the type A personality who is *driven* to compete in every situation; we suspect the relaxed, sensibly paced person. (See Chapter 5, "Self-Awareness: A Means of Taking Charge of Yourself," for a self-assessment exercise on the type A personality.)

We need to stop seeing relaxation as a sign of laziness, narcissism, or self-indulgence and begin to appreciate it as an essential ingredient in a healthy life-style, an ingredient just as important as meaningful work. Again, the important issue is balance.

NUTRITION

American people know more about what their cars need than what their bodies need. The result is an American public tempted by unhealthy food on one hand and weight-reducing gimmicks on the other. The result is a physically unhealthy nation (U.S. Senate, 1975).

We Americans, for the most part, eat too much overly processed foods, caffeine, additives and preservatives, fat, sugar, and sodium. Many of our diets lack fiber, vitamins, minerals, and balance (food at each meal from the four food groups). Myths and misinformation about nutritional needs abound, and their effects are potentially dangerous in the long run. Every month or so some new diet fad comes along and becomes popular, and is later found to be substantially deficient in meeting the body's nutritional requirements. As nurses all of us have taken nutrition classes and are familiar with basic nutritional standards. Most of us probably also had mothers who encouraged us not to eat between meals, packed fresh fruits in our lunch bags, promoted vitamins, and attempted to give us well-balanced, attractive meals. (Mothers have a way of doing these helpful things for their children even if they are not caring for themselves the same way.) It is unlikely that my attempts to persuade you of the importance of meeting your body's nutritional needs will succeed any more than your nutrition teacher's or mother's did. However, I will present some information on dieting, although a willingness to change must come from within.

Nearly everyone is familiar with the agonies of dieting—being obsessed with and craving food to the point that it becomes difficult to think of anything else. The type of food we are usually preoccupied with is "bad food"—sweets and greasy fast-foods. Most are also familiar with "psyching" up for the diet—imagining yourself in a swimsuit or attracting some desired person's attention. Then there is the almost inevitable let-down once you have failed—the public shame when your friends realize you don't have the willpower to succeed. You feel like a spineless person who doesn't have the strength to resist temptation. The final step in this pathetically predictable process is accepting (usually temporarily) that you are just going to have to live your life as an overweight person. This acceptance usually leads to wearing baggy cover-up clothes, trying to camouflage your weight with big prints, big jewelry, or scarfs, and always looking like a fat person trying to look slim.

Dieting always seems like the supreme personal sacrifice rather than a form of true self-caring. As long as you are dieting, you probably feel emotionally starved because you are denying yourself *food,* the sustenance of life. Most of us equate food with love. Getting a big box of chocolates for Valentine's day is a sign of being "loved." Mothers show how much they care for you by baking cookies, or, when you're sick, by giving you special foods to make you feel better. One of the big parts of every festival or holiday celebration is the food associated with it. Food is a well-reinforced symbol of love in most cultures. So when you are dieting, you are denying yourself love as well as food—or so it seems emotionally. You are paying the price of suffering, and it is going to be a slow, prolonged agony.

Part of the "solution" lies in the "problem" of dieting. Dieting, as usually practiced, fails in the long run because it is such a drastic *temporary* change in your eating pattern. The only people I know who don't have weight problems and, more importantly, who meet their nutritional needs are people who have an eating style that incorporates good nutritional habits on a daily basis—as a way to live and as a part of their total healthy life-style. Their food intake also is balanced by their caloric expenditure. Like them, you need to learn that self-love is giving yourself what your body needs for its well-being. Then you can begin to break the connection between seeing junk food as a treat or something nice you do for yourself.

DEVELOPING A FRIENDLY EYE

Part of what is necessary to maintain the sense of balance necessary to a healthy life-style and to manage our stress is the ability to observe ourselves at all times so we can notice our body's early warning signs of overstress and imbalance. I call this ability to be self-observant the "friendly eye."

In the middle of every work crisis, we need to have some part of our observing ego present for us to remain centered, outside the fracas, and able to take note of how we are responding. The friendly eye is an essential part of our ability to do reality-testing that can give us perspective on a stressful situation and an awareness of our imbalance. It also helps us prevent stress buildup. If stress is not managed when it initially occurs, it will accumulate—distress creates more distress. We've all experienced days where nothing seems to go right. When this happens, we say something like, "It's just not my day," or, "I must have gotten up on the wrong side of the bed today." What has probably happened is that we were experiencing stress buildup. We get swept up in the stress and are unable to stop the escalation of distress because of our inability to pull back long enough to identify what is happening. We lose our ability to intervene and control the initial distress, thus making ourselves susceptible to further stress. We then switch to operating on our automatic, uncontrolled fight-or-flight response.

By helping us observe the situation, the friendly eye allows us to avoid responding in a habitual fashion based upon our attitudes, memories, and sense of inadequacies that frequently distort present realities. Once you recognize you are experiencing distress, you can begin to utilize a problem-solving approach to determine whether or not your subjective sense of the situation is accurate and the stress you are experiencing is appropriate.

For example, if you are handling a cardiac arrest or another emergency medical situation, it is appropriate and adaptive for you to experience physiologic excitation. If, however, you notice yourself experiencing distress because someone did not say hello to you, you can tell you are creating unnecessary stress. Once you use the friendly eye to do reality-testing, you can choose to control your responses to consciously enhance your body's self-regulatory feedback system. You can catch your imbalance in the early stages.

HEALTHY LIFE-STYLE PRACTICES

The following health-enhancing practices are essential ingredients in maintaining high-level wellness (Ardell, 1977). This inventory of healthy life-style practices, compiled by the Institute for Life-Style Improvement, is not all-inclusive. This list presents only a selection of healthy life-style practices.

BALANCED LIFE-STYLE

Directions:

Place a check in the blank preceding any description of a healthy practice in which you are presently *not* engaged. Once you have completed the inventory, review the descriptions you have checked and decide if there are any others you wish to include in your life-style.

1. _____ Get regular physical exercise.
2. _____ Include physical exertion in my daily activities (e.g., climbing stairs, moving large objects, etc.).
3. _____ Keep within 10% of my recommended weight.
4. _____ Get adequate sleep each night.
5. _____ Practice regular stress-reduction techniques.
6. _____ Avoid taking alcohol or drugs to relieve stress symptoms.
7. _____ Pay attention to my body's stress symptoms.
8. _____ Read labels on packaged foods to avoid harmful additives.
9. _____ Ingest sufficient vitamins and minerals.
10. _____ Avoid processed or refined foods.
11. _____ Abstain from caffeine (in coffee, tea, soft drinks, and chocolate).
12. _____ Limit salt intake.
13. _____ Eat well-blanced meals.
14. _____ Eat breakfast.
15. _____ Relax regularly and whenever tension/distress is present.

BALANCED LIFE-STYLE (Continued)

16. _____Get regular physical examinations; do monthly breast or testicle self-examinations.
17. _____Don't smoke.
18. _____Recognize and avoid unnecessary job hassles.
19. _____Make frequent self-nurturing statements.
20. _____Accept responsibility for a sense of well-being.
21. _____Have realistic self-expectations and objectives.
22. _____Give and receive love and respect.
23. _____Accept compliments and/or valid, constructive criticism.
24. _____Maintain close interpersonal relationships.
25. _____Maintain a supportive network at work and at home.
26. _____Have a positive outlook.
27. _____Maintain enthusiasm and excitement for living and my job.
28. _____Notice and correct safety hazards.
29. _____Avoid using pollutants.
30. _____Conserve energy.
31. _____Be involved in community and professional concerns.
32. _____Actively demonstrate my spiritual beliefs.
33. _____Be aware of political issues and political candidates' positions—and vote for those which support my beliefs.
34. _____Be aware of personal moral/ethical beliefs.
35. _____Have clear-cut personal goals and objectives.

CONCLUSION

There is no one simple way to develop a healthy life-style. You will have to become your own guide by exploring various approaches, techniques, and philosophies to learn which are best for you. Try to have reasonable expectations and don't demoralize yourself by comparing yourself to "fitness freaks." The most essential ingredient in your healthy life-style is balance—the balance within your body and between yourself and the rest of your world. "It can be said unequivocally that a significant reduction in sedentary living and overnutrition, alcoholism, hypertension and excessive smoking would save more lives . . . than the best current medical practice" (Kristein et al., 1977).

REFERENCES

Ardell, D. B. 1977. *High level wellness: an alternative to doctors, drugs, and disease.* Emmaus, Pa.: Rodale Press.

Ardell, D. B. 1979. *High level wellness.* Toronto: Bantam Books.

Ardell, D. B. 1981. The physical disciplines and health. In *Health for the whole person,* editor A. Hastings (et al.) Toronto: Bantam New Age Books.

Breslow, L., and Belloc, N. 1972. The relation of physical health status and health practice. *Prevent. Med.* 1:409–21.

Cousins, N. 1976. Anatomy of an illness. *N. Eng. J. Med.* 295(26):1458–63.

Cousins, N. 1977. The mysterious placebo: how mind helps medicine work. *Sat. Rev.* 1:8–12.

Goldway, E. M. 1979. Self-regulation through nutrition. In *Inner balance,* editor E. M. Goldway. Englewood Cliffs, N.J.: Prentice-Hall.

Goleman, D. 1982. Why resolutions fail. *Psychol. Today* 16(1):19–23.

Kristein, M. M., Arnold, C. B., and Wynder, E. L. 1977. Health economics and preventative care. *Science* 195:457–62.

Lao Tse. 1973. *Tao te ching.* New York: Samuel Weiser.

Life-Style Assessment Questionnaire of the Institute for Life-Style Improvement. University of Wisconsin, Stevens Point, Wis.: Stevens Point Foundation.

Rath, L. E. 1966. *Values and teaching.* Columbus, Ohio: Charles E. Merrill Books.

Selye, H. 1975. *Stress without distress.* New York: Signet Books.

Selye, H. 1979. Self-regulation: response to stress. In *Inner balance,* editor E. M. Goldway. Englewood Cliffs, N.J.: Prentice-Hall.

U.S. Department of Health, Education, and Welfare. 1976. *Public health services: forward plan for health*, 1977–1981.

U.S. Senate Select Committee on Nutrition and Human Needs. 1975. Washington, D.C.: U.S. Government Printing Office.

CHAPTER 7

Focusing on the Possible: A Problem-Solving Approach

MICHAEL Z. WINCOR AND EMILY E. M. SMYTHE

WHY PROBLEM-SOLVING?

"OK, I'm overstressed. I admit I have a real problem managing my job and life stress. . . . So what do I do about it? How do I get rid of this unpleasantness NOW?" you may be saying to yourself.

When I tell you there is no one right answer and that no magical solutions exist for stress management, you may become frustrated, and think, So why am I reading this book, anyway? I want THE answer to solve my stress dilemma.

As with psychotherapy, there are no absolute answers that are correct or applicable for everyone. What you can learn is how to approach the problem of stress in a systematic way so that you develop your own answers and determine your own direction. What you will need to learn is how to manage stress by learning a problem-solving approach. Once you understand the problem-solving process, you can then apply it to any stressor that comes along.

Many people want cookbook solutions to complex life problems. "Just tell me what to do and I'll do it," they say. When we realize that we are experiencing stress and stress-related symptoms, many of us begin a frantic search for magical answers to immediately resolve the discomfort we now recognize—especially once we appreciate the relationship between stress and illness or premature death. It seems to be human nature to want quick and painless solutions to complex life situations. Rather than accepting the fact that we all need to struggle to find our own answers and directions, we look to others for their solutions.

Some stress-related problems such as alcoholism, drug addiction, or impulsive job-hopping actually stem from an attempt to handle difficult life stressors with simplistic, immediate solutions. As a nurse once told me, "I started taking Valium® because it helped me cope with the job pressures I experienced in the ICU. At first they really worked. When I started to get upset, I'd take one and then I'd feel in control again. Then it got to the point where I had to have two or three or more just to get through my shift. Finally, I just couldn't cope with or without the Valium®. I wish the doctor who prescribed them for my anxiety would have given me a lecture on how you can't cope with life's problems by taking pills. Now my simple solution is one disastrous nightmare!"

There just aren't any easy ways to avoid stress. Magical solutions all too often produce their own problems or additional stressors. Each of us, however, can learn to manage our job and personal stress without too much pain. In fact, ideally, any stress-management approach you undertake should also be fun and a growing and learning experience.

I've also noticed that, unfortunately, with stress management, many people impulsively jump into approaches that do not fit their personality, available time, or even interests. They then are unable to stick to the approach for long and become discouraged, only to quit and decide that stress management is not possible after all. Some people seem susceptible to any fad that becomes popular. Recently, stress-reduction fads have proliferated—tennis, handball, jogging, meditation, acupressure, and biofeedback to name but a few. Each of them can be helpful in stress reduction, but you need to first determine which will work best *for you.*

The trick is knowing yourself well enough to determine what your needs and interests are and then selecting the techniques and coping styles that will best match your life-style. Also, you need to recognize that stress is a multifaceted problem. Each of the techniques described in this book is aimed at different types of stress-related problems. You need to become familiar with each one if you are serious about wanting to control your job distress and promoting your optimal sense of wellness. No one approach is going to meet all your needs in every situation.

Because rapid and continual change is inherent in everyday living and the nursing profession has an unending array of potential stressors, what we each need to learn is not how to adapt to the *existing* stressors of the moment but how to adapt to stress in general. We need to learn one approach to manage all stress. The problem-solving approach is actually a process that can be applied to any problem; it can also help formulate an action plan in meeting life and career goals. Adapting to stress, personal and professional, is a lifelong process. Each "solution" or answer will need to change as your life and circumstances change. What you need to learn for stress management is not an answer or solution but a way of finding solutions and answers.

Unfortunately, instead of using a systematic problem-solving process to approach distress, most of us get into the bad habit of simply reacting to stressors on a haphazard trial-and-error basis. We frequently base decisions upon what feels right at the time rather than upon careful evaluation of available options and interventions. Some may avoid problem-solving because of a fatalistic belief that "whatever is meant to be will be." They end up abdicating the ability to control their lives or to determine their "destiny."

Problem-solving offers an alternative to being in a reactive position in which your sense of well-being is constantly battered by circumstances. With a problem-solving approach, you can switch from crisis intervention to a planned strategy that not only decreases distress but can also prevent it altogether.

Problem-solving is nothing more than a systematic process for decision-making. We have all learned this process in nursing education under the name of "nursing process" (Yura and Walsh, 1978). We need to realize that the same process we use so successfully to help our patients deal with their problems can also be utilized to help us deal with our own problems.

STEPS IN THE PROBLEM-SOLVING PROCESS

Although authors use different terms to describe the steps of the problem-solving process, they all agree on what the process involves (Murry, 1976). I use the following five-step approach to problem-solving:

1. Assessment (observation or data collection).
2. Problem identification (nursing diagnosis or hypothesis).
3. Goal setting (objectives or outcome criteria. This also includes prioritizing).
4. Action planning (implementation, approach, or interventions).
5. Evaluation (revision or feedback).

It is important to see each of these steps as interrelated and to recognize that each step also constantly provides ongoing feedback for every other step in the process. Thus, problem-solving is not a linear equation but instead involves a feedback cycle (Wolff et al., 1974).

You can develop your own personalized stress-management program by utilizing the problem-solving approach. To create your own tailor-made stress-management program, you will need to go through each of these five problem-solving steps and apply them to your own unique circumstances and needs.

Assessment

Assessment is not something you do once and then forget about. You need to continually assess your physical and emotional signals and notice your self-talk and patterns of responding. The more information you have, and thus the more self-awareness you develop, the better able you will be to develop self-control over your job distress. Ideally, you recognize your distress at its earliest stages before it escalates into a more disruptive pattern. Of course, not every nurse develops burn-out or is dissatisfied with her or his job. In fact, many of us get a lot of satisfaction from our work because we have learned to manage job stressors and promote our optimal sense of well-being. To do this, however, you need to recognize your personal signs and symptoms of stress.

The Paradoxical Nature of Change   Your ability to change and make effective life decisions can only come about when you fully understand where you are at the moment. There is a paradoxical nature to change. Positive, self-enhancing change is more likely to occur when you become fully aware and accepting of who you are. Change doesn't occur from trying to deny or ignore who you are or from trying to become something you are not (Beisser, 1970). The more you are able to appreciate what you are, the more you will be able to discover what you can become—and give self-support for your desired changes. When you abandon struggling to become what you think you should or must be and instead become more aware of what you are, then change almost automatically occurs. Instead of trying to deny or avoid what you are, begin to increase your self-knowledge and understanding.

Effective Coping Responses   Use this self-awareness as your beginning. No one can be other than what they are at the moment. For example, let's say you are actually angry with a co-worker but instead of acknowledging this anger to yourself, you tell yourself, "I really shouldn't be angry." You will then be unable to use the anger to change or grow and you will have difficulty controlling the angry feelings. You may, for instance, start ignoring the co-worker or you may start getting headaches, to name two possible responses. If, however, you accept your anger, you can work constructively with that feeling. You can handle the feeling and make whatever changes seem reasonable.

In developing your personalized stress-management program, it is important not only to assess what your problems and difficulties are but also to identify your positive coping styles and resources. Your program should continue, or in some cases increase, your usage of these adaptive styles.

From the information presented in Chapter 5, "Self-Awareness: A Means of Taking Charge of Yourself," and Chapter 6, "Balance: A Way of Developing a Healthy Life-Style," list your adaptive, positive coping strategies and responses in the next exercise. For example, if you accept personal responsibility for your reactions to stress, engage in regular physical exercise, and have a sustaining spiritual sense, you have three positive adaptive practices you would want to continue as part of your stress-management program.

EXERCISE I· EFFECTIVE COPING RESPONSES

Directions:

In the space below, list your effective coping responses, such as engaging in physical exercise, accepting responsibility, etc.

1. _____
2. _____
3. _____
4. _____
5. _____
6. _____
7. _____
8. _____
9. _____
10. _____

Everyone has many things they do well, so don't stop until you have written down *at least* five! If you are unable to come up with any positive coping responses, you might want to proceed to Chapter 9, "Unrealistic Expectations: The Set-Ups for Failure." Maybe you are being too harsh on yourself by expecting perfection or striving for absolute self-control in all situations. Remember, what you are attempting to do is enhance or supplement your present stress-management skills—not become a totally new and different person. You are not aiming to avoid stress altogether but to learn how to effectively manage stress and use the adaptive energy generated by stress in a productive fashion.

Identification of Problems

In this section, you are asked to do more than simply identify and list stress-related symptoms. Go one step further and recognize the contributing factors that have influenced your experience of distress. (See Chapter

2, "Origins of Stress"). For example, instead of simply saying you have "headaches," identify the cause and say, "headaches caused by my in-ability to express anger." You list both the symptom and the *influencing factors* or stressors. When you come to the evaluation step of problem-solving, you will measure your effectiveness in dealing with the symp-tom—headaches. Your main focus of intervention, however, will be in manipulating the contributing factors—the ability to express anger—and the stressors that produce the anger. You may also state only contributing factors in your problem list, for example, rescue fantasies.

Whether you state symptoms *and* contributing factors or contributing factors alone, the clearer and more specific you can be about identifying the problem, the easier it is to explore the possible interventions. For ex-ample, if you simply say "anxiety," it is more difficult to pinpoint the prob-lem than if you say "anxiety caused by inability to say no" or "anxiety caused by difficulty in asserting my beliefs to authority figures." You then have a clearer idea of what the problem is. How you define your problem helps determine the solutions you look for. It is not as important to force yourself to state problems in behavioral terms as it is necessary to identify

EXERCISE 2: PROBLEM IDENTIFICATION LIST

Directions:

In the exercise that follows write down your stress-related problems as they come to your mind. List the stress symptoms you have identified and the contributing factors or stressors.

	Priority	Symptoms of Stress	Cause of Symptoms
1.	( )	_____	_____
2.	( )	_____	_____
3.	( )	_____	_____
4.	( )	_____	_____
5.	( )	_____	_____
6.	( )	_____	_____
7.	( )	_____	_____
8.	( )	_____	_____
9.	( )	_____	_____
10.	( )	_____	_____

the problems in a way that makes sense to you and helps you pinpoint your difficulties in managing stress.

Review your problem list. Are there any problems you identified that you are not willing to tackle at this time? Although a problem exists, you may not necessarily want to commit yourself to resolve it. However, if you recognize a problem and decide not to attempt to resolve it—for whatever reason—you also need to acknowledge that *you* have made this choice. In deciding not to work on a recognized problem, you have also forfeited your right to complain about it or to feel guilty about it (Edelwich and Brodsky, 1980). For example, if a colleague of yours is constantly complaining about the job and you decide her griping is a problem you need to handle assertively, you may also decide you are not yet willing to address it. You may decide not to handle it because you have other more important problems requiring your energy and attention or because another problem, such as getting collective support for a work-related change, seems in direct conflict. The important thing is that your decision to ignore a problem should be a conscious choice. The next time you hear her griping, let it roll off you—you don't need to feel guilty for not "handling it." You have made a decision about the problem and are now acting upon your problem-solving solution. Not acting is actually acting. Your action is deciding *not* to act. You have thus made a choice.

Part of problem-solving is making decisions about what issues are important to you. Experiencing powerlessness in a situation contributes significantly to the perception of distress. One study of stress found that people who believed they could control their stressors or had a choice about controlling their stressors experienced less distress— even if, in fact, they did not choose to use their control (Glass et al., 1969). Just believing you have choices and are able to control stressors that affect you decreases your perception of distress.

Prioritizing your problem list and deciding which problems you will address is a necessary step in problem identification. You cannot successfully fight "battles" on all fronts. Each of us needs to decide what problem is of greatest concern to us. In the parentheses next to each problem you have identified, rank the problem in order of its priority or importance to you.

A word of caution. Rather than deciding to address or forget a problem, many people choose to fence straddle by gathering more and more information about what the problem is. They thus avoid committing themselves to any decision. I'm sure you have been in situations in which the plan is to get more and more information before you ever (or never) do anything. If you do this, you only prolong the sense of stressful arousal and will experience additional frustrations. I'm not suggesting that you rush into decisions blindly without understanding the problem, but I am cautioning you against using prolonged data collection as a procrastination technique. Take active responsibility for your sense of well-being, or you will ultimately feel powerless.

Goal-Setting

Your goals help you decide how you wish to allot your time. Without clear goals, circumstances and other people end up making decisions about how you will spend your time and ultimately *your* life! You may have personal goals that are focused on resolving a specific problem, and you may also have goals that allow you to meet important personal objectives or life plans.

Goals derived from life values and goals intended to resolve your stress-related problems can both be called long-term goals. Unfortunately, day-to-day demands may interfere with concentration on these long-term goals, especially if the goals seem vague and distant. However, you also can develop short-term goals that help to give clearer direction to your daily life. Short-term goals shape your daily behavior by breaking down the long-term goals into step-by-step progressions toward the desired outcome. They operate on the concept of "divide and conquer"—breaking down overwhelming tasks or seemingly monumental life goals into obtainable, reachable, and smaller stepping stones. Short-term goals also make it easier to appreciate your smaller successes and your progress toward achieving the bigger goals, thus providing reinforcement and maintaining your incentive.

How do you define a goal? Ask yourself, "If there weren't a problem, what would I be doing or experiencing?" Your answer is your goal. For example, if I didn't have a problem with lack of physical exercise, I'd be exercising for 30 minutes every day—my goal.

Goals do not have to be derived from problems only! Goals also develop from commitment to beliefs and values. For example, if you believe friendships are valuable, a goal might be to take more time to be with friends. Goals can help to keep you on course despite the frequent detours and obstacles we all face in our lives.

Not having goals is like taking a trip to some unknown place without directions. There is no telling where you'll end up. Sure, it might be fun occasionally to have a few side trips or unexpected adventures, but living your life in such an unpredictable, haphazard fashion soon produces the often heard complaint "Where did my life go? I never seem to get around to the important things."

Time Management   Time management is a process for determining the best use of your time in order to meet personal goals. "Time management means the efficient use of your resources, including time, in such a way that you are effective in achieving important personal goals" (Ferner, 1980). It is learning to work smarter, *not* harder. One complaint stressed people seem to share is, "I don't have enough time to do all the things I need to do." Or, "If I only had more time, I wouldn't feel so pressured and stressed." Poor time management and poor life or self management produce a constant sense of being rushed, missing deadlines, and being overwhelmed by demands.

Life is a constant series of decisions that eventually shape our lives. Unfortunately, many of us get caught up in meeting unimportant goals and manage to let the more valued, essential goals slip by (Applebaum, 1981).

Think for a moment about a normal day in your life. How much time in this day gets eaten up by unnecessary demands and activities? How many important tasks are left undone because you just don't have time to do them? All too often irrelevant decisions and activities take priority over more meaningful goals. This lack of time management and prioritizing can become a work problem and lead to serious complications. For example, if you spend your time filling water pitchers, passing out mail, and reorganizing supplies when IVs are running out, orders are not being noticed, and medications are neglected, then you have a serious work problem. Although this example is exaggerated, it illustrates how you squander time on less important activities when you do not base decisions on clearly established priorities.

An interesting thing about time is we each have all the time we will ever get. There is no way to beg, borrow, or steal more time. Time is doled out to all of us regardless of our qualities or virtues (Linden, 1970). You end up spending time whether you choose to or not. Time also becomes the only real boundary or limit; all else is flexible in one way or another. Time also controls and limits how we use all our other resources (MacKenzie, 1972).

With time management, you are using a problem-solving approach to move toward goals you value in the same way as you use a problem-solving technique to manage stress problems. Believing your life has meaning and value and that you are moving toward what you believe is important is one way of avoiding getting sidetracked by job hassles. It is also possible, with the time management approaches, to change your perspective about previously stressful events. You may decide something is stressful *but* you have more important, more relevant interests you wish to put your energy into and thus decide to ignore the problem. I see this frequently with part-time nurses who are going back to school. Issues that used to upset them no longer do so because they are now involved in something they value, something that requires their time and energy.

This Sanskrit proverb sums up the importance of time.

Look to this day,
For it is life,
The very life of life,
In its brief course lie all
The realities and verities of existence,
The bliss of growth
The splendor of action
The glory of power–

For yesterday is but a dream,
And tomorrow is only a vision,
But today, well lived,

Makes every yesterday a dream of happiness
And every tomorrow a vision of hope.

Look well, therefore, to this day.

Unfortunately, many of us do not even realize what our life values and goals are, let alone how these values and goals influence our daily lives and decisions. Stop for a moment and answer the following questions, which are helpful in identifying life and career goals based on personal values (Lakein, 1973; Kaplan, 1981).

- What would you like to accomplish in your life?
- If you knew you were going to die in the next five years, how would you spend your time?
- Given only six months to live, how would you like to live them?
- What basic life values do you believe are most important (independence, education/achievement, spiritual values, physical well-being, family/friend relationships, career development, etc.)?
- What are your life responsibilities—things you believe are expected of you by society or yourself (financial support of family, caring for children and relatives, responsibilities to religion/church, professional involvement, civic responsibilities, etc.)?

Additional exercises for identifying life goals and values are found in Chapter 11, "Perceptions: Believing Is Seeing," under the value clarification exercises.

Adams (1980) has suggested some guidelines for setting stress-management goals. You may wish to incorporate some of these into your goal-setting.

- Build your resistance through healthy life-style habits.
- Establish and maintain all the social support you can.
- Learn to withdraw from or ignore hopeless situations.
- Compartmentalize your work life and your private life; don't let problems of one spill over into the other.
- Develop a stress-management program that utilizes regular stress-reduction techniques and coping strategies.
- Learn specific stress-reduction techniques for emotionally charged situations (for example, deep breathing, visualizing the absurd).

Now you are ready to turn to the goal-setting worksheet. Remember, any of the problems you listed in your problem identification list can suggest a positive goal to work toward in order to improve your job or personal satisfaction. Turning problems into goals for personal growth is an important step in shifting your focus to a positive direction. For instance, if your problem is poor nutritional intake, turn the problem into a goal to eat well-balanced meals. This focuses your attention on a self-enhancing, self-supportive goal. Don't put your goal in negative terms such as "stop eating junk food," or you will feel as if you are now disciplining or punishing yourself for your "bad" behavior. See if you can address your problems by turning them into long-term, positive, self-supportive goals. On the goal-setting worksheet, rewrite your top priority problems in order of their importance. Next to each problem write in a goal that would eliminate that problem, focusing on a positive outcome. Write several short-term goals for each of these long-term goals. Do the same thing for your important beliefs and values. Devise goals that will help you realize them. Study the examples that follow.

SAMPLE GOAL SETTING WORKSHEET

I.	Problems	Priority	Long-Term Goals	Short-Term Goals
	Inability to relax	(1)	Learn relaxation techniques	1. Read chapter on relaxation techniques.
				2. Attend workshops on selected technique.
				3. Arrange for regular practice of technique.

II.	Values		Long-Term Goals	Short-Term Goals
	Career advancement	(2)	Obtain promotion	1. Develop support network.
				2. Read two articles on. . . .
				3. Discuss career opportunities with. . . .
				4. Attend in-service class on. . . .
	Family stability	(1)	Maintain family relationships	1. Increase amount of quality time spent with daughter.
				2. Arrange family reunion.
				3. Arrange regular evening/weekly get-together with sister.

EXERCISE 3: GOAL-SETTING WORKSHEET

I. Problems	Priority	Long-Term Goals	Short-Term Goals
1.	( )		1. 2. 3. 4. 5.
2.	( )		1. 2. 3. 4. 5.
3.	( )		1. 2. 3. 4. 5.
4.	( )		1. 2. 3. 4. 5.
5.	( )		1. 2. 3. 4. 5.

Prioritizing   Many people experience stress and pressure from job demands because they are not establishing clear priorities or setting limits on
requests. They end up feeling like failures because they are struggling to
be all things to all people or trying to accomplish all their varied personal
goals at once. Part of the problem-solving approach to stress management
involves prioritizing your goals to insure that you acknowledge important
values and solve personal problems.

It is important to prioritize both life-values goals and problem-gener-
ated goals in order to determine how best to spend your most valuable

EXERCISE 3: GOAL-SETTING WORKSHEET

II. Values	Priority	Long-Term Goals	Short-Term Goals
1.	( )		1. 2. 3. 4. 5.
2.	( )		1. 2. 3. 4. 5.
3.	( )		1. 2. 3. 4. 5.
4.	( )		1. 2. 3. 4. 5.
5.	( )		1. 2. 3. 4. 5.

imited resource—time. Most experts suggest there are three categories of priority (Nebber, 1972; Lakein, 1973).

. Top priority goals—vital ones with highest values; things that *must* be done.
. Important but not essential goals; medium-value goals that will improve your performance or life but will not cause disaster if they are not accomplished.
. Nice to do but not critical goals; get around to them sometime.

In the brackets next to each goal on the goal-setting worksheet, prioritize the goal in order of its importance to you using 1 as highest priority; 2 as important but not essential; and 3 as nice to do but not important.

Select one #1 "life values" goal and one #1 "problem" goal to define an action plan that will help you work toward meeting these two goals. You are not ignoring the other goals. You are simply deciding that these two goals are of greatest importance to you at the moment. There is nothing more stressful than trying to tackle all of your goals at once; somehow nothing gets accomplished when you have too many irons in the fire. After selecting these two top priority goals, you are now ready to plan out action to meet these goals.

Action Plan

Planning for action is a way of prescribing, as specifically as possible, what it is you are going to do on a daily and weekly basis to accomplish your short-term goals. Unlike goals that tell you where you are going, action plans tell you how you're going to get there. Action plans need to tell you *exactly* what you're going to do *by when*. An action plan is the series of interventions you are going to put between your problem and your goal.

Osborn (1973) suggests that before settling on a specific action plan, you first "brainstorm" the problem. When you brainstorm, you are expanding your thoughts to include new and unexpected interventions or ways of handling problems. You are looking for quantity of approaches rather than necessarily the best-quality answer. Be careful not to evaluate or reject each answer as it pops up in your mind—just let the ideas flow. The more expansive and open to new approaches you can be, the more likely you will come up with some creative options that can substantially alter a seemingly hopeless problem or reach a far-fetched goal. Problems frequently persist because we get stuck trying to solve them by using the same old, ineffective approaches or interventions.

Look over your two priority long-term goals and brainstorm possible approaches to attain one of the short-term goals for each of these. Jot down these action possibilities on a sheet of scratch paper. You may even wish to involve friends and co-workers in this brainstorming. The more brains involved, the more possibilities. Once you have written down as many plans of action as you can come up with, go over the list, crossing off any that are too far-fetched or that do not interest you.

Take the following points into consideration when planning out activities to meet goals or to intervene in stress-related problems:

- Avoid impulsive, radical changes. (They tend only to increase you stress and are difficult to maintain.)
- Take small steps toward your desired end goal.
- Select coping behaviors that offer long-term rewards such as friendship increased knowledge, and others.

- Develop "positive addiction." For example, instead of being "hooked" on smoking or coffee breaks, get hooked on meditation or herbal tea breaks.
- Plan out what you're going to do every day, making sure you allot time for important tasks or goals. Ask yourself what's the best use of your time.
- Do it now. "A journey of a thousand miles begins with but one step."
- Get someone else's help with hard problems. Brainstorming and "many hands make light of work."
- Specify your plans and better your chances of accomplishing the task.

At this point, you are ready to commit yourself to take action. Develop an action plan for each of the two goals. It might help to sign a self-contract for each of these action plans. With self-contracting, you are saying to yourself, "I am willing to put my good intentions into hard action." You certainly won't solve any problem and are unlikely to reach goals by simply thinking about them. You have to do something to insure reaching the goals.

You need to set deadlines for each action plan. Exactly when are you going to do _____ ? The word *deadline* comes from a military term. Prisoners were told if they crossed over a line drawn on the floor, they would be shot—hence, deadline (Moskowitz, 1982). Deadlines motivate behavior. For example, there is a big difference between saying I plan to get _____ done, and saying I will get _____ done by Wednesday. Somehow the deadline changes the whole nature of the activity, giving it clear expectations. Setting deadlines is also helpful whenever you are requesting something of someone else. Saying I'd like you to do _____ doesn't get the same results as I want you to do _____ by this evening. Whenever you delegate tasks, be sure to attach a deadline.

Fill out the following self-contract for each action plan. Establish a deadline for your action by putting in an exact date on the line "by." If you need someone else to help you or you need special equipment, indicate this on the line "I will need/use the following resources. . . ."

ACTION PLAN

Self-Contract

   I will: _____

               _____

   by: _____

   I will need/use the following resources:

   _____

   _____

                    Signed: _____

For example, if one of my values was to maintain my personal health (as a long-term goal) and a stepping stone for this was getting regular exercise, my action plan might be to jog three times a week. I might need my husband to watch my daughter or a friend to help me keep up my momentum. My contract would read something like this.

SAMPLE ACTION PLAN

I will: jog two miles on Monday, Wednesday, and Friday
by: starting 11/10/82 through 12/10/82.
I will need/use the following resources:
My husband to watch my daughter.
Jane to run along to report my progress.

Signed: _____

If one of my stress problem goals was to plan reasonable use of my time to avoid overcommitting myself, my short-term goal might be to keep a weekly calendar that lists all existing commitments and to plan my use of time on a daily basis. My contract might read:

SAMPLE ACTION PLAN

I will: 1. consider each request for my time by consulting my
            daily calendar before I make any new promises.
          2. not make any new decisions until I have given myself
            at least one day to think it over.
by: starting Monday for one month.
I will need/use the following resources:
          1. Weekly calendar that indicates all commitments.

Signed: _____

It may seem silly to fill out a self-contract, but it is one way to commit yourself to action. If you want to increase the likelihood that you'll fulfill your self-contract, tell someone else about your plan. Or make a copy of your contract and place it where you are bound to see it frequently—on your calendar, on your dashboard, or on your refrigerator.

Once you have accomplished each of these two contracts, go over your goal-setting worksheet again, selecting other goals you wish to work on. Since each of the self-contracts is made for small "do-able" action plans, you should be able to see marked progress on an almost weekly basis. Don't become frustrated because you are working on only one small piece of the overall stress problem. Remember, you are selecting solvable pieces that together add up to a more healthful way of living; you are not simply resolving a stress problem.

Evaluation

Too often we are so busy rushing around trying to accomplish all our goals and tasks that we miss one of the most important steps in the problem-solving approach—the evaluation step. Evaluation involves not only seeing what went wrong but reinforcing our successes. Evaluation, like assessment, needs to be an ongoing, integral part of problem-solving—not just the step you do at the end. As you are selecting goals, you need periodically to review and revise them—even life goals. Monthly short-term goals need rechecking to see how you are progressing and to determine, based on further self-knowledge, if they are still relevant to the direction you wish to go. There is nothing more ridiculous than getting stuck on a course of action that might have been appropriate years ago but has since lost its relevance.

Success for most of us is what occurs on a daily basis. As the old adage goes, "It takes 20 years to make an overnight success." There is only one grand prize winner of the Irish Sweepstakes each year; the rest of us must be content struggling daily toward the jackpot. If we evaluate only the final gain as "success," we will miss our entire lives. Evaluation and self-reinforcement need to focus on the process of growth as well as on the ultimate goal. The doing is as important as what's done. Evaluate your little successes and hold onto them. If you are failing at a task, be realistic—evaluate the problem and start the problem-solving process all over again. There's no disgrace in starting over—it is a new opportunity.

One way to notice your small, daily successes is to mark down on your calendar only the things you have to do each day. Then, as you accomplish each one, check it off. At the end of the week, you have a calendar that witnesses your successes. You can see tangible signs of all you have done. Another way to evaluate your successes is to save your self-contracts for a few months. Soon you'll have a stack of accomplishments that reaffirms your ability to meet important personal goals.

CONCLUSION

We all have the choice of how our lives will be spent. We can get caught in a reactive, helpless position of responding to whatever circumstances or external demands place upon us or we can become "proactive." We can decide to utilize the problem-solving approach, not only to manage our daily stress but to determine the direction of our lives based on personal values and life goals. Stress management is not just learning how to deal with negative events or experiences in our lives; it is learning how to enhance our optimal sense of well-being by accomplishing personal goals.

The problem-solving approach systematically attacks problems or life goals by evaluating alternatives that can lead to attaining these goals and reaching viable solutions. It allows you to be in control of your life, time, and emotional responses. Once you have decided upon a course of action, most problems seem manageable and less stressful. Whenever you face a problem, it is important to go through each step of the problem-solving process. After a while, the problem-solving process becomes a natural way to approach any situation. You are then free to learn and grow from each experience. You also develop a sense of self-support because you know that, no matter how unfamiliar or frightening a situation is, you can plan an attack that will insure the best chance of success.

The final decisions you reach and action plans you choose are not as important as determining your own plans and gaining control over situations rather than remaining a helpless victim. You may not like the options or solutions you come up with, but at least you have a choice. You may decide to leave a job that is causing you unmanageable stress, or you may decide to engage the help of others in a collective approach to solving a job problem. Instead of being a victim of stress, incorporate stress into the growing process. Problem-solving is a way to focus on the positive and the possible in every situation. It is a way of determining your own solutions.

REFERENCES

Adams, J. D. 1980. *Understanding and managing stress.* San Diego, Calif.: University Associates, Inc.

Applebaum, S. H. 1981. *Stress management for health care professionals.* Rockville, Md.: Aspen Publications.

Beisser, A. 1970. The paradoxical theory of change. In *Gestalt therapy now,* editors J. Fagan and I. L. Shepard. New York: Harper Colophon Books.

Berni, R., and Fordyce, W. E. 1977. *Behavior modification and the nursing process,* 2nd ed. St. Louis: The C. V. Mosby Co.

Edelwich, J., and Brodsky, A. 1980. *Burnout: stages of disillusionment in the help-*

ing profession. New York: Human Science Press.

Ferner, J. D. 1980. *Successful time management.* New York: John Wiley & Sons.

Glass, D. C., Singer, J. E., and Friedman, J. N. 1969. Psychic cost of adaptation to environmental stressors. *J. Personal. Social Psychol.* 12(3):200–210.

Kaplan, J. 1981. *Time management.* Lecture given at University of Southern California, Continuing Education for Nurses Program, November 8.

Lakein, A. 1973. *How to get control of your time and your life .* New York: Peter H. Wyden.

Linden, S. 1970. *The harried leisure class.* New York: Columbia University Press.

MacKenzie, R. A. 1972. *The time traps.* New York: McGraw-Hill.

Moskowitz, R. 1982. Make the most of your time. *Nurselife* Jan–Feb (2):21–8.

Murry, M. 1976. *Fundamentals of nursing.* Englewood Cliffs, N. J.: Prentice-Hall.

Nebber, B. 1972. *Time management.* New York: Van Nostrand Reinhold.

Osborn, A. J. 1973. *Applied imagination: principles and procedures of creative problem-solving,* 3rd ed., New York: Scribners.

Tubesing, D. A. 1981. *Kicking the stress habit.* Duluth, Minn.: Whole Person Associates, Inc.

Wolff, L., Weitzel, M. H., and Fuerst, E. U. 1974. *Fundamentals of nursing,* 6th ed., Philadelphia: J. B. Lippincott.

Yura, H., and Walsh, M. B. 1978. *The nursing process,* 3rd ed., New York: Appleton-Century-Crofts.

3

Self-Awareness: Tools to Develop Personal Stress Awareness

Each of the self-assessment tools and approaches provided in this section is designed to increase your self-awareness of stress symptoms and healthy or unhealthy life-style practices. The self-knowledge you derive from these tools becomes an important basis for developing your stress-management program. Assessment is always the first step in a problem-solving approach to change. The more you know about yourself, the more able you are to take responsibility for self-care. (There are also numerous additional self-assessment tools and exercises throughout the book.)

Most of the assessment tools provide subjective information rather than a statistical score. There is a type of false reassurance that can occur in taking any self-assessment tool's final score and living your life based upon that score. Stress management is a process of healthy living. It should not become a game of balancing negative odds—for example, saying to yourself, "Well, I smoke and eat junk food, but I get eight hours of sleep every night and exercise regularly, so my health score must balance out." Nor should self-assessment tools be used to tally up the number of stress-related symptoms and give a cumulative score that suggests the more symptoms you have the worse off you are. Being an alcoholic or having an ulcer, for example, are serious enough problems in and of themselves. You don't need to accumulate several more symptoms before you take action to handle your stress. The same is true of unhealthy life-style practices—even one bad habit can be a severe health risk. For example, eating large quantities of salt when you have a cardiac problem is a form of slow suicide.

When you get an annual health checkup, your doctor doesn't take all the factors and add up a score for your health status and tell you, "Well, let's see now, you're in the fiftieth percentile of healthy people." This information would be useless. Instead, the doctor identifies problem areas and symptoms that indicate your health could be in jeopardy. Ideally, your doctor will identify and encourage health-enhancing practices for you to engage in and will discourage unhealthy ones.

Self-assessment and self-knowledge are essential ingredients in any stress-management program. These tools should be used in an ongoing manner as part of your healthy life-style, not just at the beginning of your stress-management program. The more aware you are of your early stress responses, the better able you will be to intervene before your stress escalates to an unhealthy level.

Once you have completed Part 3, you will have the knowledge necessary to begin developing a personal stress-management program using the stress-reduction coping strategies and techniques discussed in Parts 4 and 5.

CHAPTER 8

Stress Assessment Tools

EMILY E. M. SMYTHE

By the time you have completed the assessment tools included in this chapter, you should be well aware of your current stress level, how a healthy or unhealthy life-style contributes to your sense of well-being, and what life events and daily hassles place stress on you. These tools should not only provide you with a baseline from which you can measure your progress with stress management but also should help sensitize you to signals of stress. Stress awareness allows you to become more attuned to your responses to potential stressors and can thus become part of a self-regulating feedback system that keeps you in balance.

(The data sources upon which each assessment tool is based are identified in the reference section.)

READING YOUR BODY'S SIGNALS

By producing muscular tension, your body records stress before your conscious mind may be aware of it. In fact, paying attention to bodily aches and pains is a good way to start identifying stress. Stop seeing these aches and pains as symptoms that need to be medicated; acknowledge them as your body's signals to you that you are overstressed.

Unfortunately, many of us ignore our body's early signals, only noticing when we develop advanced symptoms. For example, you may not notice that you are contracting your neck or head muscles until you have a migraine headache. The more aware you are of your body's early warning signals, the easier it is to correct the tension before it progresses to stress-related illnesses (discussed in Chapter 1). In addition, you can more quickly begin a stress-management approach to handling distress.

The most common cause of these body aches and pains is prolonged contraction of your muscles. An easy way to demonstrate how prolonged muscle contraction can cause muscle pain is to do the following (Sehnert, 1981):

1. Hold either arm over your head.
2. Rapidly open and close your raised hand while slowly counting to 30.
3. Make a tight fist and hold it for another count of 30.
4. Bring your hand down in front of you.
5. As you open your fist, notice the skin color of your hand as well as the numbness and stiffness

The sensations you have just felt came from muscle contractions that decreased the blood and oxygen flow to your hand, producing muscle tension and maybe even pain. This same process can cause skeletal-muscular pain and tension anywhere in your body. All too frequently, the moment we notice our body's discomfort, we are conditioned to think of taking medication to relieve the pain. This reaching for a pain reliever the moment you feel stressed has gotten so out of hand that aspirin commercials now boast their products have greater and greater strength geared for "today's modern headaches."

Instead of running for the pain killers, listen to your body's subtle early signals; use these signals to increase your awareness of stress and initiate stress-management techniques or coping styles. Of course, if you are unaware of or ignore your body's early warning signs until your body's stress responses are overloaded and have produced cellular damage such as an ulcer, myocardial infarction, or migraine headache, you will have to intervene with medication. Think of your body signals as warning lights alerting you to possible system overload.

Most of us have target muscles where we store our tension. Typical examples are tightening the jaw, knitting the brow, squinting the eyes, raising the shoulders, bracing forward, constricting the rib cage by shallow breathing, tightening the lower back muscles, and clenching the hands into fists. Indeed, numerous other body areas also experience tension.

One way to become aware of and release this tension is by doing what I call a head-to-toe physiologic check. Start at the top of your head and work down to your toes, paying attention to each part of your body in order to notice where you are experiencing tension. Also notice if your hands and feet are cold and if any areas of your body are moist or perspiring. The sympathetic nervous system produces cold and moist skin during times of stress (Travis, 1978). This type of body check should be done frequently throughout the day—especially in conflict-laden or stressful situations. Doing a head-to-toe check encourages early recognition of your body's warning signals and thus prevents the symptoms of tension from becoming more severe or uncomfortable. The moment you notice tension, you can use the progressive relaxation technique described in Chapter 17, "Relaxation: An Active Process," or you can shake loose the tension the same way you shake out writer's cramp by rapidly flexing and contracting or by stretching the tensed muscle. Instead of holding the tension throughout the day while it slowly builds, you can correct the problem at the start.

Reading your body's early stress signals also facilitates your recognition of stressful situations that you may be blocking from consciousness. The head-to-toe check (see following list) becomes an important feedback mechanism that increases your awareness of stress response patterns and gives you the ability to start controlling stressors and alter your unhealthy responses (Samuels and Bennett, 1973).

Head-to-Toe Check

1. Take a few moments to close your eyes and focus your awareness on your entire body, from your head to your toes. Slowly focus on each part of your body and notice where you are holding tension, if there are parts of your body that feel cold or numb, or if any part of your body is moist or perspiring.
2. On the body outline provided, shade in any areas where you experience tension. Shade darker the areas with the greatest tension or discomfort (see Figure 8-1).
3. Rate your body tension using a subjective rating scale from 1–10: 1, extremely relaxed; 5, moderately tense; 10, extremely tense. Put your subjective rating for each part of your body onto the figure.
4. Check your general body flexibility.
   a. Bend forward and try to touch your toes without bending your knees. You should be able to touch the floor comfortably with your fingers; ideally, you should be able to touch the floor with your palms.
   b. While holding your shoulders stationary, see how far you can comfortably bring your chin toward your chest. You should be able to rest your chin on your chest without straining.

   If you are unable to touch the floor or rest your chin on your chest, you are stiff due to chronic muscle tension (Samuels and Bennett, 1973).

At the end of each day over the next week, do the head-to-toe check as described so that you can begin to recognize your body tension. Also try to

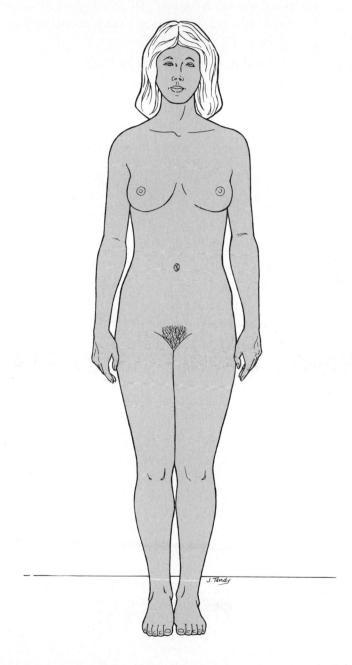

FIGURE 8-1.

Head-to-toe body check.

do periodic body checks throughout the day; release tension whenever you notice it. After doing this for a week, you will begin to notice more readily where you are storing tension and when you are under stress.

STRESS CHECKLIST: PHYSICAL AND EMOTIONAL STRESS SYMPTOMS

Each of the following symptoms may be stress-induced. If you are unsure of how each symptom is related to stress, refer to Chapter 1, "Stress and the Nurse." It is not important to add up the number of symptoms you are experiencing for a total score. What is important is recognizing the presence of any of these stress symptoms and paying attention to your body's warning that you need to manage your stress. Each of the symptoms listed can be a physical or emotional response to stress and one of your body's ways of indicating that you are having trouble managing stress (Pelletier, 1977; Selye, 1978; Davis et al., 1980; Flynn, 1980). Pay attention to this communication.

STRESS CHECKLIST

Directions:

In the blank provided next to each symptom, place the number of times per week that you experience that symptom. When physical illness has been ruled out as a cause, the presence of more symptoms and/or more frequent symptoms indicate how serious your stress problem is.

Physical Symptoms

1. _____loss of appetite
2. _____indigestion, heartburn
3. _____nausea or vomiting
4. _____diarrhea
5. _____constipation
6. _____overeating from anxiety
7. _____peptic ulcer pains
8. _____headaches
9. _____muscle stiffness/tension
10. _____lower back pain
11. _____muscle spasms or twitches
12. _____muscle weakness (not due to physical exercise)

STRESS CHECKLIST (Continued)

13. _____high blood pressure
14. _____racing heart/heart palpitations
15. _____dry mouth
16. _____perspiration on hands and/or feet
17. _____cold hands or feet
18. _____hives or allergy problems
19. _____fatigue or exhaustion
20. _____low-grade infections
21. _____skin problems: acne or dermatitis
22. _____menstrual irregularities
23. _____asthma
24. _____decreased sexual interest or sexual problems
25. _____colds and/or flu
26. _____feeling faint or dizzy
27. _____urinary frequency
28. _____teeth grinding
29. _____breathing difficulty
30. _____hyperventilating

Emotional Symptoms

31. _____minor accidents
32. _____difficulty falling asleep
33. _____early morning awakening
34. _____frequent nightmares
35. _____feeling tired after adequate sleep
36. _____feeling depressed
37. _____worrying
38. _____nervousness
39. _____irritability
40. _____crying spells
41. _____shaking or halting voice
42. _____blushing
43. _____inability to concentrate or remember things
44. _____difficulty making decisions
45. _____procrastinating

WEEKLY STRESS SIGNAL RECORD

To begin noticing what triggers your stress, it is useful to keep a weekly stress signal diary. This record will help you to pinpoint stressors, both events and people, that cause your distress, as well as to identify thoughts

BASELINE STRESS SIGNAL RECORD (see p. 114)

Directions:

Over the next week, whenever you notice yourself experiencing stress, fill out the records. If there is not enough space available for a particular day, take a piece of paper and write down the information requested. Determine how severe your stress signal is by using a subjective stress-rating scale of 1–3.

1 = barely noticeable
2 = moderately tense (uncomfortable or disturbing)
3 = extremely tense (unable to function due to stress signal)

At the end of the week, in the comment section, write down any patterns you have noticed.

STRESS SIGNAL PROGRESS RECORD (see p. 115)

Directions:

When you decide to actively practice any stress-reduction technique or coping style, begin a weekly progress log to chart your success. You may wish to reproduce extra records to use for each intervention. Use the 3-point subjective rating scale described in the baseline record to score how tense you are before the intervention. Use the following 5-point subjective rating scale to determine how beneficial the technique was after you have completed the relaxation exercise.

1 = no improvement/change
2 = lessened my tension but still feel tense
3 = slightly more relaxed but a little tension still present
4 = relaxed
5 = extremely relaxed and calm; sense of well-being

At the end of the week write down any comments you have about your response to the technique and any problems you have identified that interfere with using the technique. The stress-reduction intervention should be practiced at least twice a day or, if possible, whenever you are aware of being stressed.

or emotions that might contribute to your stress response. Thus you will begin to understand your stress patterns.

By completing a weekly stress record before beginning your stress-management program, you will establish a baseline of your stress level. This baseline information can be compared with subsequent stress signal records after you begin to practice stress-reduction techniques and coping styles; in this way you can evaluate the effectiveness of the interventions you will be using and reinforce your progress (Wolpe, 1973). Keeping a weekly stress signal record while you are learning and practicing stress management also helps you to identify potential problem areas that might otherwise lead to your abandoning the stress-reduction interventions. The process of keeping this weekly record also forces you to pay attention to your body's signals and your coping style. You will begin to recognize stressors when they occur and will identify feelings or thoughts that contribute to your sense of distress.

There are two types of stress-rating records: the baseline record, which is formulated before starting stress-reduction interventions, and the progress record, which is formulated while practicing the techniques and coping styles that will be treated in Parts 4 and 5 (see boxes on left).

SOCIAL READJUSTMENT RATING SCALE

In the mid 1960s, Thomas Holmes and Richard Rahe began research that statistically supported a relationship between stress caused by major life changes or events and an individual's physical illnesses or accidents over the subsequent one-to-two years (Holmes and Rahe, 1967). Their research has been duplicated numerous times, with various populations always demonstrating positive statistical correlation between life events and health outcomes (Rahe, 1969; Komaroff et al., 1968).

At times we tend to forget the intense impact of life changes because we have "adequately coped" with the situation or have been unaware of the cumulative effects of the event. Also, we may not be aware that life changes affect our health, especially when we associate these changes with pleasant events, such as holidays, vacations, marriage, or birth. Many life changes are pleasant and are usually not considered stressful despite the fact that they require a certain amount of adjustment and expenditure of adaptive energy. To appreciate how much stress is involved in a pleasant life change, consider the following example. You are getting ready for a much desired vacation that, due to a staffing shortage, you had to fight like crazy to get approved. You worried that your friend or children or spouse might not be able to get off at the same time. Now that everyone's vacation request has been approved, you start booking reservations and arranging for animal and house sitters. You stop delivery of your mail and newspaper; you buy travelers' checks. You refill prescriptions and have yourself

BASELINE STRESS SIGNAL RECORD

	Monday	Tuesday	Wednesday	Thursday	Friday	Saturday	Sunday
Time							
Where body signal noticed							
Subjective rating of signal							
Where you were							
What was happening							
Anyone with you							
Thoughts and feelings before stress signal occurred							
How long signal lasted							

Comments: _____

_____

_____

STRESS SIGNAL PROGRESS RECORD

Coping style or technique used: _____

	Monday	Tuesday	Wednesday	Thursday	Friday	Saturday	Sunday
Time intervention began							
How long practiced							
How tense did you feel before practice? (1–3)							
Where were you practicing?							
How relaxed did you feel after practicing? (1–5)							
Thoughts or feelings about intervention							
Anything interfere with or detract from practice?							

Comments: _____

THE SOCIAL READJUSTMENT RATING SCALE*

Life Event	Mean Value
1. Death of spouse	100
2. Divorce	73
3. Marital separation from mate	65
4. Detention in jail or other institution	63
5. Death of a close family member	63
6. Major personal injury or illness	53
7. Marriage	50
8. Being fired at work	47
9. Marital reconciliation with mate	45
10. Retirement from work	45
11. Major change in the health or behavior of a family member	44
12. Pregnancy	40
13. Sexual difficulties	39
14. Gaining a new family member (e.g., through birth, adoption, oldster moving in, etc.)	39
15. Major business readjustment (e.g., merger, reorganization, bankruptcy, etc.)	39
16. Major change in financial state (i.e., a lot worse off or a lot better off than usual)	38
17. Death of a close friend	37
18. Changing to a different line of work	36
19. Major change in the number of arguments with spouse (i.e., either a lot more or a lot less than usual regarding childrearing, personal habits, etc.)	35
20. Taking out a mortgage or loan for a major purchase (e.g., for a home, business, etc.)	31
21. Foreclosure on a mortgage or loan	30
22. Major change in responsibilities at work (e.g., promotion, demotion, lateral transfer)	29
23. Son or daughter leaving home (e.g., marriage, attending college, etc.)	29
24. Trouble with in-laws	29
25. Outstanding personal achievement	28
26. Wife beginning or ceasing work outside the home	26
27. Beginning or ceasing formal schooling	26
28. Major change in living conditions (e.g., building a new home, remodeling, deterioration of home or neighborhood)	25

*From Holmes, T. H., and Rahe, R. H. 1967. The social readjustment rating scale. *J. Psychosomat. Res.* 11:213–218. Complete wording of Table 3, page 216.

THE SOCIAL READJUSTMENT RATING SCALE* (Continued)

Life Event	Mean Value
29. Revision of personal habits (dress, manners, association, etc.)	24
30. Troubles with the boss	23
31. Major change in working hours or conditions	20
32. Change in residence	20
33. Changing to a new school	20
34. Major change in usual type and/or amount of recreation	19
35. Major change in church activities (e.g., a lot more or a lot less than usual)	19
36. Major change in social activities (e.g., clubs, dancing, movies, visiting, etc.)	18
37. Taking out a mortgage or loan for a lesser purchase (e.g., for a car, TV, freezer, etc.)	17
38. Major change in sleeping habits (a lot more or a lot less sleep, or change in part of day when asleep)	16
39. Major change in number of family get-togethers (i.e., a lot more or a lot less than usual)	15
40. Major change in eating habits (a lot more or a lot less food intake, or very different meal hours or surroundings)	15
41. Vacation	13
42. Christmas	12
43. Minor violations of the law (e.g., traffic tickets, jaywalking, disturbing the peace, etc.)	11

vaccinated; you buy new clothes, film, cosmetics, and equipment. You worry about what to take; then you pack, unpack, and repack. You make lists for whomever is caring for the house, pets, and plants; you pack up the car and dash to the airport. All this and a lot more just to get ready to relax on your vacation!

Vacations can be exhausting, not only as a result of all the preparation but because most of us feel pressured to squeeze in everything to enjoy each moment of the vacation. In addition, we drastically alter our normal patterns of living, and doing so requires energy to adjust. Don't get the wrong idea. Vacations can be restful and are necessary, but they do require an expenditure of energy. How much more stressful, then, are changes such as a marriage, divorce, or a death in the family! The important point to remember is that change is stressful and your body needs time to adjust to it. Now look at the Social Readjustment Rating Scale to evaluate the amount of change you've undergone during the last year.

PREVENTIVE MEASURES

Suggestions:

The following suggestions are for using the Social Readjustment Rating Scale for the maintenance of your health and prevention of illness*:

1. Become familiar with the life events and the amount of change they require.
2. Put the Scale where you and the family can see it easily several times a day.
3. With practice you can recognize when a life event happens.
4. Think about the meaning of the event for you and try to identify some of the feelings you experience.
5. Think about the different ways you might best adjust to the event.
6. Take your time in arriving at decisions.
7. If possible, anticipate life changes and plan for them well in advance.
8. Pace yourself. It can be done even if you are in a hurry.
9. Look at the accomplishment of a task as a part of daily living and avoid looking at such an achievement as a "stopping point" or a "time for letting down."
10. *Remember,* the more change you have, the more likely you are to get sick. Of those people with over 300 Life Change Units for the past year, almost 80% get sick in the near future; with 150 to 299 Life Change Units, about 50% get sick in the near future; and with less than 150 Life Change Units, only about 30% get sick in the near future.

So, the higher your Life Change Score, the harder you should work to stay well.

*Copyright © 1976 by Thomas H. Holmes, M.D., Department of Psychiatry and Behavioral Sciences, University of Washington School of Medicine, Seattle, Washington 98195.

Whether or not life changes cause distress and contribute to the probability of illness depends on many factors. You need to take into account the following questions:

- What is the meaning of the change to you? How well prepared are you to deal with the change?
- What type of support do you have to cope with the change?
- Have you had experiences with similar changes? How well did you cope with those changes?
- What was your general stress level before the change occurred?
- How healthful is your ongoing life-style?

For example, moving to a new home within the same city may or may not be a stressful experience, depending on these considerations.

Let's look at two nurses, Jane and Sue, who are facing an identical house move. Jane is in good physical shape and takes pride in her self-care. Having moved several times in the past, she has developed a systematic approach to moving. She knows what to do to minimize the hassles. Jane is pleased that she is moving to a nicer place that she can easily afford. She has decided to have a moving party for her friends who are helping. The move is a success thanks to many cheerful helping hands and is celebrated at the end of the day.

Sue, however, doesn't like the idea of moving one bit. She has made only one previous move, when she left home after college, and that was a disaster. She has no idea how to tackle the job of packing and has to rely on professional movers, who she feels are charging an unreasonable price. Recently, she has been sick with various minor colds and feels depressed, lonely, and overstressed by her job. Her closest friend moved recently, and no one offered to help her move, and she didn't feel comfortable "imposing" on anyone. At the end of the move, Sue is sitting in her living room amid unpacked boxes, crying her heart out.

Both women made moves, had to expend energy, and will have to readjust to new surroundings and the loss of a familiar environment. However, Sue is far more likely to experience negative health consequences.

HASSLE ASSESSMENT

It has recently been found that "the petty annoyances, frustrations and unpleasant surprises that plague us every day may add up to more grief than life's major stressful events. . . . Hassles are more direct predictors of—and may therefore have a greater immediate effect on—physical and psychological health than major life events" (Lazarus, 1981).

Any daily occurrence that is frustrating, distressing, or annoying qualifies as a hassle. What is experienced as a hassle is highly subjective. As with life events, it is the cumulative effect of daily hassles, as well as the meaning we attach to these occurrences, that determines their effect upon our health and sense of well-being (Delongis et al., 1982). However, unlike many life events, such as a death in the family, hassles may be prevented or avoided if they are recognized.

HASSLE ASSESSMENT RECORD

To examine the number of hassles you experience and your reactions to them, keep a weekly hassle assessment record. At the end of the week, look over the information you have recorded. Are there any hassles that occur on a regular, almost predictable basis? Begin to explore whether

WEEKLY HASSLE ASSESSMENT RECORD

	Monday	Tuesday	Wednesday	Thursday	Friday	Saturday	Sunday
Time							
Type of hassle							
How intensely you experienced it (slightly moderately, extremely)							
How often it occurred							
Your reaction to it							

	Monday	Tuesday	Wednesday	Thursday	Friday	Saturday	Sunday
Time							
Type of hassle							
How intensely you experienced it (slightly moderately, extremely)							
How often it occurred							
Your reaction to it							

there is anything you can do to prevent these hassles. Also, ask yourself if there is anything you can do to change your responses to them. Certainly, some hassles are unavoidable, but you can reduce their frequency and change your reactions to them. (See Chapter 13, "Recognizing the 'Givens': Accepting What Can't Be Changed.")

MALADAPTIVE COPING STYLES

The following methods of coping with stress have been found to be unhelpful or even, in some cases, self-destructive. At best, they may only temporarily decrease stress symptoms while doing nothing to decrease the

MALADAPTIVE COPING STYLES

Directions:

As you read over the list of maladaptive coping styles, place a check in the blank next to any that you currently employ. Each check should be seen as a warning signal or red flag, indicating that you are only adding to your present level of distress.

1. _____ Using drugs or alcohol regularly to relieve tension or stress.
2. _____ Blowing off steam by putting co-workers and patients in their place in an attempt to get them off your back.
3. _____ Smoking.
4. _____ Avoiding any hassles by going along with everyone.
5. _____ Blaming other people for your job stress.
6. _____ Avoiding co-workers or patients so that you won't feel burdened with their problems.
7. _____ Taking work home, trying to read up on everything related to your job, in an attempt to solve work problems.
8. _____ Using up sick time to avoid facing work stress.
9. _____ Conserving your energy for work by not socializing with friends, exercising, or engaging in hobbies.
10. _____ Switching jobs without carefully evaluating what you're going into and why you're leaving.
11. _____ Withdrawing your interest in your job, not putting yourself into your work, as a way of protecting yourself from being overstressed.
12. _____ Becoming overly involved with work in an attempt to solve work problems.

MALADAPTIVE COPING STYLES (Continued)

13. ____ Playing the "ain't it awful game"—constantly complaining about work hassles.

14. ____ Worrying or being obsessed with work all the time.

15. ____ Taking out your frustrations behind the wheel by driving carelessly or aggressively.

16. ____ Seeking support or intimacy through careless sexual relationships.

17. ____ Coping with unpleasant emotions by eating.

18. ____ Spending most of your free time with co-workers.

19. ____ Avoiding commitments as a result of feeling exhausted.

20. ____ Retreating into sleep—sleeping more than you physiologically need.

21. ____ Constant daydreaming or fantasizing about being someone else or somewhere else.

22. ____ Beating yourself into the ground for failures or shortcomings—being overly self-critical.

23. ____ Neglecting your physical health or, conversely, being preoccupied with your physical health.

24. ____ Using sleep medications.

25. ____ Continually criticizing yourself while not noticing personal strengths and achievements.

stressor or alter your personal response to the stress. This list is designed to alert you to potentially unhealthful coping styles. Once you are aware that you use any one of these, you can decide what changes you wish to make in your life-style. The greater the number of unhealthy practices you engage in and the more frequently you use any or all of them, the more you increase your likelihood of becoming ill or having a shorter life expectancy (Ferguson, 1980; Applebaum, 1981; Cartwright, 1979; Goldberg, 1978).

CONCLUSION

To learn to cope with stress, you need to develop an awareness of the stressors you encounter—from daily hassles to significant life events—and the way you respond to them. You need to become sufficiently aware of your body's signals and symtomatology so you can anticipate and manage stress before it becomes overwhelming. The assessment tools in this chapter are designed to help you do this by suggesting ways to establish patterns of self-study that contribute to a healthy life-style.

REFERENCES

Applebaum, S. H. 1981. *Stress management.* Rockville, Md.: Aspen.

Cartwright, L. 1979. Sources and effects of stress in health careers. In *Health Psychology.* San Francisco: Jossey-Bass Publishers.

Davis, M., Eshelman, E. R., and McKay, M. 1980. *The relaxation and stress reduction workbook.* Richmond, Calif.: New Harbinger Publications.

Delongis, A., Coyne, J. C., Dakof, G., et al. 1982. Relationship of daily hassles, uplifts and major life events to health status. *Health Psychol.* 1(2):119–136.

Ferguson, T., editor. 1980. *Medical self-care: access to health tools.* New York: Summit Book.

Flynn, P. A. 1980. *Holistic health: the art and science of care.* Bowie, Md.: Robert J. Brady Co.

Goldberg, P. 1978. *Executive health.* New York: McGraw-Hill Book Co.

Holmes, T. H., and Rahe, R. H. 1967. The social readjustment rating scale. *J. Psychosomat. Res.* 11:213–218.

Komaroff, A. L., Masuda, M., and Holmes, T. H. 1968. The social readjustment rating scale: a comparative study of Negro, Mexican and White Americans. *J. Psychosomat. Res.* 12:121–126.

Lazarus, R. S. 1981. Little hassles can be hazardous to your health. *Psychol. Today* July, pp. 58–62.

Pelletier, K. 1977. *Mind as healer, mind as slayer.* New York: Dell Publishing.

Rahe, R. H. 1969. Multi-cultural correlations of life change scaling: America, Japan, Denmark, and Sweden. *J. Psychosomat. Res.* 13:191–195.

Samuels, M., and Bennett, H. 1973. *The well body book.* New York: Random House.

Sehnert, K. W., 1981. *Stress/unstress.* Minneapolis, Minn.: Augsburg Publishing House.

Selye, H. 1978. *The stress of life.* New York: McGraw-Hill Book Co.

Travis, J. 1978. *Wellness workbook.* Mill Valley, Calif.: Wellness Resource Center.

Wolpe, J. 1973. *The practice of behavior therapy,* 2nd ed. New York: Pergamon Press.

CHAPTER 9

Unrealistic Expectations: The Set-Ups for Failure

EMILY E. M. SMYTHE

Our beliefs and expectations directly affect our perception of what is stressful and what is not. Unfortunately, many of our expectations are on an unconscious level—we are unaware of their existence or their ability to directly influence our sense of well-being. Unrealistic personal and professional expectations are among the most significant factors contributing to our perception of distress. Unrealistic expectations are *unreachable* goals by which we measure our sense of self-worth and happiness. This is a self-defeating process (Burns, 1980a).

Unreasonable expectations are set-ups for failure, disappointment, and distress. Furthermore, the degree of disappointment and distress we experience is directly related to how strongly we believe in unrealistic expectations. The more we *expect* the impossible or near impossible, the more we are disappointed when what we believe *should* happen doesn't.

Unreasonable expectations lead to a sense of failure and frustration because we can rarely reach them and because our emotional investment in their successful outcome is significant. They become a form of addiction rather than preference; we *need* to have these expectations met to feel good about ourselves. An alternative is to *prefer* them to occur, but to not have to put our self-esteem on the line (Rubin, 1975). At times, rare though they may be, we may be able to achieve an unrealistic expectation, but the process of struggling toward the goal is far too costly.

Unrealistic expectations should not be confused with striving for high standards or attempting to pursue goals that require investing energy or personal commitment to create constructive changes. Struggling to reach impossible goals makes an emotional yo-yo of our self-esteem, causing it to fluctuate with our failures to reach the unobtainable. With unreasonable expectations, we also minimize the accomplishments we do achieve because they cannot possibly come close to our infeasible goal. If, at times, we do seem to succeed despite the overwhelming odds against us, the battle requires all our energy and attention, thus diminishing our overall sense of accomplishment and satisfaction and potentially destroying our interpersonal relationships or health. For example, a person with a type A personality that is highly associated with coronary heart disease may, in fact, succeed against impossible odds but may also die in the process. One should question the price of such "success" (American Heart Association, 1973; Ray and Bozek, 1980).

Edelwich (1980) states that the idealistic enthusiasm that stems from unrealistic expectations is the first stage on the road to burn-out. "The more one's expectations are in line with reality, the less frustration one will suffer."

Setting unrealistic expectations for ourselves, our clients, co-workers, or the health care system can only lead to disappointment and resentment. Part of what is difficult about attempting to change unrealistic expectations is that frequently when we fail to realize these goals we do not question the expectation itself but wonder what more we could or *should* have done to reach the goal. We ask ourselves, What's the hidden, magical ingredient for successfully obtaining my goal? We see the failure as a personal shortcoming, not an indication that the goal should be reexamined (Burns, 1980b). Unreasonable expectations for ourselves as nurses develop not only through the life expectations we establish through socialization in our families and society while growing up but also through professional socialization in school and during nursing practice (Freudenberger, 1980).

PUBLIC IMAGE OF NURSING AS AN UNREALISTIC EXPECTATION

From the media's presentation of nurses, the general public has come to expect so distorted and unrealistic a product that we can seldom deliver. We are the self-sacrificing angels of mercy, whose greatest personal satisfaction comes from caring for and nurturing the patient, much like idealized (and unreal) mothers. Many women, in fact, choose the profession because of the myths and images of nursing portrayed in books for adolescents (*Cherry Ames* or *Sue Barton*) or the glamorized views of nursing on TV and in movies. Needless to say, the disparity between these images and the reality of nursing directly contributes to the neophyte's distress and disappointment. She had expected a glamorous, romantic profession filled with excitement and had looked forward to the opportunity to spend a great deal of time socializing with her patients or eligible male co-workers.

Many nurses probably shared my experience. When I went to college, friends and family discussed my choice of nursing as a "noble calling"—made for a woman. No one believed I'd ever *work* as a nurse, unless of course I needed it to fall back on if my future husband died. (And, naturally, I'd probably do nursing only until I could remarry.) You can imagine the shock I experienced with my noble calling when I confronted reality!

Some individuals with degrees in other areas, such as a bachelor's in psychology, education, or humanities, enter nursing because they expect that as nurses they can get jobs using their minds rather than having to take the menial positions open to them otherwise. It doesn't take much imagination to realize how disappointed and distressed they become once they discover nurses serve food, transcribe orders, act as "go-fers" for physicians, and "babysit" patients. In their case, the expectations might seem logical, but since they do not reflect current practice, they are unrealistic and so are stressful.

Because in the public mind a nurse is caring, always available, sweet and kind, understanding, and all-accepting, our clients expect something we nurses cannot deliver. Most people don't realize they are probably not going to get much individualized attention—few, if any, backrubs or pleasant social chats, and little personalized client-centered care. It's no wonder clients complain. They've been "promised" (read: conditioned to expect) something we cannot provide. Some clients are determined to get the most for their money—"I expect good (read: idealized) care for all the money I've paid. I don't expect to get bargain-basement treatment for the deluxe charges I've been coughing up!"

Increasingly complex and technical medical care and more fragmented client care have decreased the opportunities for most nurses to perform direct personalized care (Corwin et al., 1961). It is then infeasible to have expectations of giving or getting loving, personalized nursing care. Any nurse who has ever spent a day lifting patients, emptying urine drainage, changing infected bandages, collecting stool specimens, or pouring medications knows there's a whole different world to nursing than the glamorized version presented to the public. And what happens to the neophyte nurse who expects to have romantic encounters with doctors or lengthy, significant interactions with clients that will alter the course of her life? She feels ripped off. Her frustrated cry, "No one told me it'd be like this!"

is justified. Not only didn't anyone tell her about the demands of nursing, but no one bothered to inform her of the limited scope of nursing practice. Needless to say, this creates fertile ground for frustration to blossom into distress or exodus from the profession.

RECRUITMENT PROMISES AND JOB INTERVIEW EXPECTATIONS

In addition to the unrealistic expectations of nursing provided by the media, recruitment promises and expectations developed from job interviews can also foster distorted expectations. Frequently, we don't stop to scrutinize the promises made by health care organizations but are instead enticed by clever advertising gimmicks or the wining and dining practices associated with job interviews. (Interestingly enough, many nurse recruiters may be nurses who could not tolerate practicing nursing in the institutions they are now getting other nurses to join.)

It is helpful to determine whether unrealistic expectations were generated by the recruitment or interviewing processes in your present job. These expectations may be contributing to your disenchantment with your position or the organization in which you work. If you are considering a new job, evaluate *realistically* what you consider important in a work setting and what contributes to your sense of job satisfaction. Beware of slick advertisements and seductive interviewers who promise you everything but have little to offer of real interest. A job selection should be a carefully thought out process. After all, you are going to spend a significant portion of your waking hours at work, and you want your expectations about it to be as realistic as possible. The following guide will help you achieve this.

Before you start stumbling through advertisements, looking through phone books, or attending job fairs, get a clear idea about what you are looking for in a job. Recognize that no job is going to be ideal but that certain characteristics or features are important to you. Also, ask yourself what you want from your career. Are you interested, for example, in developing your leadership skills or in continuing your pursuit of an advanced degree? Also consider what personal needs you have that might influence your work. For instance, if you are a mother with small children, you might need to work close to home with a routine work schedule or to work only part-time. A job that offers a day-care and/or an after-school program for employees might have attractions that outweigh other deficits. On the other hand, if you are more interested in furthering your education and are attending classes, having work-study or tuition reimbursement programs might be important to you. What is essential is that your job choice fit your existing commitments and personal needs.

What is the major emphasis of the recruiter or personnel officer you speak with initially (salary scale, flexible hours, model or philosophy of nursing care)? Are these features important to you? How open are the recruiters about discussing existing problems, long-range institutional plans, and what they feel are major achievements of the organization?

Be sure to interview your immediate potential supervisor as well as some of the staff you might be working with. Unless you're considering a position as a nurse recruiter, you won't be working primarily with the recruiter but with the floor staff. Who are these future co-workers? Are they people you'd like to get to know? Be sure to ask them what they see as positive features of the organization and what they see as the existing problems. If they can't identify any problems, I'd be suspicious either that no one cares enough to notice what is going on or that you are getting a "snow job," which is a definite set-up for disappointment. The more candid inside information you can get, the better. You also need to be realistic in evaluating each person's comments. No job is perfect and no job is totally horrible either. Scout out the physical environment where you'll be working and investigate the nursing tools (care plans, charting, flow sheets—and, most important, the staffing sheets). (Prospective employees may be given a staff-patient ratio that is the *ideal,* not the reality they will work with.)

Make sure you ask the tough questions that will give you an accurate picture of the situation. For example, how much "say" (power and control) do nurses have in this institution? What is the relationship, in general, with other professionals such as physicians, support services, or pharmacy? What are the channels for communication like? How available are nursing supervisory personnel and in-service, educational, or training personnel? Be sure to get a job description that clearly states expectations and responsibilities. If one doesn't exist, you might consider, depending on how confident and assertive you feel, requesting that major points of agreement be drawn up in a contract. Also consider what kind of advancement and growth potential are available to you.

Feel comfortable asking questions regarding any concern you have. Remember, job interviewing should be a two-way street. You are not just trying to sell yourself; you are also trying to see if you want what the organization has to offer. Of course, no organization is going to be ideal, and no matter how thoroughly you evaluate a prospective workplace, there will always be some disappointments and a few surprises. These little events, however, are not what usually produce the sudden awakening that makes you feel as if you've walked into a trap, that you have been grossly misled, or have blindly trusted without inquiring.

Unfortunately, what is often presented as "what it's like to work here" is pure wishful thinking, having little, if any, resemblance to reality. Although many hospitals advertise bonuses such as living in exciting cities, the romance of nursing, or the educational opportunities available in a university hospital, the day-to-day realities are what make a good job or one fraught with stressors.

An acquaintance of mine began working at a prestigious university hospital because she was impressed with the clinical research being published there and with the nursing leaders at the university-affiliated school of nursing. Her expectation, to learn and grow professionally, became unreasonable in light of the position she accepted. She agreed to work nights, which she should have realized would offer no opportunity for educational growth. Furthermore, because of an acute staff shortage, she had little opportunity to utilize her existing expertise or share it with her fellow colleagues. After eight months she quit, terribly disappointed and embittered by the negative experience. In her case, no one had promised her a different reality than what existed, but they also had not been forthright about discussing current problems. Most importantly, she had not checked out her fantasies to see if they matched what the university hospital had to offer.

As with any product, believing the advertising and sales promotion without investigating the claims and comparing the product to other products increases the chances you will not get what you expect or want. Behind the pretty packaged advertisement is the world of the 40-hour week, where you will spend about one-third of your waking hours. Many new graduates I have known just wanted to get a job offer. Rather than asking questions to see if this might be the right offer for them, they focused on selling themselves and then felt like captives having to take whatever they could get. Given the present nursing shortage, what you have to offer is a valuable commodity, whether you are a new graduate or someone returning after years of absence from nursing practice.

You have a lot of leverage when you are interviewing. Make your bargains and requests during the interviewing process, rather than once you have been hired. You don't have to make demands or get into a showdown—just state your needs and see what the organization has to offer. For example, you might say, I have small children and will have difficulty working weekends or odd shifts. See what helpful solutions your interviewers come up with. When you appear confident, as if you have something of value to sell, you will be surprised how much interest you can generate. Even if your potential employers may not be able to offer any helpful solutions, you haven't lost anything in the attempt. The manner of their response will communicate valuable information about how receptive this organization is to personal needs. If they are sympathetic, even though unable to give you what you want, their concern tells you they value individual staff more than does an organization that simply responds with, "This is our offer; take it or leave it."

I always make it a practice, no matter how good the offer I'm given, to inquire why they are not offering me the next pay step. Naturally, I must be willing to discuss what qualifications I have to justify being placed in a higher classification. In a few instances, I have moved into the higher step simply by pointing out specific education or experience I have. Once you have accepted an entry salary, it's next to impossible to get a raise out of sequence or to be reclassified.

Don't be rushed into making a decision even though many will try to pressure you into starting immediately. Take your time. Weigh the advantages and disadvantages. Make another appointment, if necessary, to discuss additional questions or concerns that trouble you. As for any significant commitment in your life, be sure this commitment is what you really want and that you aren't basing your decision on unrealistic expectations! Also, review Chapter 2, "Origins of Stress in Nursing," for guidelines about system stressors to consider when evaluating a job offer. If you decide to accept a position in a unit that has numerous personnel and system problems, you are accepting a "challenge" and should be forewarned of the hazards. You will feel as if you made the choice willingly rather than being betrayed by lies or false impressions. Unless you are willing to take personal responsibility for asking the hard questions, it is unlikely that you will get more than a superficial selling job. The "courtship" can present a picture full of unrealistic expectations that lead only to disenchantment and resentment once you are living in the day-to-day reality of the job.

EDUCATIONAL AND PROFESSIONAL STANDARDS: SOCIALIZATION FOR IMPOSSIBLE EXPECTATIONS

In the process of becoming socialized to the nursing role, we are subjected to many professional and educational expectations that are grandiose and idealized. These help us to develop unreasonable expectations, not only for ourselves and other nurses, but also for the profession in general. What occurs when these idealized standards are confronted with reality is what some experts call professional disillusionment. This process contributes to high levels of job stress and may contribute to the exodus of many new graduates. Nursing students are given a professional orientation while in school, but once they enter the work force, they are confronted by the expectation that tasks take priority over independent critical judgment or problem-solving skills (Corwin et al., 1961).

Professional Submission

Others have suggested that the contradictory expectations students are exposed to during their professional socialization also lead to distress and confusion (Bullock, 1975). Being socialized to accept professional submissiveness to physicians as part of our nursing identity is antithetical to the demands of any profession for autonomy—control over practice and education, and having distinct areas of expertise and responsibility (Simms, 1977; Richards, 1978). Thus, our implied subservience to physicians, which is reinforced by hospital administration, nursing supervisors, and the educational process, contradicts our role expectations. Are we to be professionals or are we to be handmaidens?

Authoritarian Atmosphere

Cohen (1981) believes "The origins of nursing problems . . . lie in the authoritarian atmosphere in nursing education and the entire health care field. This authoritarianism interferes with the process of professional socialization." Part of this authoritarianism produces the implicit or explicit message that everything we do as nurses has life-or-death consequences for our patients. This message, which is obviously incorrect but nonetheless powerful, gives us the unrealistic personal expectation that we must perform with perfection in *all* instances. I remember our "basics" nursing instructor who nearly "stroked-out" when she saw my first bed-making attempt. "Do you realize how painful it would be to sleep in this lumpy bed? It is our responsibility as nurses to help the patients we care for, not to make their every waking moment more miserable." Naturally, I felt incompetent, but I also began to wonder if I did not have some deep-seated sadistic tendencies. This experience seems ridiculous now. And yet, as nurses, we have been educated to feel we have our patient's lives in our hands and that our every action can cause disastrous harm, or, on the opposite and equally unrealistic side, can save patient's lives. I sincerely doubt that any single nursing act has ever ended or saved a patient's life. *Contributed* to either one, yes; *caused*, no.

Related to this impossible professional belief is the implication that a right answer exists in every nursing or medical situation. In reality, there are numerous limitations to our knowledge, as well as countless moral dilemmas for which we have no guidelines. If we expect that there is one right answer to each medical or nursing problem, we get stuck feeling like failures whenever we face a situation that exceeds our current knowledge, limitations, and ethics. Probably, at best, we in the health care community can help nature along with the curing process, but we alone do not cause a patient to recover or die. Once we begin to acknowledge these reasonable limitations of our scope of practice, we can stop feeling responsible each time a patient dies or suffers. Certainly we still must deal with our feelings about pain and death, but we do not add onto this the unreasonable expectation that if only we'd done the "right" thing, we could have saved them from their misery.

Contradictory Expectations

In the educational process we may also be given contradictory expectations regarding our responsibility. We are expected to have a rationale for every nursing action and to comply with nursing dogma without questioning its rationale. I remember, as a naive nursing student, asking a clinical instructor the reason for wearing caps and starched bibs over uniforms. After she bit my head off for my heresy, it became clear: "You just do as you are told. Don't question the rationale behind the rules, policies, tradition, practice standards, etc." Yet as nurses, we must be able to clearly state the rationale for our actions, using scientifically supported principles. Unfortunately, those who question dogma are labeled as "problem students" or, since this process continues in the work setting, as "problem employees who are always making trouble."

Another variation on this theme of contradictory professional expectations is that nurses are expected to blindly comply with existing practices rather than to respond as professionals and openly evaluate existing nursing problems or offer solutions to them. I have always found it amusing that many health-care organizations will pay outside organizational consultants or efficiency experts exorbitant fees to suggest the same changes that staff nurses may have been proposing all along. Somehow the experts' "objective" feedback seems to carry more weight than the nurses' "emotional" observations and opinions.

Obviously, the more contradictory messages we attempt to integrate into our self-expectations as functioning professional nurses, the more distress and confusion we are going to feel. The messages create unrealistic expectations because we cannot be professionally responsible and blindly conforming at the same time. For myself, I have decided to speak up whenever I question rationale, rules, or policies, risking the rejection and horror my questioning might cause. I also acknowledge the existence of the mixed message being given to me, "Speak up and contribute, if you support the status quo." Once I recognize the coexistence of these subtle messages, then I can "metacommunicate," or talk about the communication process itself rather than the actual content of what is being said. For example, I might say, "I'm sorry to see that what I said upset you. I was under the impression that you wanted my opinion on this problem, but it seems that you wanted my endorsement of your opinion, which I disagree with." At least metacommunicating stops the crazy-making process of trying to meet two opposite goals at once. It makes it possible to see that the problem isn't that you have said or done anything wrong, but that the other person is closed to any input. Also, by metacommunicating you can avoid being trapped into the unrealistic expectation that what people say is necessarily what they mean. When you comment on the process, you address their stated objectives rather than getting frustrated or distressed by their hidden (and frequently unconscious) agendas.

Doctor-Nurse Game

The "doctor-nurse game," identified by Stein in 1968, also become part of our professional socialization and is based upon several faulty as sumptions that contribute to our sense of distress. In the doctor-nurse (communication) game, nurses communicate with physicians without appearing to do so. Again, we are socialized with two paradoxical messages. On the one hand, we are taught that because the doctor is omnipotent and all-knowing, any suggestion from a lowly nurse would be insulting and possibly leave us open to public ridicule. The second message we are given is that we as nurses directly contribute to our patients' care and are morally and *legally* responsible for the patients' well-being. In the doctor-nurse game, when our judgment indicates the doctor needs to consider certain patient care recommendations, we must somehow disguise our knowledge in a way that won't offend the doctor but at the same time will influence the doctor to do what is in the patient's best interest (Richards, 1978).

There is, of course, an alternative to this stressful game; Thomstad and co-workers (1975) have developed what they call "new rules" for doctor-nurse communication. As you read over Table 9-1, which contrasts the old and new rules to the doctor-nurse game, notice the unrealistic expectations that operate within the "old rules" systems. Obviously, these unrealistic expectations cause a sense of powerlessness and dependency in the nurse that contributes to our sense of distress and resentment—not to mention conflict with physicians.

Professional Delusions

Norris (1973) discusses "delusions that trap nurses . . . into dead end alleys away from growth, relevance and impact on health care." She identifies six myths that can create unrealistic expectations for the individual nurse and the nursing profession in general. (Chapter 2, "Origins of Stress in Nursing," discusses some of these myths as well as others that contribute to our perception of distress and to job dissatisfaction.)

Delusion 1: Nurses Are in General Agreement About What Nursing Is* In case you haven't noticed, no one, including nurses, seems to know exactly what education and experience are necessary to prepare a nurse; nor do we have a clear understanding of what it is that a nurse "should" do.

The unrealistic expectation underlying this myth is that "Anyone who is a nurse must be like me. She must have the same experience, values, and abilities. She does what I do." Obviously, the result of this unrealistic expectation is anger directed toward other nurses, constant battles over values and perceptions, and role conflict.

---

*Quoted material on pages 133–135 from Norris, 1973 is with the permission of The American Journal of Nursing Company. Copyright © 1973, American Journal of Nursing Company. Quoted from *Nursing Outlook*, Catherine M. Norris, "Delusions that trap nurses . . . into dead end alleys away from growth, relevance, and impact on health care," January, Vol. 21, No. 1.

TABLE 9-1. DOCTOR-NURSE GAME*

Old Rules	New Rules
Medical care is more important than nursing care.	Good health care requires both good nursing care and good medical care.
The nurse can help the doctor as long as nobody knows about it, including the doctor.	The doctor and nurse are both there to help the patient and have to communicate directly and openly to do so.
The doctor knows more than the nurse.	Good doctors know more medicine than good nurses; good nurses know more nursing than good doctors.
If the doctor tells the patients what to do, and they don't do it, it's the patients' fault. The doctor did his best.	If a health care plan is to be carried out, it must be worked out with the patients' needs, beliefs, and capabilities in mind.
Doctors are so busy that nurses may have to take over some of the tasks.	Many doctors don't like or know much about health care. Nurses are prepared in this, like it, and are usually better at it than doctors.
Good doctors rarely make mistakes and see to it that others don't either.	Everyone makes mistakes, but open communication between doctors and nurses minimizes them.

*Copyright © 1975, American Journal of Nursing Company. Reproduced with permission from *Nursing Outlook*, July, Vol. 23, No. 7.

Delusion 2: Nurses Care for and Are Concerned About Patients   "Nursing has never raised the critical question about whether it is possible to have warm feelings, to say nothing of concern, for the hundreds of patients a nurse is responsible for in the course of a week or two." "Won't the nurse feel less frustrated if she doesn't feel she has to have a special bond with each of her patients?" (Norris, 1973).

Delusion 3: Knowledge Prevents Disease   "All around and among us the message is clear: the American people do *not* use the knowledge available to help determine their life style, to meet their basic needs or to promote their optimum health and well being" (Norris, 1973). This unfounded belief may protect us against our feelings of impotence and helplessness, but it also contributes to our sense of frustration and anger with clients who do not improve or adhere to our health teaching. With this belief, we end up feeling like professional failures whenever clients don't improve.

Delusion 4: Nurses Significantly Influence Patients' Lives   "When it comes to helping patients to cope with their illnesses or to establish new health goals or changed life styles, . . . the average patient doesn't see a nurse and does not expect this kind of assistance" (Norris, 1973). When our goal is to significantly influence patients' lives, we are doomed to a sense of defeat and resentment, as well as to devalue the realistic contributions we do make.

Delusion 5: Professional Nursing Skills Have Market Value   "Employing agencies do not define differences in technical and professional nursing, and only a few agencies pay a small differential to professional nurses. . . . In fact, professional nursing skills might be likened to luxury items for patients after technical nursing has provided what they really need" (Norris, 1973). The nurse trained for and expecting to do health teaching, psychosocial interventions, or comprehensive interventions that produce a significant impact on the patient's life-style is soon overwhelmed by the physical care demands of her patients. This, along with the short staffing that renders any of these expectations next to impossible, creates a sense of failure and disappointment for the professional trained nurse.

A closely related, infeasible expectation is that we *should* receive adequate compensation as well as respect from other professional colleagues for our contributions. Yet nursing is, to me, the epitome of responsibility without power. We are considered a low-status group within the health-care hierarchy; we are low on the pay scale of professionals with equal responsibility; we have little or no input in the decision-making that directly influences our practice. If you entered nursing expecting to receive adequate compensation for your contributions, you are probably quite embittered if you have begun to appreciate how you are valued in tangible ways—money, power, and status. I do not believe the lack of tangible rewards makes nursing any less important or gratifying, but it does mean that you need to acknowledge the low-status position of nursing—and fight to change it rather than play the "poor me" game.

Delusion 6: Nursing Is Patient-Centered   "When nurses integrate the patient-centered delusion into the system, they overlook the fact that the needs of physicians, the demands of the system or bureaucracy, the time-consuming routines, the endless secretarial duties, the supervision of countless technical and ancillary personnel as well as the urgent needs of many patients all take precedence over consideration of and concern for individual patients" (Norris, 1973). Any of these demands can become annoying stressors that interfere with what we believe is our primary focus. Belief in patient-centered care, as opposed to work-centered, hospital-centered, or physician-centered care leads to an unending sense of frustration and resentment that our true *raison d'être* cannot be actualized.

"Super-Nurse" Myth

The "super-nurse" myth, as identified by Gunderson and co-workers (1977), states, "A nurse should be able to be all things to all people.

Highly competent in all areas of patient-care, she makes no mistakes. . . . When the nurse recognizes that a multitude of needs are unmet, she tells herself she's not a good nurse because she is unable to achieve her valued nursing goals." Many of us berate ourselves when we are unable to accomplish the herculean tasks of meeting every need to the level of excellence—we forget to question whether the expectations placed upon us by others are feasible. We do not stop to evaluate whether, in fact, the problem lies in our abilities or in the unreasonable demands of the task itself. We need to accept that many of the high professional standards we are taught through the socialization process are not feasible given the realities of the typical worksetting. This does not mean these standards are not valuable, but it does mean that we need to stop judging ourselves against them on a daily basis. They are goals to be reached for, not criteria to judge against. Part of what we need to learn from our education is how to prioritize our goals and to acknowledge the limitations of our services. Most nursing students have little firsthand experience with a typical patient-care load before they graduate. No wonder they are shocked to realize that not only do they have three to five times as many patients assigned to them, but they also have few if any available resource personnel to help integrate their transition from the protective cocoon of studenthood to the harsh realities of professional nursing.

Another unreasonable belief is that patients should be grateful for all the care we give them. "Here we are killing ourselves, trying against impossible odds—the least they could do is say 'thank you,' " we tell ourselves. Here again, disappointment is right around the corner. Not only don't many patients thank us, but in reality many patients are highly critical of any and all nursing care they receive. We end up feeling angry and/or guilty because of their inappropriate expectations, coupled with our own unrealistic expectations that they will be grateful.

My favorite set-up is what I call the martyr role of nursing, the expectation that nurses are self-sacrificing, nonjudgmental, always caring. Naturally, this comes in part from nursing's early connection with religion. History tells us that martyrs suffer and are crucified. I, for one, don't plan to give up my life this easily. No educational process should dictate how people ought to feel. It is next to impossible to care for and about all of our patients. Certainly there are some for whom we develop strong attachments, but there are others with whom this type of bond simply doesn't exist—or, worse still, whom you intensely dislike. To give good nursing care, you don't have to love all your patients. You do have to *respect* their concerns—but not necessarily meet all their demands. Of course, it is wonderful when you can genuinely like and care for them.

Being nonjudgmental is next to impossible. We all form opinions and make judgments about everything from the moment we interact with a person or object. No one can dictate that you "will not perceive a stimulus once it is in your perceptual field," and yet that is exactly what the expectation that nurses be nonjudgmental implies. What we need to learn is awareness of our reactions and responses, since we all have them for everything and everyone. Then we need to develop the ability to handle and cope with our feelings, rather than to ignore or deny their existence. This crazy-making expectation encourages repressed feelings, both our own and our colleague's. We all know what happens to strong emotions that are repressed—they are acted out, either consciously or unconsciously, when they cause internal tension and anxiety. I am sure you have had the experience of disliking a patient, for whatever reason, but instead of being able to discuss this and to learn how to handle these feelings, you probably hid them and were ashamed and self-critical of your unprofessional, uncaring attitude. The more you can become aware of and accept your feelings, the less control they will have over your behavior and the less distress they will cause you.

I accept the fact that I react to all my patients. When these reactions are negative or critical, I use this information to learn more about myself and to find ways to intervene with the client. The more I accept these feelings, the more I am able to accept the client. I don't feel this internal struggle: "But you really should like this person. What's the matter with you? How can you be so self-centered?" And I can then develop nondestructive ways to relate to the person. We all have feelings, good/caring or bad/uncaring, for all patients. The issue is not how to stop having these feelings, but how to learn to work with, and in spite of, them.

Empathy has become a buzz word in the psychosocial approach to patient care. The process of empathy can be stated as, "Imagine yourself in the patient's shoes, and then care for him as you would wish to be cared for." Although I certainly endorse the basic notion of empathy, I also agree with Elder (1978) that a word of caution is in order.

> It is far more useful to ascertain how someone else feels and respond to that with your feelings. If I believe I feel someone else's feelings or treat them as I would be treated myself, what I am actually doing is imagining and projecting my own perceptions of how I would feel if I were in that situation. With regard to illness, nurses often project their personal frame of reference on patients, then treat those patients accordingly.

When the patient doesn't respond as we would or as we *expect* they should, we become disappointed and frustrated. Ultimately, this leads to a more stressful interpersonal interaction with the patient.

PROFILES AT RISK: UNREALISTIC SELF-EXPECTATIONS

Several personality styles have unrealistic expectations as part of their dynamics. These "profiles at risk" have been associated with susceptibility to stress illnesses as well as to emotional problems.

"Type A" Personality

Perhaps the most widely known profile is the type A personality, which is a predictor of coronary heart disease. As Friedman and Rosenman, two cardiologists who have published extensively on the relationship between type A behavior and heart disease, said in 1974,

> In the absence of Type A behavior pattern, coronary heart disease almost never occurs before seventy years of age, regardless of the fatty foods eaten, the cigarettes smoked, or the lack of exercise. But when this behavior pattern is present, coronary heart disease can easily erupt in one's thirties and forties.

Type A behavior is a psychologic profile of a personality style that is characteristic of approximately 60% of American managers, as well as other individuals who are recognized as "hard-driven strivers." People with the type A personality feel they are going to achieve, even if the struggle kills them. It frequently does. As nurses, we've all seen type A individuals who, even in the coronary care unit, are unable to ease up—some even conduct business at their bedsides. Although this personality style is closely associated with business managers, other people with the same profile are found in health care professions as well as any other profession.

Type A's are "workaholics," people who get their "kicks" or "highs" from overworking. They are just as dependent and hooked on their craving to work as an addict upon drugs or alcohol. Even when their driving work interferes with their relationships, happiness, or health, they still cannot seem to put work into a more reasonable perspective (Suojanen and Hudson, 1981). Even vacations, if they get around to taking them, are approached in the same hard-driving style. They are known to have obsessive-compulsive characteristics that trap them into an escalating, compulsive striving for perfection in anything they undertake, whether it be a sport, hobby, relationship, or work (Oates, 1972). Type A individuals also have what is referred to as "hurried sickness." Everything feels as if it has top priority and must be done as quickly as possible in a literal race against the clock. But once they reach their goal, instead of being able to slow down for a while, they feel an even greater urgency to do more in less time (Glass, 1977). Another characteristic of this personality style is polyphasic behavior—doing several tasks or having several thoughts at once (Burke and Weir, 1980).

Type A's are also unable to work with other people and feel a sense of furious competitiveness in every situation. This contributes to their inability to delegate tasks or work in a collaborative way with co-workers as well as to their aggressive behavior. Part of what is motivating their behavior is, in fact, an overwhelming sense of insecurity and inferiority. If they do not excel beyond all reasonable expectations to the level of perfection, then they are worthless (O'Flynn and Cominskey, 1979).

It should be remembered that type A behavior is not a stress response to a stressful situation but a style of behavior that constantly elicits the stress response, which to a large extent consists of cardiovascular system arousal (Girdamo and Everly, 1979). To see if you have type A behavior characteristics, take a moment to do the next exercise.

SELF-TEST FOR "TYPE A" PERSONALITY

Directions: As you can see, each scale below is composed of a pair of adjectives or phrases separated by a series of horizontal lines. Each pair has been chosen to represent two kinds of contrasting behavior. Each of us belongs somewhere along the line between the two extremes. Since most of us are neither the most competitive nor the least competitive person we know, put a check mark where you think you belong between the two extremes.

1 2 3 4 5 6 7

1. Doesn't mind leaving things temporarily unfinished. - - - - - - - Must get things finished once started.

2. Calm and unhurried about appointments. - - - - - - - Never late for appointments.

3. Not competitive. - - - - - - - Highly competitive.

4. Listens well, lets others finish speaking. - - - - - - - Anticipates others in conversation (nods, interrupts, finishes sentences for the other).

5. Never in a hurry, even when pressured. - - - - - - - Always in a hurry.

6. Able to wait calmly. - - - - - - - Uneasy when waiting.

7. Easygoing. - - - - - - - Always going full speed ahead.

8. Takes one thing at a time. - - - - - - - Tries to do more than one thing at a time, thinks about what to do next.

9. Slow and deliberate in speech. - - - - - - - Vigorous and forceful in speech (uses a lot of gestures).

10. Concerned with satisfying him- or herself, not others. - - - - - - - Wants recognition by others for a job well done.

11. Slow doing things. - - - - - - - Fast doing things (eating, walking, etc.).

12. Easygoing. - - - - - - - Hard driving.

SELF-TEST FOR "TYPE A" PERSONALITY (continued)

13. Expresses feelings ------- Holds feelings in.
    openly.
14. Has a large number ------- Few interests outside
    of interests.   work.
15. Satisfied with job. ------- Ambitious, wants quick
                                 advancement on job.
16. Never sets own ------- Often sets own deadlines.
    deadlines.
17. Feels limited ------- Always feels responsible.
    responsibility.
18. Never judges things ------ Often judges performance
    in terms of   in terms of numbers (how
    numbers.   many, how much).
19. Casual about work. ------ Takes work very seriously
                              (works weekends, brings
                              work home).
20. Not very precise. ------ Very precise (careful about
                             detail).

Scoring: Assign a value from 1–7 for each score. Total them up.

Analysis of Your Score

Total score=110–140: Type A_1.
    If you are in this category, and especially if you are over 40 and
    smoke, you are likely to have a high risk of developing cardiac
    illness.
Total score=80–109: Type A_2.
    You are in the direction of being cardiac prone, but your risk is not
    as high as the A_1. You should, nevertheless, pay careful attention to
    the advice given to all the Type A's.
Total score=60–79: Type AB.
    You are an admixture of A and B patterns. This is a healthier
    pattern than either A_1, or A_2, but you have the potential for slipping
    into A behavior and you should recognize this.
Total score=30–50: Type B_2.
    Your behavior is on the less–cardiac–prone end of the spectrum.
    You are generally relaxed and cope adequately with stress.
Total score=0–29: Type B_1.
    You tend to the extreme of noncardiac traits. Your behavior
    expresses few of the reactions associated with cardiac disease.

SELF-TEST FOR "TYPE A" PERSONALITY (continued)

This test will give you some idea of where you stand in the discussion of type A behavior. The higher your score, the more cardiac prone you tend to be. Remember, though, even B persons occasionally slip into A behavior, and any of these patterns can change over time. In the description of the range of scores, the most extreme "type A" personality is the type A_1, the hard-driving, overconscientious person. At the far end is B_1, the "laid-back," extremely easygoing person. Most of us, of course, are somewhere in between.

The evidence suggests that type A behavior is learned behavior. As such it can be unlearned or at least modified. Stress-reducing techniques, both specific to type A behavior and in general, are presented in Parts 4, 5, and 6.

Self-test based on research by Drs. T. H. Holmes and R. H. Rahe. Score analysis based on research by Dr. Howard I. Glazer. Reprinted by permission from Schnert, K. W., M.D. *Stress/Unstress*, copyright © 1981, Minneapolis, Minn.: Augsberg Publishing House.

Rescuer Fantasy

The rescuer complex may affect people professionally or personally. Many of us may have become nurses because we felt the need to save other people—and, in fact, feel at our best when others are dependent on and obligated to us. As nurses, we can become professional rescuers (Steiner, 1974). Certainly there is nothing wrong with caring about other people's well-being—it is a commendable quality. However, it becomes a problem when our needs for others to depend upon us get confused with a patient's needs, frequently even inhibiting the patient's well-being. When our sense of self-worth is related to the patient's recovery or adherence to our expectations, we are rescuers. Instead of helping patients become healthy and self-actualized, we foster their dependency and stifle their healthy self-exploration, not to mention the fact that our own sense of well-being becomes attached to events beyond our control (Berne, 1961).

The helper needs the patient to remain helpless in order for there to be a purpose in their relationship. When the professional nurse-rescuer repeatedly tries to save the patient from irresolvable situations, she or he is likely to feel overwhelmed and suffer a subsequent loss of energy and confidence. There is also a subtle seduction to try harder when the initial attempts to save or cure the client fails. Obviously, the more we invest in this game, the greater our sense of emotional bankruptcy will be when our expectations are not met despite our time and energy investment.

Underlying the rescuer role is the belief that we are better or wiser than our patients. The more patients can be forced to rely upon us to do things for them that they could do or need to learn how to do, the more we can cling to our belief that we are indispensable. The pitfall is, of course, that when we fail we either become angry and resentful of the patient or we feel incompetent because we failed with our impossible task (Elder, 1978).

Self-Assessment Questions

How prone are you to becoming a "rescuer"? (Each question answered in the affirmative indicates rescuer belief or behavior.)

1. Do you feel your patients aren't appreciative enough of your help?
2. Do you pay more attention to your patients' needs than to your own needs?
3. Do you feel best when you are helping other people?
4. Do you feel responsible for other people's happiness?
5. Do you have difficulty letting other people come to their own decisions or voice opinions that do not agree with your own beliefs?
6. Do you have difficulty allowing other people to take risks or try new behaviors?
7. Do you always feel obligated to respond to anyone who seems to need help?
8. Does a large portion of your job satisfaction and personal well-being depend on your patients improving?
9. Are there personal needs of yours that are being met through your job that should be met outside of work?

We can only help others when *and if* they wish to be helped. The old adage, "You can lead a horse to water but you can't make him drink" applies in the nurse-patient relationship. We need to see if our patients are interested in what we have to offer rather than operate on the often-mistaken perception that they want what we think they want. The patient's rejection of the nursing care we offer does not have to diminish its value. It simply means the patient does not want what we wish to give. At times, this can make us feel truly helpless while we watch patients behave in ways we know will kill them or reject assistance we know could help them. And yet ultimately the patient has control over and responsibility for his or her life.

CONCLUSION

The more we become aware of the unrealistic expectations we have about ourselves as care-givers, our profession, and our clients, the more we will be able to alter our perception of the stressors in nursing. Chapter 12, "Cognitive Approach to Stress Management," suggests how we can change these unrealistic expectations and thus gain more self-control and decrease our job stress. Chapter 13, "Recognizing the 'Givens': Accepting What Can't Be Changed," also offers many interventions to manage unrealistic expectations that frequently induce the fight-or-flight response.

Maintaining unrealistic expectations leads to frustration and resentment and diminishes our sense of accomplishment. Whenever you feel frustrated or resentful, stop and consider the cause of your distress. The chances are good that failure to meet some unrealistic expectation is contributing to your stress.

REFERENCES

American Heart Association. 1973. *Coronary risk handbook*. New York: The American Heart Association.

Berne, E. 1961. *Transactional analysis in psychotherapy*. New York: Grove Press, Inc.

Bullock, B. 1975. Barriers to the nurse practitioner movement. problems of women in a woman's field. *J. Health Sci.* 5 (2) 239:310–313.

Burke, R. J., and Weir, T. 1980. The type A experience: occupational and life demands, satisfaction and well-being. *J. Human Stress*, Dec.:28–38.

Burns, D. D. 1980a. *Feeling good*. New York: William Morrow.

Burns, D. D. 1980b. The perfectionists' script for self-defeat. *Psychol. Today*, November:34–52.

Cohen, H. A. 1981. *The nurse's quest for a professional identity*. Menlo Park, Calif.: Addison-Wesley Pub. Co.

Corwin, R. C., Taves, M. J., and Haas, J. E. 1961. Professional disillusionment. *Nur. Res.* 141–144.

Edelwich, J. 1980. *Burnout: stages of disillusionment in the helping professions*. New York: Human Sciences Press.

Elder, J. 1978. *Transactional analysis in health care*. Menlo Park, Calif.: Addison-Wesley Pub. Co.

Freudenberger, H. J. 1980. *Burnout: how to beat the high cost of success*. Toronto: Bantam Books.

Friedman, M., and Rosenman, R. N. 1974. *Type A behavior and your heart*. New York: Alfred A. Knopf.

Girdamo, D., and Everly, G. 1979. *Controlling stress and tension: a holistic approach*. Englewood Cliffs, N.J.: Prentice-Hall.

Glass, D. C. 1977. Stress, behavior patterns and coronary disease. *Sci. Am.* 65:177–187.

Gunderson, K., Percy, S., et al. 1977. How to control professional frustrations. *Am. J. Nurs.* July:1180–1183.

Kramer, M. 1974. *Reality shock: why nurses leave nursing.* St. Louis: The C. V. Mosby Co.

Muff, J. 1982. Handmaiden, battle axe, whore: an exploration into the fantasies, myths, and stereotypes about nursing. In *Socialization, Sexism and Stereotyping,* editor J. Muff. St. Louis: The C. V. Mosby Co.

Norris, C. M. 1973. Delusions that trap nurses into dead end alleys away from growth, relevance and impact on health care. *Nurs. Outlook* 21:18–21.

Oates, W. E. 1972. *Confessions of a workaholic: the facts about work addiction.* New York: Abingdon Press.

O'Flynn-Cominskey, A. 1979. The type A individual. *Am. J. Nurs.* Nov.:1956–1958.

Ray, J. J., and Bozek, R. 1980. Dissecting the A-B personality type. *Br. J. Med. Psychol.* 53:181–186.

Richards, R. D. 1978. The game professionals play. *Supervisor Nurse* June:48–50.

Rubin, T. I. 1975. *Compassion and self-hate.* New York: Ballantine Books.

Schnert, K. W. 1981. *Stress/unstress.* Minneapolis, Minn.: Augsbury Publishing House.

Simms, S. 1977. Nursing dilemma: the battle of role determination. *Supervisor Nurse* Sept.:29–31.

Suojanen, W. W., and Hudson, D. R. 1981. Coping with stress and addictive work behavior. *Business* 31(1):7–14.

Stein, L. L. 1968. The doctor-nurse game. *Am. J. Nurs.* 68:101–105.

Steiner, C. 1974. *Scripts people live.* New York: Grove Press, Inc.

Thomstad, B., Cunningham, N., and Kaplan, B. 1975. Changing the rules of the doctor-nurse game. *Nurs. Outlook* 23:422–427.

CHAPTER 10

Writing: The Process of Self-Reflecting

EMILY E. M. SMYTHE

You may say to yourself as you begin to read this chapter, "Keeping a journal? Writing observations? What boring exercises these are! Writing is nothing but a tedious chore."

Many of us approach the idea of writing with painful memories of unpleasant experiences in school. The task of writing conjures up old associations of critical evaluations by unsympathetic, rigid authority figures—our teachers. If you had this experience, writing may not have resulted in self-exploration or self-expression; instead you may have found yourself trying to guess what the teacher wanted to read and then trying to produce it for a favorable grade.

What I'm suggesting here, however, is writing solely for yourself—your own exploration and growth. No grades or judgments attached. Unless you plan to publish your writing, forget the fear of a critical evaluator tearing apart each sentence you write. Imagine the writing process simply taking you where it will—a type of written free association.

The writing formats suggested in this chapter are designed to help you become more familiar with yourself by carrying on correspondence with yourself. The writing is definitely not meant to be an exercise in proper grammar.

Perhaps you are uninterested in the notion of keeping a diary or journal because you feel that your life isn't important enough to record. As one participant said, in a workshop I led, "What's there to write about? I get up at the crack of dawn, work as a nurse for eight exhausting hours, return home, and just collapse."

Another said, "I'm too stressed with all my other responsibilities. How can you expect me to squeeze in time to write every evening? That sounds more stressful to me." My response to these concerns is that writing is a tool for your personal use. Don't let it become another reason for feeling guilty or stressed.

"I really should have written in my journal today," you say, punishing yourself with guilt. Write when you wish. This writing is for you to enjoy— for growth and self-appreciation. It should not become something you dread doing. I firmly believe that you need to select stress-management techniques and assessment tools that interest you; otherwise, the chances are very good that you'll not use them regularly. They'll just become additional burdens. Part of what is so useful about writing is that it can help you to take a look at yourself from a different perspective. Write whenever the interest arises or as a specific exercise to help resolve a particular crisis.

BENEFITS OF SELF-WRITING

But why should you write about your life? What can the writing do to help with your stress?

The focus of any personal writing is to develop intimacy with yourself. This intimacy may be a personal awareness of daily events, images and dreams, behavioral patterns, values and beliefs, or a combination of any or all of these. This type of self-knowledge is important for stress management.

Most of us are not only alienated from other people; we are also alienated from ourselves. Frequently, I see clients who say they have no idea what their problems are, how they react, or what direction their lives are taking. They are truly out of touch with themselves. They may be spending their lives rushing around at a hectic pace with little awareness of why they live in this fashion; indeed, they have no idea that their life-styles are their own conscious or unconscious choices.

Many terminally ill cancer patients I work with make statements like, "If I'd only known I was going to die, I would have lived my life so differently. There are so many important things I didn't find time to do. Where did my life go?" Somehow events get into motion and we lose track of ourselves; we forget our ability and our responsibility to make choices about our lives. We're all going to die. Does someone have to constantly remind us of the closeness of death before we stop to evaluate our lives? Writing about our lives gives us the chance to slow down long enough to look over how we are living. The process of writing about our lives and paying attention to our use of time offers us the opportunity to decide if we are living the way we want to.

Have you ever gone in for a health evaluation that included filling out a self-assessment evaluation form—the type that asks for detailed information about your life-style, as well as your medical history? Did you suddenly notice things about yourself that were unfamiliar? Perhaps the profile you were describing seemed like someone else's. You may have asked yourself, "Is this really me? How did I get to be this way?"

What happens in the process of filling out the health self-evaluation is that you must stop for a moment to reflect upon yourself. You also may make connections between your life-style and your medical complaints that previously, even with your nursing knowledge, you didn't recognize. Seeing parts of our lives condensed into concrete black-and white responses to questions gives us self-knowledge.

Keeping a journal or diary that recounts daily events and reactions to or thoughts about these events is a written format that allows you to see yourself in more depth. When you review this type of writing, you begin to reflect on how your emotional states relate to the events in your life. You can develop a sense of connection with the world you live in so that these events seem less haphazard and random. The process of reflecting on your journal is similar to what occurs in therapy. The therapist is a reflective observer with whom we share our lives, our fears, our hopes, and our memories. Rarely does the therapist give his or her personal evaluation of our lives or ourselves; instead the therapist helps us to gain our own perspective by asking questions that stimulate us to reflect upon ourselves and arrive at our own solutions.

Writing in a journal can accomplish the same purpose. The process of putting your thoughts and feelings onto paper allows you to separate yourself from the feelings and thoughts. Once you are able to distance yourself, you can begin to examine what you have been feeling and thinking. Have you ever written a letter describing your concerns about an issue and started objectively to ask yourself, "Does this make sense? Do I really feel this way?" Keeping a journal will have the same effect.

Writing may also help to clarify your thoughts and feelings by offering you the chance to describe and sift through relevant information. Have you ever had this experience when writing a nursing note on a patient whose behavior has you confused? By the time you gave a detailed description of the patient's behavior, you noticed you were gaining some insight into the problem. The vague impressions you had became clear as you forced yourself to describe them logically and concretely.

Reflecting about our self-notations may provide different meanings and significance each time we read them. How we interpret the information will depend on our current needs and focus. This experience is similar to what happens when you read a book at one time in your life and reread it later, only to find a completely different message in it.

We see more complexity and richness in ourselves by studying ourselves the same way we would study any subject matter. The more you know about the artist, the style, the period in which the piece was produced, and the symbolic meaning of the work, the greater your appreciation will be. This is true of ourselves as well. The more we observe and learn about ourselves, the richer our appreciation of ourselves becomes.

Writing for yourself allows you to integrate various parts of yourself. By writing about contradictory feelings and beliefs, you can begin to have a dialogue with yourself; this allows you to explore and repossess parts of yourself you may have forgotten or never fully explored and acknowledged. We often tell patients to jot down their questions so that they won't forget important things. The same holds true for us. At times we become aware of something that is important but that gets lost in the rush of daily events. The thought's getting lost does not mean it is unimportant—despite the adage, "If it's important, you'll remember it." What is forgotten is perhaps so important and such a revelation that it is difficult for our minds to hold onto it because of its unfamiliarity.

Self-writing also helps you identify repeating themes in your life and your patterns of behavior. The process of writing heightens your awareness of what is happening around you. The connection between seemingly unrelated events begins to become apparent, and your whole perception changes as a result of this awareness. If we only respond to the present content of our lives, we are like ships at sea without anchors. We are tossed around and carried off with every passing emotional wave or situation. Every breeze of change potentially alters our course. Self-writing allows you to see patterns in your life and to look at the process of your life—the underlying themes and motivating dynamics. This appreciation and self-understanding can become the anchor allowing you to weather the storm, secure in your own inner purpose and direction. The lines of your anchor let you rise and fall with the changes and demands as needed, without leaving your safe harbor until you are ready. Self-writing is one of the ways you can achieve self-knowledge and self-support that provides the anchor. Experiment with each of these four different writing formats to see if any are useful in increasing your self-awareness.

FORMATS FOR SELF-WRITING

Self-Notes: "To Do" and Other Reminders

Often when you want to remember something important, you jot it down. Nurses are great list keepers. We have to be, we are always trying to do so many things at one time. One way we manage to keep everything straight is to write ourselves little reminders.

Have you ever caught yourself running around with many little scraps of paper, shuffling through them in an attempt to organize information or messages to yourself? Sometimes rather than making our lives simpler and less stressful, the way we keep lists makes us more confused and pressured. Once you make organized self-reminder notes, you can forget a task until it is time to do it, rather than being uptight about the many things you have to do. Most people who are able to accomplish a great deal in a day without feeling pressured use some type of self-reminder system; this helps them to compartmentalize the many aspects of their hectic activity schedules. When they are in the middle of doing one thing, they do not need to worry that they are neglecting something else. Ideally, some day we'll all have personal computers that do this organizing and reminding without our needing to pay much attention to such concerns. But until then, here are a few hints on how to use self-reminders to their best advantage.

Calendars In addition to reminding you what to do, a calendar can be helpful for recording information about how you spend your time and money (for tax records), names you want to remember, or information to be included when you update your curriculum vitae or resumé. I use my personal calendar the way many people use a diary to record the external events of their lives. I also use it for self-notes—to remember to take in drycleaning, make phone calls, arrange health checkups, and so on. That way I not only know when something is due, I also need not worry about forgetting something important or cluttering my mind with a million details.

Personal Feedback Systems Self-notes can also become a part of a personal feedback process. Use them daily to check off what you have accomplished toward meeting your personal goals. But be aware of the endless list syndrome. Most of us write a list and keep adding to it. We begin the day with 20 things that need to be done, and at the end of the day 20 things still need to be done. You forget the fact that you've already accomplished 20 tasks; there are still 20 more unfinished, high-pressure demands that require your attention. The result of these endless lists is a constant, nagging sense of pressure—"There are so many things I need to do"—without the feeling of accomplishment. Instead of an endless list, write a daily list on which you can cross off each task as you do it. At the end of the day you should have an empty list. You'll be able to appreciate all that you have done because it's down in black and white. You'll also avoid the need to beat yourself for all those unfinished tasks you should do. Making endless lists is an easy trap that can put a hole in your emotional piggy bank.

To improve your awareness of how much you actually do accomplish in a week and how complex your life may be, try saving these daily "to do" lists for a few weeks. Examine a two-week collection. Do these lists alter your view of your life?

Many of us are totally unaware of how demanding our lives are. When you look over your list, do you see anything you are doing that can be omitted or simplified? For example, do you go to the grocery store three times a week? Do you drive all over town on different days but in the same general direction? You can save gas and travel time by coordinating these trips. Are there things you do that someone else in your family or circle of friends can help you with? For example, do you pick up your children every day from the same school attended by other neighborhood children? Could you share this chore with other mothers? Or do you cook a dinner from scratch every day? Can you reduce your cooking to only three or four days a week by cooking a quantity of food and freezing it or by making meals for two or three days at once? *Anything* you can do to simplify your life and coordinate your demands and tasks will reduce needless distress. Until you start to explore what you do with your time, you will never be able to identify how to make the best use of it.

Be creative. Your time is valuable. Can you turn an unpleasant chore into an enjoyable experience? Part of a stress-management approach to life is trying to turn boring, tedious chores that cannot be avoided into enjoyable, less stressful events. Or can you avoid stressful chores altogether? The more you know about how you spend your time, the better you will be able to make choices about your time expenditures. Writing down and re-evaluating what you do offers you the opportunity to make such an assessment.

Self-notes as Change Agents   For years, nurses have been doing all sorts of ridiculous tasks that have little to do with nursing. Until we start to write down what we do and how long it takes us, we are not going to have the needed documentation to convince others of a need for change. I question the rationale for having a nurse order stock supplies, transport patients, prepare or serve meals, fetch equipment, or organize paper supplies. What are some of the tasks you do that have nothing to do with nursing care?

I am sure you have heard the adage, "The pen is mightier than the sword." It would be helpful for you to record how much time is spent in these tasks; multiply it by the hourly wage of the average nurse in your institution and present the data to administration. How do they feel about spending so much money for these tasks? Nurses need to realize that the business community of which hospital administrators are a part is accustomed to having ample data presented to support the need for a change. We in nursing all too frequently rely on the good will of others to understand our felt needs without providing the documentation necessary to make the need for change apparent. Frequently, a problem described in terms of its cost to the organization will be recognized more clearly than one described from the standpoint of professional standards or principles of patient care. Money is more persuasive than feelings and concerns.

Writing down self-notes whenever a problem bothers you at work gives you the chance to identify the patterns involved; it also provides the documentation you'll need to support your belief. You will find that you receive a very different response from administration when you document problems. If, for example, you are chronically short staffed, going to your supervisor and stating, "We are always short-staffed," will probably not have as much impact as going to her to talk about the staffing problem—supported by documentation of the number of staff on each day over the last month, the number of patients, and the type of patient care required. This type of documentation is hard to ignore or sweep under the carpet. If you want to make changes in your system to decrease your job stress, do your homework: document the problem over time.

I have also found that noting, or threatening to note, unsatisfactory physician responses in the patient chart is a great way to force the physician to respond more appropriately. "Dr. Jones, I feel it's important for you to see Mrs. Smith due to the changes I've just described. Since you don't feel it is necessary to do anything in light of this, I'll simply note my observations in the chart, indicating that I discussed the problem with you and requested that you evaluate it further. I will also note you felt this was unnecessary." Dr. Jones usually rethinks his or her decision if for no other reason than fear of possible litigation. One physician told me he felt I was blackmailing him by stating I'd write his response in the chart. If clear documentation of nursing observation and judgment is blackmail, then he was being blackmailed. Our primary concern is for good patient care, not protecting uninterested or incompetent physicians.

Emotional Letters: "Letting Go"

Another value in writing is that it enables you to let go of unpleasant feelings. Writing an emotional letter that will never get mailed is a much safer form of emotional catharsis than letting out all your feelings in public. When you write down all your feelings—really "spit it all out" onto paper—you can release the built-up emotional tension. You may have experienced something similar in writing a consumer complaint letter about a defective product that made you furious. Sometimes when you start writing such a letter, you feel like stating that the company is horrible, that none of its products are any good, that the personnel are incompetent, and on and on and on. You may generate several pages of angry accusations as you begin to unwind. Throughout this process your anger decreases as you release the frustration you are feeling. You may still be upset about the defective product and continue to demand satisfaction, but you become a little more rational in how you plan to go about getting it.

You can get the same kind of emotional release by writing sad letters that need not be mailed. Such letters can allow you to release tension and may provide a sense of closure to partings. Writing a good-bye letter to a loved one who has just died or separated from you can provide a means of letting go of the pain you feel and repossessing the parts of your relationship that are cherished. Many meaningful relationships end without closure, for example, with sudden death or unexpected departures. The person who remains is left with strong, unresolved feelings that need an outlet. Writing a letter to the loved one can help release the emotions while clarifying the meaning of the relationship.

Whenever our emotions become overwhelmingly strong, they can paralyze us unless we can slowly release some of the pressure. Once you let go of the emotion and are no longer paralyzed, you can begin to decide what else you want to do about the situation. Then you can begin to engage in problem-solving.

Journals

Personal journal writing is one of the best ways to increase your self-awareness; to learn to listen to your thoughts, images, and emotions; and to pay attention to the processes and patterns of your external realities (Miller, 1975). The process of writing one's dreams—daydreams as well as dreams during sleep—helps the writer understand the unconscious motivations and dynamics of his or her behavior; in addition, it helps to identify the relationships between seemingly unrelated emotional events. Unlike a diary, in which the writer records events in a chronologic sequence, journal entries focus on internal dialogue and personal responses to life without respect to time. For example, an entry in your journal may focus on images of your self. The images may come from the past, present, or future but all be related to the various ways in which you perceive yourself. Using a journal can become a lifelong self-development process that allows you to understand your internal themes more deeply.

Ira Progoff (1980) has developed the *Intensive Journal* method by creating structured exercises that focus on interrelated aspects of life in the process of seeking self-wisdom.

> Context and continuity are two basic aspects of the work that the *Intensive Journal* structure makes possible, enabling us to draw our lives into focus at a given moment in the midst of the pressures of a crisis so that we can resolve the immediate issues. . . . In addition to providing perspective, [the *Intensive Journal*] acts as a self-adjusting compass, seeking the 'true-North,' the special meaning and direction of each individual's life (Progoff, 1980, p. 17).

Two of his books, *At a Journal Workshop* and *The Practice of Process Meditation*, provide all the necessary information on how to set up and use your own *Intensive Journal* workbook. *Intensive Journal* workshops are also offered throughout the United States. (See Resource Section for further information.)

The following is my summary of Progoff's beginning exercises, "The Period Log" and "Period Images" (Progoff, 1975). This summary is included to permit you to sample Progoff's approach to the use of the *Intensive Journal* method and to assess the potential of this tool for your further development of self-awareness.

For your thoughts and feelings to emerge, you must first become relaxed. Let go of your conscious monitoring of thoughts and events in your environment. One of the easiest ways to become deeply relaxed is by using the breathing exercise described in Chapter 17. Allow yourself ample time to complete this exercise without being hurried or distracted by other concerns.

As you begin to relax, let your mind float over recent events; ask yourself, "Where am I now in my life?" Do not attempt to think about events. Simply relax and let the feelings and thoughts emerge as they will. You do not need to evaluate or interpret the thoughts and feelings that emerge; just note them in a passive, open manner as you might watch leaves float by in a stream or clouds drift across the sky.

The "now" period may extend back for several months or years, or it may encompass only a few weeks. It includes whatever past events remain actively present in your life at this moment, as moving forces are considered a part of the now period.

Once a period of time begins to define itself, jot down brief descriptions of the feelings, images, or thoughts you have experienced as they relate to the following questions. (Do not judge or attempt to explain and clarify the meaning of your answers. There is no need for literary accuracy or even complete sentences. Just jot down your responses to these questions.)

1. When did this period begin? Was there any special event that started it or did I seem to enter it without being aware of it until later?
2. Who were the significant people involved with this period? What made them important to me?
3. Were there special events or interpersonal situations that occurred during this period?
4. What were my normal daily activities during this period?
5. Were there any persistent dreams or memories from this period?
6. What memories of loving and sharing are there in this period? What memories of anger and resentment are there?
7. Are there any spiritual or artistic experiences from this time?
8. What was my physical health like at this time? What was I feeling about my body?
9. Were there any people whom I admired, identified with, or tried to emulate?
10. What was my experience of the world around me and of my physical environment like during this period?

After you have answered the questions, begin again to enter a relaxed state, beginning to drift into a "twilight" level of consciousness where all conscious thoughts are suspended. Turn your attention inward to a deeper, more relaxed awareness of yourself. Begin to experience the period you have just described as a whole. Images will begin to emerge as you focus only on the feeling quality of the period. Assume a passive, meditative position of simply noticing but not evaluating the images that form. You cannot force images to appear by conscious choice; rather they are unconscious creations of your brain's right hemisphere. The more you allow yourself to experience the feelings of this period, the more likely it is that images, impressions, and symbols will begin to surface on their own. Record these inward perceptions as they come.

Begin to compare your period memories of outer events with your period images of your inner life. Are the two similar or opposite? As Progoff asks, "Does the information that comes to us from our nonconscious depth confirm the opinion we have in our consciousness?" Refrain from analyzing the two awarenesses; again, simply experience them in an undirected fashion. The two pictures of the period create your whole of this time that recombine on their own. Avoid the temptation of looking for quick interpretations of the information you have gained. Appreciate your awareness. "The two memories and images run parallel to one another, each reflecting the other. . . . The imagery gives us an additional awareness, an interior perspective by which we can recognize the integrative principle that is present beneath the surface of our lives and is the connective thread of our existence" (Progoff, 1975).

Dialogue Writing

You can carry on a dialogue with almost anything, People, parts of yourself, feelings, or objects can become part of a dialogue, and it doesn't matter if the person or thing with whom you are conversing is even present.

All of us talk to ourselves constantly about all sorts of things. We rehearse what we are going to say in important situations. We imagine what others will say and how we shall respond to their behavior. We talk to ourselves about how we are performing. In fact, we are talking with ourselves all of the time. Most frequently, these dialogues occur outside of our level of awareness. How this type of self-talk can influence your emotional state and general sense of well-being is discussed further in Chapter 12. By writing down these dialogues with ourselves, we can make the conversations conscious and purposeful. The process of writing out our dialogue can help to resolve problems, integrate various aspects of the personality, and provide new perspectives. You can also write imagined dialogues between yourself and other people that help you to understand the other person's point of view and possibly clarify your relationship with that person.

Gestalt therapy uses the verbal dialogue process to help integrate disowned aspects of the client's personality or past. Instead of talking about how someone or something makes you feel, you talk with that person or thing. You reenact the conversation in the here and now. This type of direct communication forces you to take responsibility for your feelings and decreases gossiping. Such a dialogue is a safe experiment that allows you to explore various responses to see how they fit.

Dialogues with Another Person   When you are writing imagined dialogues with another person, you avoid the trap of not listening to the other person. Often in actual interactions you are not relating to the other person at all. Imagined dialogues provide a special type of relating. You are making contact with others by actively listening to and understanding their points of view. To really listen to others, you must quiet your own thoughts— clear your mind sufficiently to hear what they are saying. This is hard to do if you are worried about what you will say in response to their statements or when you are experiencing unpleasant emotions as a result of the interaction. The following steps will help you imagine a dialogue with another person:

1. Think to yourself: Is there someone at my job toward whom I am having a lot of feelings? What do I imagine I'd like to say to him or her? Close your eyes and try to experience as vividly as possible the setting where this conversation will take place. Imagine what you'd like to say until it seems so real that you can almost hear yourself talking.
2. Open your eyes and, on a piece of paper, write down what you'd like to tell the other person.
3. Close your eyes again and begin to imagine the other person until his or her image is clear. Try to feel what it would be like to be that person. Wonder about how he or she would experience your remarks. Wonder about that person's needs, values, or motives until you can appreciate his or her reference point.
4. Open your eyes. On a separate sheet of paper write down the other person's responses to your statements.

By writing down real or imagined dialogues with other people, you can unhook yourself from many stressful interpersonal problems. One of my former clients provides an example of this. The client, a nurse, was having difficulty working with her supervisor. The problems had become so unbearable for my client that she was having repeated tension headaches. The client believed that her nursing supervisor was unfeeling, rigid, and authoritarian. I asked the client to write down, over the next week, what she imagined the supervisor would say in response to the client's raising her specific work concerns. At our next session the client described having difficulty writing the supervisor's response. No matter how hard she tried, she kept rejecting all the cold and insensitive replies she'd imagined the supervisor might offer because they seemed unrealistic. She also described being unable to see herself in a totally blameless, untarnished position. She began to realize that most of her concerns had never been discussed with the supervisor because she had arbitrarily decided the supervisor would respond negatively.

This exercise helped the client become more aware of her own behavior; in addition, it made the supervisor a more complete person in the eyes of my client. As a result of the exercise, the client sought out real communication with the supervisor. She never ended up liking the supervisor, but she did establish an open line of communication that allowed them to work together despite their differences.

Dialogues with Parts of Yourself   There are many facets to all of us. We may experience ourselves as strong in one situation and weak in the next. We may feel very open toward and accepting of other people most of the time, and yet we may have an absolute blind spot with respect to some group of people toward whom we are prejudiced.

As with dialogues with other people, you can write dialogues with these different parts of yourself. Again, try to imagine these aspects of yourself as clearly as possible until they become distinct subpersonalities. Then write down a conversation between them. As you are writing each position try to experience it as vividly as possible.

All of us have a number of opposing but coexisting parts to ourselves. The more familiar we can become with these, the more we can integrate the polarities of our lives and appreciate ourselves more completely.

CONCLUSION

As nurses, we are constantly rushing around attending to everyone else's problems and needs to the point that we may become anesthetized to ourselves. Ideally, we should be the experts about ourselves. Unfortunately, the opposite may be true for some of us; we may know least about ourselves. Writing gives us the opportunity to get in touch with ourselves and to notice the patterns of our lives.

REFERENCES

Miller, S. U. 1975. Keeping a psychological journal. *Psychosynthesis Workbook* 1(2).

Progoff, I. 1975. *At a journal workshop: the basic text and guide for using the intensive journal process.* New York: Dialogue House Library.

Progoff, I. 1980. *The practice of process meditation: the intensive journal way to spiritual experience.* New York: Dialogue House Library.

4

Thinking Your Way Out of Distress

Much distress is self-generated—a product of how we perceive stressors and how we talk to ourselves. Our experience of distress is not so much a direct result of external stressors as it is how we interpret these stressors. Our perceptions and self-talk create our reality. Our minds can think us into distress or can provide us with a way out of distress and into a sense of well-being.

The critical variable in experiencing distress and in our ability to control the stress response is our perception—of the stressors and our ability to influence these stressors. At times, what we perceive as most stressful in a job are givens—realities of everyday life that are not going to readily change. All too frequently we allow these givens to have powerful control over our lives by feeling powerless when we cannot change them. Many of the nursing stressors mentioned in Chapter 2 are unpleasant givens. Learning to accept these givens need not imply a hopeless resignation to job stressors. Accepting the givens involves a conscious decision to maintain self-control by determining what issues are worth our energy and attention.

Since perception is the critical variable in determining which stressors cause distress, it is important to become aware of and to control our self-talk, which influences our perceptions. The automatic, constant self-talk usually occurs outside our level of awareness; this can frequently lead to unpleasant emotional consequences and self-defeating pessimism. Using cognitive therapy we can become aware of our self-talk; then we can begin to use it constructively for stress management.

In this section, we shall explore the relationship between perception and distress; in addition, we shall identify ways to alter our negative, stressful perceptions so that we can begin to gain control over and enhance our sense of well-being.

CHAPTER 11

Perceptions: Believing Is Seeing

EMILY E. M. SMYTHE

WHAT ARE PERCEPTIONS?

For demonstration purposes, pretend for a moment that on a certain day two nurses, Meghan and Heather, both cared for the same patients at the same time; hence, both had identical interactions. As you read each person's description of the day, remember that they both saw and did exactly the same things during their time at work.

Meghan: Hopefully, I'll *never* have another day like this one! It was unbelievable. I'm just exhausted. First off, there was that damn Mrs. Smith with all her demands! Call light on constantly, asking one question after another. . . . Then Dr. Black came along and changed nearly every order on each of his patients. Took me half the day just to sign off the orders, let alone trying to carry them out. He's impossible! No matter how hard you knock yourself out, he'll manage to find something to scream about. To top it off, remember I told you about Brenda, the new head nurse? Well she's absolutely incompetent! She kept asking me questions about how to do things, where things were kept. She's more trouble than having ten student nurses on the floor pestering you!

Heather: Really wasn't a bad day today. Lots of interesting patients. I felt so good about doing the pre-op teaching with Mrs. Smith. She really was frightened about the surgery; she had a lot of questions to ask. I think the chat helped prepare her and allay some of her anxiety. . . . Dr. Black is certainly conscientious! He always carefully reviews each patient's chart on morning rounds. If I ever get sick, I hope I have a doctor who's as thorough as he is. Unfortunately, we couldn't get all the supplies on the floor by the time he was ready for the dressing change. So he got understandably upset since he was due in surgery. . . . You know, I think Brenda, the new head nurse, is going to work out well. She spent the morning trying to familiarize herself with the floor, asking all the staff for their input about how the unit ought to be. . . .

Their accounts are as different as night and day. It's impossible to believe that they are describing the same situations. Yet they both were subjected to the same experience and potential stressors. Meghan left work angry and exhausted, feeling everyone she had encountered had been totally unreasonable. Heather, on the other hand, seemed very satisfied with her productive day and pleased with how she performed as a nurse. She saw her interactions with others as positive. The disparity between their descriptions of the day is amazing. So what accounts for this difference? Their *perceptions* of what was happening to them affected their appraisals of the day, how they behaved, and the amount of stress each subsequently experienced. It is clear that if Meghan continues to perceive her work in such a negative fashion, she will end up hating her job, feeling put upon and overstressed and probably wanting to flee the nursing profession. After all, who would want to go through weeks of misery like what she described in her day?

What *really* happened during this shift? Which nurse is telling the truth?

Interestingly enough, each nurse is accurately describing *her view* of the same situation, based on her perceptions of the events. There is no one truth. Each view of "reality" is correct, that is, from each nurse's perspective. You might be thinking to yourself, "Now wait a moment. There must be a more objective view of the events. Look at it in behavioral terms. How many times did Mrs. Smith put on the call light? How many orders did Dr. Black write? How many questions did Brenda, the head nurse, ask? That is the objective reality!''

Not exactly. Both nurses were in the same external situation; however, how each experienced the situation, based on her cognitive appraisal of the stimuli from the day, ultimately created each nurse's subjective reality.

WHAT AFFECTS OUR PERCEPTIONS?

Most of us maintain that there is only one reality—the reality we see, hear, touch, smell, or taste. This reality is based on our sensing external stimuli. These sensations are absolute and definite as far as we are concerned. After all, we reason, we've been taught that two things cannot occupy the same space at the same time. Therefore, there must be only one reality. If you can't believe what you see with your own eyes, then what can you trust?

But then how are we going to account for the fact that two honest witnesses in a murder trial vehemently swear that they both saw exactly the same event in completely opposite ways? Or how can it be that you experience telling a doctor or co-worker something that they later swear you never mentioned? Is someone lying? Maybe, reality isn't *reality!* Could whatever happens change depending upon whose eyes (or other sensory organs) perceive it? Is it all in the eyes of the beholder?

Selective Attention

To some degree reality is something different for each of us. In fact, we all create our own reality from the vast array of available stimuli that bombard us constantly. Partially due to our anatomic limitations, we are aware of only a portion of the physical phenomena around us. For example, we cannot simultaneously watch three cardiac monitors, nor listen to a nurse talk about a patient while we receive telephone orders from a physician. What we see or hear is a limited version of objective reality that is based on that portion of the events around us that our sensing organs perceive.

In addition, we are not passive targets bombarded by environmental cues. We continually structure the stimuli around us by selectively attending to input; our selectiveness is based, in part, upon our needs at any given moment. For example, you've probably driven to work on the same route each day and not noticed every gas station along the way. However, if one day you notice that you are low on gas, you suddenly see gas stations you had never noticed before. When we chart nursing notes, for instance, we hope we can block out all the noise around us and focus only on the task at hand. At times, however, our focus is more on personal need than on the task at hand. The need may be so pressing that it interferes with our current professional task. Have you ever been extremely hungry and at the same time tried to concentrate on the task at hand? Chances are good that your need for food continually interfered with your ability to concentrate, thus causing you stress.

We also impose order on the world around us as a means of reducing the overwhelming amount of stimuli impinging upon us. We would literally go crazy if we attended to everything around us. Instead we protect ourselves through selective attention. This helps to prevent sensory overload. Have you ever noticed, for example, that when you are performing a task, such as administering a medication, you don't think through—or attend to—every step of the process? Most of the process of giving a medication is automatic and habitual. (Hopefully you are aware of getting the correct drug and you focus your attention on giving it to the right patient!) Once we are proficient with procedures, we no longer need to be aware of each step of the process. It would be exhausting if every time we tied a shoelace we had to think about each part of the process. The habituation allows us to tune out mastered skills and perform them by rote.

The process of selective attention can have detrimental effects, as in the process of stereotyping. *Stereotyping* is, among other things, a way of selecting which data will receive one's attention. When certain characteristics suggest that a person fits a familiar category, we overlook his or her other traits and immediately attribute a behavior pattern to that person. Meghan, in the above vignette, saw any patient who had many questions as being a "difficult patient." Difficult patients are demanding, impatient, self-centered, intentionally irritating to the nursing staff, and so on. At times, we may group together *all* elderly patients: they're senile, grouchy, uncooperative, and most likely to make ridiculous requests. Medical and nursing students are always "the same." I've exaggerated these typical prejudicial views to point out how, once stereotyping occurs, we attribute many qualities to others with whom we interact; in cases such as these we make our interactions far more stressful than they need to be.

Also as a result of stereotyped views that alter our perception of events, we may ignore or misread subtle changes in our patients. I recall occasions when, because of a patient's unexpected emotional response to an illness, the doctor suspected mental illness and requested a psychiatric consultation. Idiosyncratic responses to medications may be misread or overlooked because, again, we don't expect the reaction; and thus we do not pay attention to the patient's response. Medical complaints of psychiatric patients are frequently ignored because we have labeled the patient as "crazy"; we then believe that all this patient's concerns are phobias or somatic delusions. This process of ignoring information also occurs in medical situations when a patient is labeled as a chronic complainer; following that, we no longer listen to his or her concerns (even if some of the complaints are real).

The process of selective attention can help us pay attention to relevant stimuli, or it can hinder us by causing us to ignore relevant stimuli. Obviously, then, it is important for us to become more aware of when we are selectively attending to environmental input; whenever possible we must make this process a conscious choice rather than an incomplete focus on reality.

Attitudes Toward Life

Our general attitudes toward life also significantly affect what we perceive. Two people can look at the same glass of water. To one person it is half full; to the other it is half empty. Their views are based upon their different attitudes toward life—optimism or pessimism. We've all heard someone described as having "a chip on his shoulder." Like the pessimist, this person tends to see everything that happens in a negative light. As a result, this individual experiences much more stress and tension than is tolerable. Nurses with negative attitudes toward their jobs or the nursing profession will tend to see each patient's request as an unreasonable demand, and experience an undue level of job stress as a result. Our past experiences and the attitudes we develop as a result of these experiences become like tinted glasses that darken all that we perceive.

On the other hand, I would not suggest that we put on rose-colored glasses that blind us to existing problems within nursing! Becoming a Pollyanna, by ignoring all personal awareness, needs, and beliefs, will do little to advance the profession. Being blindly optimistic and living in a fantasy world will be no more adaptive than walking around with a chip on your shoulder. Neither attitude allows you to perceive your work in a realistic manner. If you have a positive attitude, however, you can maintain some degree of optimism while squarely facing problems. A positive attitude also protects you from stress by helping you avoid personalizing situations and perceiving events as an unending succession of tragedies. Most of us are familiar with "terminal" patients who undergo miraculous cures or patients who are able to overcome incredible physical obstacles. One of the main ingredients in such success is always a positive mental attitude. Much recent work being done with cancer patients employs visualization techniques to utilize the mind's creative powers for developing positive and optimistic attitudes toward recovery (Simonton et al., 1978). (See Chapter 18, "Creative Imagination.")

Your general attitude toward life has been developed and reinforced throughout your entire lifetime. It takes a great deal of energy to alter it. Yet many of us could learn to "destress" ourselves, our profession, and our work by changing our attitudes. Perhaps you find yourself now saying, "So what's the point? If my attitude is that ingrained, it'll never change!" If so, you are seeing an example of your pessimism in action. This negative, de-featist attitude will certainly be an obstacle on your road toward learning how to change and manage your stress!

Anxiety Level

As you probably remember from your early nursing education, one's anxiety level directly affects one's ability to perceive external events. Peplau (1963) showed that perceptual capabilities are one of the main in-dicators of a client's anxiety level.

In first-level anxiety (+), we have a heightened sense of awareness. We feel more alert, more able to recognize relationships between events and to utilize a problem-solving approach. This level is usually subjectively as-sociated with a positive "high" such as what we experience when we are competing in sports or making love. With the second level of anxiety (++), however, our perceptual field narrows, and we pay attention only to the details of our immediate concerns. In third-level anxiety (+++), our perceptual field is drastically reduced to the point of acknowledging only scattered details or even a single detail. We become unaware of stim-uli in the environment and are virtually unable to utilize our problem-solv-ing skills. Of course, with the fourth level of anxiety (++++), or panic state, we are unable to perceive what is happening around us. We cannot hear or see the environmental stimuli because our anxiety level virtually blanks out our perceptual abilities. Whenever our anxiety increases above our tolerance, reality is distorted because we spend our energy and atten-tion in defending ourselves. We are unable to learn or use problem-solving skills and thus cannot grow from the experience.

We are all familiar with patients who say that they know the doctor ex-plained what he was going to do but that once he said the word surgery they couldn't hear anything else. Their anxiety interfered with their per-ception. Or try to remember times when you were very anxious about tak-ing an exam; even though the teacher told you how to complete the exam and the directions were clearly printed on the text booklet, your anxiety level completely deafened and blinded you. When anxiety climbs suffi-ciently high, what we are probably most aware of is feeling confused—as if we were in a daze.

It is my belief that one of the main factors that makes nursing so difficult and causes so many problems in our interpersonal relationships with pa-tients and co-workers is that we are continuously dealing with others who are anxious or we, ourselves, are experiencing unmanageable anxiety. Whenever you interact with others in an anxiety state, the dice are loaded against you. The chances are very good that reality will be distorted; peo-ple will come from a defensive position that significantly decreases the probability that they can accurately perceive what is happening. Anxiety, like selective attention and attitude, can be controlled. Numerous tech-niques for managing anxiety are discussed in Chapters 16, 17, and 18.

HOW PERCEPTIONS AFFECT OUR STRESS LEVEL

Believing is seeing. Based on our perceptions, reality is literally whatever we make it. "What we perceive depends on what is there, what we have been told is there and also on our needs and projections of the moment. Generally speaking, the salient figure in our field of perception is always related to our immediate needs and goals. When we perceive . . . we always give it meaning" (Jourard, 1974). Of course, there is an objective world from which we all create our own subjective worlds. But the two realities are not necessarily the same. As Fritz Perls stated, "The reality which matters is the reality of interests—the internal reality and not the external reality" (Perls, 1969). We have a choice in how we wish to perceive our world.

"Stress is not necessarily caused by stressor agents; rather, it is caused by the way stressor agents are perceived, interpreted or appraised in each individual case" (Roskies and Lazarus, in press). If when given a potential stressor you evaluate it as a positive event, you will experience what Selye calls eustress, or good stress. Your positive perception of the event will cause you to feel pleasantly excited with a heightened sense of awareness, increased performance capabilities, and an increased energy level. If, however, you perceive the same potential stressor as threatening, you will experience distress, which depletes your adaptive energy, focuses your attention on defensive strategies, and precludes the opportunity for learning or growing from the situation (Selye, 1975). Reaction to stress depends on the eye of the beholder.

VARIABLES THAT INFLUENCE OUR PERCEPTION OF STRESSORS

Personal Control

There are, of course, certain variables that affect how most people perceive events as distressful. Personal control is one. You may have noticed that the more control you have over a situation the less you experience the situation as stressful (Lazarus, 1971). For example, suppose you have a job in which you can control the number of admissions to your unit. At a critical point you can give significant input that leads to closing admissions. You would feel much more like an active participant, rather than a helpless victim. The more direct control we feel that we have in deciding policies, procedures, and patient care issues, the more we feel a shared responsibility and motivation; rather than viewing our work as filled with potential causes of distress we see it as filled with manageable challenges. As another example, consider the difference between choosing to work a double shift because you need the money and being forced to work a double shift because of staff shortage. You probably will not feel as distressed in the first case as the second.

"Feeling helpless and feeling a lack of sufficient power to change one's environment may be a fundamental cause of distress. . . . Anything that adds to the feeling of self-control is likely to reduce the severity of the stress reaction" (Girdona and George, 1979). In nursing, one of the major stressors is that nurses frequently have little or no voice in decisions that directly affect their work. Thus our perceptions of stressful stimuli are heightened.

Familiarity and Predictability

Think, for a moment, of all the environmental stimuli—pollution, some would call it—present in your work. The constant traffic of personnel, visitors, and patients, obnoxious odors, sounds of various monitoring equipment, call buzzers, and voice paging systems are only a few of these stressors. For the most part, you are probably somewhat oblivious to all these potential stressors because they are predictable occurrences in your daily work setting. If, however, you were suddenly switched to a new work environment and faced with different environmental stressors, you would probably experience many of the same environmental stressors—odors, traffic, and noise—as jarringly unfamiliar and stressful. Our brain activity is able to habituate itself to expected stressors in our work environment. Once this habituation has occurred, these environmental stressors are only perceived as distressing if they are stopped or if the rate of the stressors is changed (Blattner, 1981).

You may even have experienced this effect on perception when you began your present job. You felt exhausted after a day of orientation that wasn't all that demanding. You paid a high price in energy because each stimulus was unfamiliar and therefore required your attention. Now that you are accustomed to these environmental stressors you probably don't even notice them. However, when you return from a vacation you may be struck by how busy and noisy your unit is.

Familiarity and predictability, then, tend to neutralize these potential environmental disturbances so that you do not experience them as distressing. It is important to realize, however, that even though you are not consciously aware of these familiar environmental stressors, your body is continually having to adjust to them.

Social Supports

The old saying "misery loves company" refers to the need we all have to pass along our burdens to supportive associates, particularly those who share our experiences. Numerous studies indicate that social support affects our perceptions. In *Work Stress And Social Support*, House (1981) cites research indicating that "social support can buffer the effects of work stress on health but has primarily main effects on perceived stress." The role of social support in decreasing stress and ways to begin developing and maintaining adequate interpersonal support are discussed in depth in Chapter 15, "Developing Social Support: We're All In This Together."

Past Experiences

Our present view of the world is directly related to our past history and the values and assumptions we have developed as a result of these previous experiences. All of our perceptions are based on cognitive processes learned through experiences. It is precisely because our perceptions are learned that we can alter them through additional, corrective education.

Past experiences do not *cause* us to behave in a certain way, nor do they force us to perceive events as distressful. They simply *influence* our present perceptions of the here and now. Too often, as a mental health consultant, I encounter nurses who feel destined to failure and distress as a result of previous negative experiences. They feel helpless to deal with current work stress because in the past they have been unsuccessful; now with damaged self-esteems, they are unable even to imagine themselves as successful in making a change. "It obviously makes a difference whether we consider ourselves as pawns in a game whose rules we call reality or as players of the game who know that the rules are 'real' only to the extent that we have created or accepted them, and that we can change them" (Watzlawick, 1978).

A buildup of past major life changes does not result in subsequent illness, although the Holmes and Rahe measurement of recent life change units (discussed in Chapter 8) has frequently been misused as "proof" that it does. What must be kept in mind in using this assessment scale or any other psychosocial stress scale is that the average person is more vulnerable to illness given certain stressors, but the likelihood of illness is directly influenced by a number of factors, including how the individual perceives changes, the amount of ongoing social support, previous experience with similar stressors, personality style, and the current health status of the individual (Grout, 1980).

"REFRAMING" AS A WAY TO DECREASE OUR STRESSFUL PERCEPTIONS

Seeing the Opportunity

An old Buddhist teaching maintains that one-third of human suffering is inevitable, but the rest we create ourselves. In many nursing situations we cannot change the external realities—those awful "givens," the unpleasant realities of people and things—that exist (see Chapter 13, "Recognizing the 'Givens': Accepting What Can't Be Changed"). There will always be, for example, difficult and ungrateful patients, patients suffering and dying, interpersonal conflicts, insufficient time to accomplish needed tasks, and many, *many* other potential sources of stress in nursing. We can choose, however, to change how we view these stressors. We can alter the signifi- cance we place upon these external events and thus change the degree to which we experience them as stressful. We can also decide to be self-nur- turing rather than self-doubting or self-punishing and thus eliminate self- imposed stressors. Our work satisfaction is based less on being confronted by these givens and more on how we perceive and ultimately cope with them (Grout, 1980).

Stress isn't reality. Stress is how your mind reacts to objective reality based upon your perceptions. The critical variable in whether a situation will be experienced as distressing or enhancing is our perception of the external and internal realities (Selye, 1979). The Chinese word for crisis is made up of the characters for the words danger and opportunity. We can choose to feel threatened or excited whenever there is a change in our job or when demands are placed upon our adaptive energy. We can force our- selves to examine where the growth and opportunity in a new situation might be; or we can choose selectively to focus on the negative aspects. The choice is ours.

Questions to Ask Yourself

As you answer these questions, try to determine how your responses affect your perceptions of your job and the people with whom you work.

1. When there is a change in your work environment, do you see it as a challenge or a crisis?
2. When someone asks you a favor at work, do you automatically see it as a stressful demand or as a request to which you can choose to re- spond?
3. In your work environment, are there events that regularly upset you despite the fact that they are predictable and you have no way of con- trolling them?
4. Do you notice a difference in how you perceive your job when you feel supported by your co-workers?
5. Thinking back over stressful events in your life, do you feel that you grew and learned from them or do you feel scared and frightened by them?
6. When you are involved in a conflict with a co-worker, are you able to listen openly to the other person's side or do you already have your mind made up about what he or she thinks, feels, or wants?
7. Are there particular groups or types of people toward whom you auto- matically have a negative response? (For example, do you believe that most doctors are self-centered or that most hospital adminis- trators aren't concerned with the quality of patient care?)

8. Are there certain co-workers you feel are *all* bad, with no redeeming qualities?
9. Are there particular types of patients with whom you automatically assume it will be impossible to work?
10. Would you describe yourself as generally positive/hopeful or negative/pessimistic about events that happen at work and in your life?

Altering Your Perception of Disaster

Are there times when you experience a crisis at work and feel that you simply can't take it any more and that something disastrous is about to happen? Here are a few questions you might want to ask yourself in order to reframe your perception of how important the event really is.

Which Hill to Die On?   Many stressful events happen daily in nursing. At times we may feel that each problem or stressor in our environment requires an all-out battle with someone or something. Unfortunately, we think that we must be knights in shining armor, attacking any and every evil in our path. If your goal is really to decrease your stress level and make significant contributions toward improving health care, you'd be better off deciding which hill to die on. What problems or issues are sufficiently important that you need to make an all-out attack? If you determine that your perception is that everything is a problem, you should begin to wonder if your all-out, do-or-die attitude is really helping you or exhausting you. On the other hand, choosing your battles and deciding what the most important issues are will allow you to disconnect from the less urgent while you first address the more relevant. Being selective about the issues we wish to address is necessary for accomplishing goals and for maintaining sanity. You may alter your perception of a stressor by deciding that the problem is important but, for the moment, will have to be placed on the back burner.

Time Perspective   Have you ever been in the middle of an argument and really felt you needed time to think it over? Yet somehow you felt you just couldn't say, "Well, I need some time to think about it. We don't seem to be able to reach an understanding now." Time is a wonderful healer. Today's crises are often tomorrow's boring history. One helpful way to get a clearer perspective on a problem is to step back by giving yourself time to think over the problems when you're less anxious and have adequate time.

For example, is the fact that Dr. Jones screamed at you really going to be a big issue in your life next week? Probably not. You may have some residual feelings about it, but it probably won't be so important that you want to quit your job. At the moment he screams at you and you experience the stress response, you might feel awful, as if you're going to quit on the spot. But stop at that moment and ask yourself, "By tomorrow, next week, or next month is this really going to be such a big deal?" If it is, then by all means give yourself enough time to decide how you want to solve the problem rather than losing control and giving your immediate response. If it isn't such an important concern, then you're probably going to wonder, "Why am I allowing this minor event to upset me so much?" Once you've altered your perspective on the situation, use one of the quick stress-reduction techniques discussed elsewhere in the book. Slow down when it is possible. People working under relentless time pressures do not perform at their best; in fact, they frequently make mistakes that have more disastrous effects than if they had taken a moment to think about what they're doing.

In nursing we frequently don't really *have* the necessary time available to sort out all the information and reach what seems like the best solution. But we also often don't *ask* for time. We make the assumption that any request is a demand for immediate action. For example, your supervisor asks you to work "a double." You probably feel on the spot to decide at that instant. Yes or no. You may need to give yourself a few moments to really think it over. What's so awful about saying, "I need to think about it *alone* for a few moments. Where can I reach you to tell you my answer?" Whenever possible, reduce the immediacy of decision-making.

I often wonder how many "emergencies" in our profession are really emergencies. Certainly there are medical emergencies, but not every medical problem is a matter of life and death.

What If?   When a crisis seems like the end of the world and you are positive you can't survive it, ask yourself, "So, what if _____ happened? What's the worst possible thing that could occur?" Frequently, we add to our perception of a stressful event by scaring ourselves with all sorts of imagined horrors; no one knows how to scare you better than you do! Now not only are you dealing with your reactions to the stressor but also your reactions to all the awful things you've imagined. By stopping this process of scaring yourself and asking, "What if _____ happened," you can make your fears conscious. Once your fears are conscious, you can then evaluate how real your perceptions are. If there's a chance that something bad might happen, you can do some problem-solving about the issue rather than sitting around immobilized. This technique of imagining the worst possible outcome of a situation is similar to the behavioral modification technique of implosion. Your immobilizing fear causes you to avoid the threatening situation; thus you have no opportunity to do reality testing. The avoidance produced by the fear actually contributes to maintaining your anxiety. By imagining a "full blast" of the fearful situation you will soon realize that, although it is neither pleasurable nor desirable, you do not suffer any disastrous consequences (Stampfl and Levis, 1968).

Desensitization   You have probably on occasion thought to yourself, "I'll never be able to cope. It scares me to death. I'll just have to avoid dealing with it." If there is a situation in your job that makes you feel this way, desensitization may be useful. You can learn how to alter your perception of the situation and increase your mastery of it.

Desensitization, a behavioral approach, is useful when you realize your fearful perceptions of a particular situation inhibit your behavior. These perceptions are, in part, based on anxiety responses that we previously learned to associate with the situation. One way to change our stressful perceptions is to dissociate the negative response from the situation. Desensitization is the dissociating process. It is based upon the concept that you cannot experience relaxation and anxiety simutaneously, the two states being incompatible.

You have learned to perceive events as stressful, in part, by associating the event, or stressor, with unfavorable outcomes or anxiety. Through the technique of desensitization, you substitute deep muscle relaxation for the anxiety response, thereby gradually decreasing your sensitivity toward the fearful event (Agras, 1978).

Although desensitization has been successfully used in the treatment of everything from phobias to sexual problems, the approach is most useful in treating specific fears that result in inappropriate avoidance behaviors. Examples in nursing would be fear of a patient dying or fear of working with a patient who may have a cardiopulmonary arrest.

This technique is not intended to change your attitudes or personality structure. Nor should you use it when anxiety is appropriate and when you need to eliminate the problem rather than eliminate its effects on you. For example, anxiety is appropriate when a unit is dangerously understaffed or when you are assigned to a specialty unit for which you have insufficient training or knowledge (Wolpe, 1973). You may also want to use desensitization in conjunction with assertiveness training (Chapter 16) or cognitive approaches (Chapter 12).

The following suggestions, based upon theoretical concepts of desensitization, have been adapted for use with stressful nursing situations—typical situations that your anxiety causes you to avoid.

1. Identify as specifically as possible what the fear or stressor is by asking yourself:
   ● What is the anxiety-evoking situation?
   ● How anxious does it make me feel?
   ● When does it occur?
   ● Where does it occur?
   ● With whom does it occur?
   Also, attempt to identify what meaning the fear has. For example, being afraid of working with a cancer patient may actually be a fear of working with any terminally ill patient or it may be a fear of working with patients suffering severe pain.

2. Make a detailed, step-by-step hierarchy of the anxiety-evoking situation; break down the fear into a sequence of concerns from the most to the least anxiety-evoking. Base the hierarchy on *your* personal concerns; do not base it on what you *think* you should fear or what you believe *other* people might feel.

As an example, if you have a fear of working with dying patients, your hierarchy of fears or concerns might be as follows:

Most Anxiety-Provoking

- I die.
- I'm blamed for the patient's death.
- My assigned patient dies while I'm working with him.
- I'm told that a patient I'm working with is not expected to live through my shift.
- I'm assigned to a patient in the terminal stage of cancer.
- My patient talks about dying.
- My patient says that he's afraid he might die.
- I'm told that a patient with whom I had worked has died at home.

Least Anxiety-Provoking

3. Meanwhile, begin practicing deep muscle relaxation as described in Chapter 17. Surprisingly, many people are anxious so much of the time that they have never enjoyed a truly relaxed state. Once you've experienced deep muscle relaxation—a parasympathetic, skeletal muscular, relaxation technique—you will readily recognize the difference between relaxation and anxiety. It is essential that you be able to make this discrimination.

4. Once you are able to experience deep muscle relaxation, return to your list of items. Begin to imagine the least anxiety-evoking concern on your hierarchy of fears. Try to visualize the fear in a scene as graphically and as realistically as you can. (If you have difficulty with imagery, see Chapter 18 for suggestions to improve this skill.) If at any time during your imaginary creation of the anxiety-evoking scene you begin to experience anxiety or tension, stop the imagery and again focus on the process of deep muscle relaxation. Once you are able to imagine the scene without becoming anxious, move on up the hierarchy to the next anxiety-evoking scene. It will probably take you at least one day for each scene. You may find yourself stuck on a particular scene; if several attempts at relaxation fail, stop the process and break the scene down into progressively less stressful experiences.

   For example, if a scene concerning talking with a dying patient about his fear of dying continually makes you anxious, you might create a hierarchy of related anxiety-producing scenes and practice relaxation techniques from easier to harder.
   - Talking with a supportive co-worker about how I feel when I'm assigned to a dying patient.
   - Talking with my peers about what dying patients may experience.
   - Talking with my patient's relatives about their concerns (one of which is the possible death of my patient).
   - Talking with my patient about his dying.

Another way to approach this step in desensitization is to place yourself in the feared, anxiety-evoking situation. Provide yourself with an in vivo experience as you go up each step of your hierarchy of fears. If you plan to do an in vivo experiment, be sure you have some control over the situation and can terminate the experiment whenever you become anxious. It is also helpful to have available a good support such as a trusted colleague who is aware of what you are doing and who can take over the task if you should become too anxious.

Whichever approach you choose, imagining or an in vivo experiment, be sure to go at your own pace; allow yourself as much time with each anxiety-evoking scene as you need. This process of desensitization occurs constantly in any learning situation; however, you probably are often unaware of it.

CONCLUSION

Distress is how your mind reacts to reality. Stressors in nursing are numerous, but whether you allow them to affect your sense of well-being and job satisfaction is up to you. The critical variable in experiencing distress and your ability to control your stress response is your *perception*—of the stressor itself and your ability to influence the stressor.

REFERENCES

Agras, W. S. 1978. *Behavior modification: principles and clinical applications.* Boston: Little, Brown and Co.

Blattner, B. 1981. *Holistic nursing.* Englewood Cliffs, N.J.: Prentice-Hall, Inc.

Girdona, P., and George, E. 1979. *Controlling stress and tension: a holistic approach.* Englewood Cliffs, N.J.: Prentice-Hall, Inc.

Grout, J. W. 1980. Stress and the I.C.U. nurse: a review of nursing studies. In *Living with stress and promoting well-being: a handbook for nurses,* editors K. E. Claus and J. T. Bailey. St. Louis: The C. V. Mosby Co.

House, J. S. 1981. *Work stress and social support.* Reading, Mass.: Addison-Wesley Pub. Co.

Jourard, S. M. 1974. *Healthy personality: an approach from the viewpoint of humanistic psychology.* New York: MacMillan Pub. Co.

Lazarus, R. S. 1971. The concepts of stress and distress. In *Society, stress and disease,* editor L. Levi. London: Oxford University Press.

McLean, A. A. 1979. *Work stress.* Reading, Mass.: Addison-Wesley Pub. Co.

Peplau, H. E. 1963. A working definition of anxiety. In *Some clinical approaches to psychiatric nursing,* editors S. F. Burd and M. A. Marshall. New York: MacMillan Pub. Co.

Perls, F. S. 1969. *Ego, hunger, and aggression.* New York: Vantage Books.

Roskies, E., and Lazarus, R. S. In press. Coping theory and the teaching of coping skills. In *Behavioral medicine: changing health life styles,* editor P. Davidson. New York: Brunner/Mazel.

Selye, H. 1975. *Stress without distress.* New York: Signet Books.

Selye, H. 1979. Self-regulation: the response to stress. In *Inner balance: the power of holistic healing,* editor E. M. Goldwag. Englewood Cliffs, N.J.: Prentice-Hall, Inc.

Simonton, O. C., Simonton, S. M., and Creighton, J. 1978. *Getting well again.* Los Angeles: J. P. Tarcher, Inc.

Stampfl, T. G., and Levis, D. J. 1968. Implosive therapy—a behavioral therapy? *Behav. Res. Ther.*

Watzlawick, P. 1978. *The language of change.* New York: Basic Books.

Wolpe, J. 1973. *The practice of behavioral therapy.* New York: Pergamon Press.

CHAPTER 12

Cognitive Approach to Stress Management

EMILY E. M. SMYTHE

THINKING AND DISTRESS

Despite what you have been told, talking to yourself is not a a sign of craziness. What you say to yourself may drive you crazy, but talking to yourself isn't a sure sign of insanity. The fact is that we all talk to ourselves *all* of the time. Unfortunately, a lot of our self-talk may be crazy talk in that it is illogical or irrational (Ellis and Harper, 1975).

We all have a basic need to create order out of our world and the events we experience. When we notice something, immediately our minds begin to evaluate the stimulus to determine its meaning. This process is occurring constantly. One reason you may not be aware of talking to yourself is that frequently this self-talk occurs as what Beck (1970) calls "automatic thoughts." Your internal dialogue occurs so rapidly that it seems almost like a reflex, out of your control. If you are aware of your self-talk, it probably just seems to appear without any conscious reasoning or intent. You may even say things like, "The idea just popped into my mind," or "I couldn't get rid of the idea that. . . ."

As we have seen, the critical variable in what you experience as stressful is your perception of the stressor. In experiencing distress your perception is related to your thoughts—what you tell yourself about the events that happen. Your experience of distress is produced not by the stressors themselves but by your thoughts about the stressors (Lazarus, 1966).

> The research on the role of cognitive variables in stress reactions indicates that how one responds to stress in large part is influenced by how he appraises the stressor, to what he attributes the arousal he feels and how he assesses his ability to cope (Meichenbaum, 1974).

Your thoughts alone can initiate the stress response in the absence of any external stressor. You can literally worry yourself sick by playing a "what if . . ." game. "What if I don't get all my patient care assignments done?" "What if I make a mistake and harm a patient?" "What if . . .?" This type of obsessive anticipatory self-talk can make you feel anxious and physically aroused although nothing even happened in the external environment. As much physiological arousal and body tension are produced by this type of negative self-talk as by any actual threat or external stressor (Rimm and Litvak, 1969).

Our thoughts also determine how we will evaluate physiologic arousal. For example, if you experience a racing heartbeat, sweaty palms, dry mouth, and "butterflies" in your stomach but you tell yourself these are "good" sensations because you are with someone you find interesting or physically attractive, you will not experience distress at all but will in fact call this experience wonderful and exciting. Schachter and Singer (1962) term this process of interpreting your physiologic arousal labeling. Your emotional reaction to any stimulus depends upon how you label your physiologic response.

Other researchers have found that your emotional response also depends on what you think your physical reaction is, regardless of what it actually is (Velten, 1968; Childress and Burns, 1981). If, for example, someone you trust tells you you seem angry and then substantiates his impression with objective information, such as your face is red or you are clenching your fists, you are apt to experience anger. In nursing situations you may experience emotions that are suggested by other people. Another nurse might tell you a certain situation is anxiety- or anger-provoking. "Boy, that must make you feel furious," she might say. Sure enough, you start to feel the anger build up whether or not you had previously experienced anger or had labeled yourself as angry. You may simply have been confused or frustrated before your colleague made the comment. (See Chapter 14, "Controlling Contagion: Disturbing the Stagnant Quo," for further discussion of this process.)

The stress response creates a negative feedback loop between your mind and body. What you tell yourself influences what you feel emotionally and physically. How you label your physiologic arousal influences your emotional response. The self-talk and labeling each escalate the pattern of arousal (McKay et al., 1981).

> In other words: people not only partly create (or conceptualize) the original "stressors" they experience, but they also bring about their over-reactions to these "stressors." Then to crown their self-imposed inequity, they damn themselves for damning themselves and thus immensely escalate their "stress." A vicious circle—or endless spiral, if you will—that seems to have no finish line! (Ellis, 1978).

ABCs of Distress

Albert Ellis, the founder of rational emotive therapy (a cognitive therapy), has described the ABCs of emotional responses: *A, a*ctivating event or stimulus, *B, b*elief and self-talk, and *C,* consequence and emotional response (anger, guilt, depression). With few exceptions the emotions we feel have little to do with the events or stressors we face but have everything to do with the things we tell ourselves about these events based upon our beliefs (Ellis, 1962). Most of us, however, believe the exact opposite to be true. We believe that events directly cause us to feel certain emotions. We make statements like, "I'm upset because Dr. Jones yelled at me." "Mr. Smith's death depressed me." "I feel so guilty because I should have known better." "Whenever I'm in situations like this I get anxious." What we are saying over and over again is that A (the stressor or activating event) causes C (the consequence or emotional response). But what actually causes the emotional responses of anger, depression, guilt and so on is what we say to ourselves about the events, that is, our belief about the event. B causes C. A does not cause C.

Let's see how different self-talk can produce different emotional consequences for the same activating event or stressor. Most of us may believe that when someone yells at us we become angry. Right? Well, possibly. Or we could end up feeling depressed, guilty, anxious, or anything else, depending entirely on what we say to ourselves about the yelling. Let's see how different self-talk can change the emotional consequence of being yelled at. For each example of self-talk on the next page, guess the consequence or emotional reaction.

These examples demonstrate that what you feel as an emotional consequence usually is directly related to what you tell yourself about the events. There are, of course, a few extreme exceptions to the principle that beliefs cause emotional consequences. For example, extended sleep deprivation, starvation, or prolonged extreme pain can cause fear or despair regardless of your beliefs (Ellis, 1973). Although we sometimes find

SELF-TALK: BELIEFS AND CONSEQUENCES

Example 1: Who the _____ does he think he is talking to me like that? I don't need this kind of abuse and I'm certainly not going to stand for it!

Consequence_____

Example 2: I can't handle this. I just don't know what to do now. I've got to say something. I can't just stand here looking like a fool.

Consequence_____

Example 3: I feel so bad. I should have known better. What an awful mistake. He certainly has a right to yell at me. It's all my fault.

Consequence_____

Example 4: It doesn't matter what I do. I can't seem to do anything right. I'm such a failure. I don't know why I even bother to try. How is anyone ever going to respect me when I'm so stupid?

Consequence_____

Answers: The most likely consequences are Example 1, *Anger;* Example 2, *Anxiety;* Example 3, *Guilt;* and Example 4, *Depression* or *Decreased Self-Worth* (now return to page 177).

it hard to admit, few, if any, of the job stressors in nursing fall into these extreme categories. Most nursing stressors, then, do not directly cause our distress or emotional responses. Obviously the stressors initiate the process and contribute to it, but they do not *cause* our distress; our beliefs do.

The idea that thoughts influence behavior and emotions is certainly not new. Greek, Roman, and Buddhist philosophers identified this principle centuries ago (Ellis, 1973). Plato described self-talk as an internal dialogue. Small children provide a good example of this internal dialoguing process when they talk out loud to themselves while playing. For example, my daughter will say things like "No, Meggie. Don't do that. Bad girl. . . . But I want it. Please. . . . No, Meggie, don't do it." Both of the conflicting positions she vocalizes are parts of her. She is instructing herself based on her internalized self-monitoring. The dialogue is between two "Meggies," who each want different things.

Self-Talk

If self-talk is so natural, why is it that many of us are unaware of how influential it is in producing the stress response? We are mainly unaware of our self-talk because it is so automatic and constant. Beck (1976) describes these automatic thoughts or self-talk:

> They are specific and discrete. They occur in a kind of short hand . . . as in a telegraphic style. Moreover these thoughts do not arise as a result of deliberation, reasoning or reflection about an event or topic. There is no logical sequence of steps such as in goal-oriented thinking or problem-solving. The thoughts "just happen" as if by reflex.

I am sure you are familiar with the experience of having a bad day at work, only to come home and have your mind go over and over the day's events much like a stuck record. It often feels impossible to shut off these ideas once they start. It might seem that the thoughts are controlling your mind rather than your mind controlling your thoughts.

Another familiar example of self-talk occurs when you anticipate something you expect to be difficult or stressful. All of a sudden your mind starts racing over the most disastrous images—you'll be a total failure, no one will accept you, your nursing career will end. No matter how irrational these automatic thoughts are, for the moment you probably believe them. Ellis calls this type of self-talk catastrophizing—imagining the worst about anything and everything. Of course, since you alone know your own worst fears, who better than yourself can scare you into paralysis? In both of the preceding examples the self-talk seems to begin on its own accord and, once started, feels uncontrollable.

How you talk to yourself differs significantly from how you talk to other people. If you said aloud what you say to yourself unconsciously, you would probably begin to question the validity or reasonableness of your self-talk.

In some situations you may have an illogical self-conversation while you simultaneously carry on a controlled and rational conversation with another person. McKay and co-workers (1981) describe self-talk as an intercom that is constantly on, monitoring everything that occurs while also talking back and forth.

For example, in a disagreement with someone, your internal and verbalized (public) conversations might go something like this:

Verbalized comments: I disagree with your evaluation of this situation.
Internal talk: Why did you open yourself up for attack? You'll make a fool of yourself! You look so silly. No one will ever respect you after this. Don't say another word or your career is ruined.

These illogical self-statements cause you to feel vulnerable to rejection and overcome with self-doubt simply because you voiced your disagreement.

Once our faulty self-talk has continued over a long period, not only does it become automatic and involuntary but it also produces visual images that reinforce the faulty underlying belief. As with self-talk, negative self-images seem plausible and reasonable despite their absurdity (Beck, 1970).

Thus, to elaborate upon the previous example in which you voiced your disagreement, you may now visualize yourself eating alone in the cafeteria—a social outcast. At this point both the right (visual) hemisphere and the left (verbal) hemisphere are self-talking in destructive, self-defeating ways. The negative self-talk and self-images become anxiety-generating, self-fulfilling prophecies of defeat.

To appreciate experientally how this occurs, stop for a moment and try to vividly remember the last time you got really upset, depressed, or anxious.

- Did your self-talk dwell on how horrible or disastrous this situation was?
- Did you project negative images of your future as a result of this situation?
- Do you remember questioning the reasonableness of these thoughts or images?

Our beliefs about reality and about ourselves, which underlie our self-talk, can be based either on rational or irrational thinking. As used here, rational beliefs are ideas that help us meet our life goals or realize basic values and needs. Irrational beliefs are attitudes and values that sabotage our sense of well-being and inhibit us from reaching our goals. Our rational beliefs will not protect us from feeling appropriately upset when things go wrong, but they can keep us from allowing appropriate emotional responses such as irritation or sadness to escalate into immobilizing and distressing symptoms such as depression, rage, or protracted anxiety. Establishing rational beliefs can also help us defuse situations that previously caused stress.

Irrational Beliefs

Ellis (1974) has suggested four unforgettable terms that he feels encompass all other irrational beliefs.

"*Must*erbation is the devout and quite untenable belief in some absolutistic or dogmatic form of should, ought or must" (Ellis, 1974). Naturally the belief that things that should, ought, or must be a certain way is based on our own inflexible rules about what is right and good. When anyone doesn't do what is right in our eyes, then of course they are bad. With musterbation it becomes difficult to see the exceptions to every rule. We also fail to appreciate the uniqueness of other people—we miss their value if they don't conform with our own inflexible values. Things get polarized into extremes with no middle ground. When we apply this type of polarized—good or bad, for or against—distorted reasoning to ourselves, every action may seem to have disastrous consequences attached. The following statements are examples of musterbation:

- I *must* be perfect.

- I should always be calm and relaxed.
- I ought to be loved by everyone.
- The world ought to be different.
- People shouldn't do things like that.

The logical consequence of musterbation is *"awfulizing."* Because things aren't what they ought to be or must be, things are absolutely awful. We lose our perspective and make catastrophic interpretations of an event, jumping immediately to the conclusion that it is awful. When we awfulize, we can no longer logically evaluate what has just happened. We develop a type of tunnel vision, only seeing one part of the situation to the exclusion of everything else. "You can't see the forest for the trees." One bad event becomes a disastrous day, one mistake becomes a total failure, and so on. We might say to ourselves things like:

- This is the worst thing that I've ever done!
- Her disapproval of my decision means she'll never speak to me again.
- Because of this I will never succeed.

Once we have decided a situation is this awful, we quickly come down with a case of *"can't-stand-it-itis."* We convince ourselves that the awful situation is completely unbearable. If it continues much longer, we will surely go mad or die. With this "illness" not only is there distress caused by failing to accomplish the impossible "must, should, ought" but there is also additional pressure and distress because something even worse is about to happen unless we take drastic corrective measures. We tell ourselves:

- I've got to do something about this.
- No one can live like this!
- This job is driving me crazy. I've got to leave it.

"In a world in which you must get what you want and in which awful things are happening that you just can't stand, clearly someone is to blame. That's where *'damning yourself and others'* comes in" (Donnelly, 1981). Whoever you decide is the cause of the mess is now damned to suffer. You tell yourself things like:

- He's horrible. I hope he gets caught.
- I'm always failing at everything.
- It's all his fault—so let him suffer!

Recall once again the disturbing incident you analyzed when we were discussing self-talk in the last section. What was the "must" underlying the problem? What drastic measures were you convinced needed to occur because of your "can't-stand-it-itis"? Who did you pin the blame on? If you fingered yourself for the blame, you probably felt depressed or guilty, or a diminished sense of self-worth. If you couldn't decide who was to blame but knew someone must be and believed the situation was overwhelming, you experienced anxiety or frustration. Or if you were able to find someone else to foist the blame upon, then you probably felt righteous indignation or anger.

Remembering the incident, was there any reasonableness to your beliefs? Probably not. Few work events are essential to our sense of well-being or cause disasters if they occur or are really unbearable. Maybe someone was responsible for what happened, but did they or you really deserve blame for the exaggerated perception you had of the event or for your distressed feelings?

Underlying all irrational beliefs and self-talk is the assumption that things are done to you. Because of this, you end up feeling like a hopeless victim who is constantly battered around by other people's malice and lack of consideration or by uncontrollable events. So what can be done to control our faulty beliefs and irrational self-talk? The following sections concern this issue.

COGNITIVE STRESS MANAGEMENT APPROACHES

All cognitive approaches to stress management are based upon the premise that stress is caused by distorted thinking. By using a cognitive approach, you can break the negative feedback loop escalating your stress response, either by changing your thoughts or by changing your interpretation of the stimulus. Cognitive coping strategies for stress management are based upon identifying and changing distorted thought patterns that produce and perpetuate distress. The aim of cognitive coping strategies is to substitute self-enhancing rational thoughts for negative assumptions and irrational thoughts that lead to disatisfaction and distress (Goldfried and Merbaum, 1973).

Guidelines for Rational Thinking

Goodman (1974) has proposed guidelines for promoting rational thinking that are useful as cognitive stress management techniques.

- *It* doesn't do anything to you. The way you feel is caused by what you think, not by situations or people.
- Everyone makes mistakes. As human beings we are all fallible. Expecting yourself or others to be perfect only creates disappointment or resentment.
- It takes two to fight. If you are engaged in conflict, you are contributing to it, and thus you are not totally blameless. By walking away from a disagreement or ignoring it, you don't add fuel to keep the fire burning.

Looking for "the cause" of distress, determining who's to blame, or who started the mess is basically a waste of time. Your energy is better spent deciding how to change your behavior now.

Attacking Irrational Beliefs

The first step in learning to create less stress for yourself is to recognize your ABCs. Whenever you experience any unpleasant emotion, stop and identify what was the activating event or stressor (A), what you told yourself about this based on your beliefs (B), and the feeling you now have (C). Using the stress response diary discussed in Chapter 8, Stress Assessment Tools, will help you recognize when you are experiencing a stress response that involves irrational beliefs. It is useful at first to write down the ABCs in a column across the page.

A	B	C
Activating event	Beliefs	Consequence

Spend most of your energy focusing on your self-talk. What did you say to yourself? At first this will be hard to do because you probably have not paid attention to it. When you can recall your self-talk from a previous experience, you will soon be able to catch yourself in the process of self-talk. Write down all your assumptions, worries, judgments, and expectations about the activating event under the beliefs heading.

The next step is to dispute (D) any irrational beliefs you have identified that contributed to your distress.

Ask yourself the following (Ellis, 1971; Davis et al., 1980):

- Is there any rational basis to my beliefs?
- What is so awful about this situation?
- Is there any basis for the must, should, or ought I'm telling myself or is it just my *preference* that things be a certain way?
- What really is the worst thing that could happen to me?
- Is there anything good that might happen as a result of this?
- Is there any evidence or objective data available that refute this irrational belief?

Beck (1976) refers to this process of disputing irrational beliefs as learning to regard self-thoughts as hypotheses rather than facts and then testing out each hypothesis against reality. Because our self-talk occurs outside our conscious level of awareness, we do not test its reasonableness—we automatically assume its validity. Using a cognitive approach, however, forces us to debate the pros and cons of our beliefs, much as Socrates suggested the truth could be found by debating opposite positions. By determining the worst thing that could happen from this situation, we weigh the inherent risks to determine whether they exist and are as serious as we might have imagined.

Lastly, according to Ellis (1974), by disputing your irrational ideas you acquire a new cognitive effect (E) and develop alternative emotions and thoughts in place of the old irrational ones.

Rational Emotive Imagery

It is difficult to do something differently if you are not even able to imagine doing the new behavior. Fantasizing yourself in a new activity changes your outlook and belief system, thus helping you to adopt the desired behavior. As I said previously, negative images are usually associated with irrational thoughts; they produce distress and pain. Maultsby and Ellis and Harper developed the technique of rational-emotive imagery to be used in conjunction with rational-emotive therapy; its purpose is to short-circuit the negative images that reinforce irrational thoughts (Maultsby, 1971; Ellis and Harper, 1975). (The theoretical concepts and supporting research upon which imagery operates is discussed in Chapter 18, "Creative Imagination.")

Exercise: Pushing Your Feelings   Begin by imagining as vividly as you can an unpleasant situation (an activating experience, A). Recreate the experience until it seems to come alive again, to the extent that all your senses experience the details of the situation. Do not try to stop the unpleasant emotions that you associate with this scene (consequences, C); instead, get in touch with these feelings—feel them again.

Once you have reexperienced the stressful emotion, push your emotion—force the emotion to change. For example, if you experience depression, force yourself to feel disappointment. Or if you experience anger and resentment, push your gut feeling until you feel irritation or annoyance. Push whatever distressing emotion you are feeling until you have turned it into a different, less stressful, response. Don't let negative thoughts creep up by saying, "You can't change your feelings like this." Research has proven over and over again that in fact you can do exactly this! You can and will change your negative experiences into less stressful ones by consciously forcing yourself to decrease and alter the emotion (Maultsby and Ellis, 1974; Stampfl and Levis, 1967; Wolpe and Lazarus, 1966).

Examine how you were able to change your feelings. What did you do to alter your feelings of anxiety, anger, depression, or whatever? You will notice that what changed was your belief system (or as Ellis puts it, your "bullshit")! Changing your belief system was done in a way unique to yourself. No one can give you exact directions on how do it. This also appears to be true of self-learning through biofeedback.

Practice recalling a vivid, disturbing emotion and then changing it to a less crippling emotion such as displeasure, annoyance, or disappointment. When you can do this, you will automatically tend to experience the milder form rather than the strong emotional consequences you previously felt.

Exercise: Positive Imagery or Covert Modeling   Take another unpleasant work situation that "always" makes you feel upset. Imagine this situation vividly until you can reexperience the situation as if it were happening right now.

Immediately imagine yourself successfully handling the situation. Focus your attention on how you would behave if this situation didn't bother you. Try to create your own movie of yourself behaving in this different, successful way. Allow your imagination to vividly enact the whole drama. Or you might find it useful to imagine someone else whom you've seen successfully perform the desired behavior. By recreating the image of another person's successful behavior in the distressing situation, you are able to identify the steps that are necessary to accomplish the behavior.

This technique of imagining a positive behavior as modeled by someone (including yourself) is called covert modeling (Cautela, 1966). It is in fact part of how we all naturally learn to behave. Small children dressing up like grown-ups are imitating adult behavior and thus learning how to behave a certain way. In practicing this technique, it is important to imagine yourself or the model struggling to master the situation. If you imagine someone effortlessly performing a task, you will feel overwhelmed. What will most likely happen then is that you will further handicap yourself by seeing the model's smooth performance as beyond your capabilities. As you imagine the successful completion of the behavior, include some realistic effort and struggle. We learn from mistakes as well as from success. By including the struggle, you prepare yourself to experience normal anxiety and resistance when you try to do the behavior. Since you have included some strain or floundering in your image, you see the anxiety and difficulty as expected components. Since in your image this didn't stop the successful behavior, you will believe you can also overcome it in real life. And, in fact, you can (McKay et al., 1981).

Thought Stoppage

Thought stoppage is a useful technique when obsessive thoughts produce distress or paralysis that prevents you from doing things you'd like to do. What happens both in obsessional rumination and phobic behavior is that you concentrate on upsetting and unwanted thoughts that seem to control your mind. But as I've said before, all thoughts *can* be controlled, no matter how automatic and powerful they seem to be (Rumm and Masters, 1974).

THOUGHT STOPPAGE

Exercise: Begin to think about some particularly upsetting things. Elaborate on these thoughts. For example, if you are worried about failing at something at work, allow yourself to think about this. Tell yourself all the scary things you know only too well; how disastrous this failure would be; how awful it would be if anyone discovered your mistake. And so on.

After you have allowed your mind to begin its obsessive, counterproductive thinking, do something that will either startle you or cause you pain. I usually bite the inside of my mouth or dig my fingernails into the palm of my other hand. Other people will shout "stop" or snap a rubberband they have on their wrist. *Anything* that will interrupt the unpleasant ruminative thoughts! These interrupters are aversive stimuli that distract you from the counterproductive thoughts.

As soon as you have stopped thinking your distressing thoughts, immediately force your mind onto some pleasant thought. This is called thought substitution. Of course, at first the unpleasant thought will try to creep back. When this happens again, interrupt your thinking with whatever device you have found works for you. Again, immediately focus on your pleasant thought. This technique can work immediately, but for well-established obsessive or phobic problems you will have to practice over and over again. Once you have been doing it for awhile you will soon notice that the unpleasant, intrusive thoughts begin to lose their control and force. Now instead of "controlling" your mind they just seem to "sneak in" and can be shoved out with a little will power and conscious refocusing of your thoughts.

Stress Inoculation

Meichenbaum (1975) created the stress inoculation process to teach clients what they should tell themselves in order to cope with stressful situations. This coping strategy teaches you a way to approach any type of stressful event; you thus learn a positive head set, a way of talking to yourself that is helpful in any situation. With this strategy you learn how to modify your appraisal of the stressful situation and change your belief about being able to cope with it (Meichenbaum, 1975). There are four categories of self-statements that need to be modified and rehearsed as positive self-talk: (1) Preparation statements before the event, (2) statements during the stressful event, (3) calming statements, and (4) self-reinforcing statements (Meichenbaum and Cameron, 1977).

STRESS INOCULATION

Exercise: Select a particularly stressful work situation you have to deal with frequently. As you begin to think about the situation and start to imagine you are going to face it again, make statements to yourself that diffuse the situation's ability to cause you anticipatory anxiety. These are called preparation statements.

The following are examples of what you might say to yourself before an upcoming stressful event:

- Don't worry, I'll be able to handle it.
- I've handled worse things than this. It'll be OK.
- Just think it through. Plan how to attack it and soon it'll be over with.
- Other people have lived through it and come out fine. So will I!

Next, imagine the steps necessary to get through the stressful events—what actually must be done. Imagine the situation as clearly and vividly as possible. This time instead of imagining you are *going* to do something, imagine that you are actually doing it. Think of things to tell yourself that will calm you as you confront the situation.

- I'm in control here. Just take a few deep breaths and relax.
- All I have to do is take one step at a time.
- Focus on what I'm doing. If I don't pay attention to my fears, they can't stop me.
- Hey, I'm doing it. It's coming along fine.
- No need to be perfect. Just do the best I can.

As you imagine yourself doing the dreaded thing, you will probably notice uncomfortable feelings associated with the stress response syndrome. At this time you need calming statements. Here are a few suggestions:

- Yes, I feel a little anxious. That's normal and can help me think more clearly.
- I don't need to be totally relaxed; a little fear is OK. This is a new experience.
- Pay attention to what I'm doing. That will stop these scary thoughts.
- This will be over in a second.
- If I really get overwhelmed, there is always _____ to bail me out.

Once you've survived the situation and it's over in your fantasy, reinforce your accomplishments by making self-reinforcing statements such as:

- Wait till I tell _____ how I handled this!
- I was great! Give me an A for the attempt.

STRESS INOCULATION (continued)

- Practice makes perfect. Sure I was a little uncomfortable, but I'm just beginning.
- Only goes to show I can do anything I put my mind to.

Once you've imagined yourself through all four steps with the supportive self-statements, pick a few more upsetting, stressful situations and go through the same process until the coping self-talk comes naturally and feels familiar. Now you're ready to take on a live situation, to practice stress inoculation in vivo. As you encounter the situation, say the self-statements. If you notice tension or signs of anxiety, see these as signals alerting you to use one of your relaxation techniques. If you feel over your head at any point, give yourself permission to re-trench and leave if necessary. Above all else see the exercise as a learning experience—you don't need to be perfect. You are unlearning negative thought patterns that have developed over a long period of time. You'll need to be patient and kind to yourself as you slowly unlearn the stressful habits of irrational disturbing self-talk.

CONCLUSION

Since we all talk to ourselves, we might as well learn how to talk in ways that are helpful. The more you are aware of your distorted thinking and irrational beliefs and how these beliefs influence your self-talk, the better you will be able to control your unpleasant emotional responses to stressors. As with any of the stress management approaches presented in this book, you have to be willing to assume personal responsibility. In this case, you have to control your self-talk. Sometimes I have to laugh at the crazy things I used to tell myself. Before I began to pay attention to what I was saying to myself, these self-statements would have been accepted as reasonable and rational. "You must always be right." "If he raises his voice again, I'm going to die!" "I'm too dumb to write a book."

What are your crazy self-statements? Don't let them cause you pain or stop you from becoming the best you possibly can. Don't talk yourself into misery! There are enough stressors in life and in nursing without your creating more personal stress from the way you talk to yourself.

REFERENCES

Beck, A. T. 1970. Cognitive therapy. *Behavior therapy*. 70:184–200.

Beck, A. T. 1976. *Cognitive therapy and the emotional disorders*. New York: New American Library.

Cautela, J. R. 1966. Treatment of compulsive behavior by covert sensitization. *Psychol. Rec.* 16:33–41.

Childress, A. R., and Burns, D. D. 1981. The basics of cognitive therapy. *Psychosomatics* 22(12):1017–1027.

Davis, M., Eshelman, E. R., and McKay, M. 1980. *The relaxation and stress reduction workbook.* Richmond, Calif.: New Harbinger.

Donnelly, G. F. 1981. Stop driving yourself crazy. *R. N.* Feb.:100.

Ellis, A. 1962. *Reason and emotion in psychotherapy.* New York: Lyle Stuart.

Ellis, A. 1971. *Growth through reason.* Palo Alto, Calif.: Science and Behavior Books.

Ellis, A. 1974. *Disputing irrational beliefs.* New York: Institute for Rational Living.

Ellis, A. 1978. What people can do for themselves to cope with stress. In *Stress at Work,* editors C. L. Cooper and R. Payne. New York: John Wiley and Sons.

Ellis, A., and Harper, R. A. 1975. *A new guide to rational living.* North Hollywood, Calif.: Wilshire Book Co.

Goldfried, M. R., and Merbaum, M. 1973. *Behavior change through self-control.* New York: Holt, Rinehart and Winston.

Goodman, D. S. 1974. *Emotional well-being through rational behavior training.* Springfield, Ill.: Charles C Thomas, Publisher.

Lazarus, R. 1966. *Psychological stress and coping process.* New York: McGraw-Hill Book Co.

Maultsby, M. 1971. Rational emotive imagery. *Rational Living* 6:16–23.

Maultsby, M., and Ellis, A. 1974. *Techniques for using rational emotive imagery (REI).* New York: Institute for Rational Living.

McKay, M., Davis, M., and Fanning, P. 1981. *Thoughts and feelings: the art of cognitive stress intervention.* Richmond, Calif.: New Harbinger Publications.

Meichenbaum, D. 1974. *Cognitive behavior modification.* Morristown, N.J.: University Programs Modular Studies.

Meichenbaum, D. 1975. A self-instructional approach to stress management: a proposal for stress inoculation training. In *Stress and anxiety in modern life,* editors C. Speilberger and I. Sarason. New York: Winston and Sons.

Meichenbaum, D. H., and Cameron, R. 1977. The clinical potential of modifying what clients say to themselves. In *Handbook of rational-emotive therapy,* editors A. Ellis and R. Grienger. New York: Springer Publishing Co.

Rimm, D. C., and Litvak, S. B. 1969. Self-verbalizing and emotional arousal. *J. Abnormal Psychol.* 74:181–187.

Rumm, C. D., and Masters, J. C. 1974. *Behavior therapy: techniques and empirical findings.* New York: Academic Press.

Schachter, S., and Singer, J. E. 1962. Cognitive, social and physiological determinants of emotional state. *Psycholog. Rev.* 69:379–399.

Stampfl, T., and Levis, D. 1967. Phobic patients: treatment with the learning approach of implosive therapy. *Voices* 3(3):23–27.

Velten, E. 1968. A laboratory task for induction of mood states. *Behavior Res. Ther.* 6:473–482.

Wolpe, J., and Lazarus, R. 1966. *Behavior therapy techniques.* New York: Pergamon Press.

CHAPTER 13

Recognizing the "Givens": Accepting What Can't Be Changed

EMILY E. M. SMYTHE

WHAT IS A GIVEN?

Have you ever felt as though you were banging your head against a brick wall? That no matter how hard you tried, you couldn't get someone else to change his or her behavior and do what you believed ought to be done? Or have you ever felt as though you were slowly sinking in quicksand? The more you struggled with an issue or problem, the farther away the solution seemed to slip. Perhaps there was a time when the mere sight of someone in your work environment made you see red. Or maybe you heard someone discuss a unit problem only to find yourself incensed. If you've ever had any of these feelings or experiences, the probability is high that you were waging war against the "givens."

The givens are simply the realities of everyday life—of people and things. We can get into serious trouble with these realities when we believe them to be contrary to our sense of well-being and thus decide they shouldn't exist. But these givens simply *are,* despite our wishing they *weren't.* People or events beyond our immediate control may seem to be immovable obstacles blocking the way to our desired goals. They ruin our day, start our adrenalin pumping, or give us those all too familiar feelings of anxiety and anger. They become our pet peeves.

Many of us allow these negatively perceived givens to achieve overwhelming power in our lives. We may fruitlessly channel our energy into correcting them. The givens can even seem to be all-consuming; they can prey constantly on our minds. Yet, despite all our time, energy, and discomfort, the givens never seem to budge. In the long run it is probably our battle with the givens that produces our greatest sense of frustration and powerless rage.

There are many givens in nursing practice that most nurses, regardless of education, experience, personality, or location, would consider problems. Anger and resentment in present-day nursing practice can come from being short staffed, not being adequately compensated for our services, physicians who are disrespectful or arrogant, co-workers who won't fairly share the work-load, budget cuts that trim necessary services or personnel, or manipulative patients. The list could become quite long. Many of the stressors discussed in Chapter 2 could be seen as unpleasant realities of modern-day nursing practice or as negative, unpleasant givens.

Then there are the more personal annoyances of everyday life that may be unique to each of us. How we see these givens depends on our personalities, past experiences, beliefs, and expectations.

Take, for example, a typical morning commute. You wake up each morning, refreshed and eager to go to work. You get onto the freeway, and there they are—those crazy drivers! Some cut across your lane; others move at a snail's pace; some choose to break down and block a lane. And, of course, there are the gawkers who can't seem to pay attention to the road. All these nuisances clog up the freeway. You start to mutter to yourself, "These people shouldn't be allowed to drive. They're dangerous. They should have to take an IQ test before they're issued driver's licenses." Your heart starts racing. "I'm really getting angry. Look at that idiot. He nearly killed me. There ought to be a law against those kinds of drivers!" Your jaw and neck start to stiffen; hands clutch the wheel; no longer relaxed, you start to vent your rage toward everyone and everything. By the time you finally arrive at work, your stress has you in knots. In this state, can you really say you're ready to start work?

What could you have done to combat this unpleasant reality? Honk your horn? Complain to co-workers? Write your congressperson? Move closer to work? Quit the job? Probably nothing. As you might imagine, this freeway scenario could be replayed each and every day. Crazy freeway commuters are a fact of life—a given.

But it doesn't stop there. After months of battling givens, all you have to do is think of the freeway and your anger swells. It becomes an automatic, conditioned response. At that point the anticipation of driving can cause the same response as the driving itself.

You're probably beginning to think, "There's something ridiculous about intelligent people allowing freeway traffic to control their emotions in this fashion. How absurd this chain of events is." But the strange thing about fighting the givens is that the battle insidiously takes over; we lose our sense of emotional control and our awareness of what's happening. The result is a conditioned response to specific stressors and a total loss of perspective.

I'm convinced that this type of experience is not unique to me. It may not be the morning freeway, but think for a moment. Isn't there something that *really* bugs you? Isn't there something or someone who you feel can ruin your day or at least pull your emotional strings and knock you off balance? Take a moment to think about your job, the people or situations that really bother you, or the things that seem to go wrong on a fairly regular basis. Think about the big or small things at work that push your emotional buttons. Some of these might even be things about yourself—for example, being a slow worker, having difficulty being assertive, or caring too much.

If you're becoming upset over these issues and feel that you're on an emotional roller coaster, you're allowing the givens to control you. There is probably someone at your job who is also thinking, "Can't she see how stupid it is to get upset over something like that?" And the answer for you, as it is for anyone who is fighting the givens, is probably not. We all tend to be blinded toward our own "craziness" of fighting over givens with anger, resentment, or loss of personal control. At the very least this tendency is a refusal to acknowledge reality; in its extreme form, this tendency becomes a symptom of mental illness.

If you're like everyone else who becomes enraged by the givens, at this point you're probably telling yourself something like this: "Well these issues *shouldn't* be this way. There's nothing wrong with me for being upset by them. They need to be changed!" And, of course, you're right. The truth is that we would all be better off if many of these givens did not exist. However, the world is far from ideal. Many of these unpleasant, "bad" givens are the unfortunate, but frequently unavoidable, hassles of our jobs. In nursing, we face a disproportionately large number of them. In the daily practice of nursing, we encounter suffering, defeat, and numerous givens that are less than ideal. Marlene Kramer, in her book *Reality Shock*, describes how many nursing graduates experience a form of shock upon first facing these givens in nursing (Kramer, 1974). However, in all fairness, any human service professional who has been living in the unreal, idealized world of the student can become shocked upon first seeing clearly the reality of his or her profession. Reality shock is experienced by teachers, doctors, social workers, police officers, lawyers, and others. We all face the same shock during the transition from student to practicing professional.

Many of the stressors in nursing discussed in Chapter 2 are givens. The unpleasant realities of daily nursing practice—the current nursing shortage, the burden of responsibility without authority, fragmentation of patient care, working with clients who are under stress, and dealing with death and suffering will not evaporate. Like the freeway traffic, they'll be there tomorrow.

I don't want you to get the mistaken idea that *nothing* can be done with these givens. Potential solutions exist for some of them, but until such solutions are possible, we cannot allow these dilemmas to control our sense of job satisfaction, emotional state, or sense of professional competence and value. As long as we do, we cannot consider ourselves in control, nor will we be able to focus on possible solutions to the problems.

IDENTIFYING WORK "GIVENS"

The first step in learning how to handle any situation is to develop awareness of its existence. In learning to manage the givens, this self-awareness involves identifying when you are becoming angry and upset with people and events beyond your immediate control.

Directions

1. In the space provided on the next page make a list of all aspects of your job that upset you. Be sure to include people you feel make your job more difficult and less satisfying. (Some of you may discover that the space provided is not nearly sufficient; feel free to use an additional sheet of paper.)
2. In the space between the brackets, to the right of each number, rate on a scale of 1–5 how much this item upsets you. Use the following criteria:
    1 = Bothers me; no fight or flight symptoms; can continue working.
    2 = Annoys me; feel uncomfortable; can put it out of my mind.
    3 = Angers me; fight-or-flight response present; can use stress reduction techniques to control.
    4 = Infuriates me; fight-or-flight response present; stress reduction techniques temporarily control but I don't feel relaxed.
    5 = Enrages me! Fight-or-flight response present; nothing helps decrease level of discomfort; can't concentrate on anything else.
3. For each item you've just rated, ask yourself if there is anything direct, immediate, and/or single-handed that you can do to change the situation or person. If there is nothing short of a miracle or a herculean expenditure of energy that could change the event or person, put a check (✓) mark in the space provided to the left of such items. Each checked item is a given.

IDENTIFYING WORK "GIVENS" (continued)

4. Look over the givens you have identified and think how much of your energy and sense of job satisfaction is drained because you get upset with the persons or events beyond your control. Do you choose to give up your self-control to these givens?
5. Look at your ratings. If you are allowing anything, givens or not, to upset you to the extent that it rates a 4 or 5, you are putting your health in jeopardy and significantly decreasing your personal sense of well-being.

Givens	Degree of Upset	Events and People That Upset Me at Work
——	1. [ ]	————————————————
——	2. [ ]	————————————————
——	3. [ ]	————————————————
——	4. [ ]	————————————————
——	5. [ ]	————————————————
——	6. [ ]	————————————————
——	7. [ ]	————————————————
——	8. [ ]	————————————————
——	9. [ ]	————————————————
——	10. [ ]	————————————————
——	11. [ ]	————————————————
——	12. [ ]	————————————————
——	13. [ ]	————————————————
——	14. [ ]	————————————————
——	15. [ ]	————————————————

THE PRICE OF BLINDLY FIGHTING THE GIVENS

The price we pay for fighting the givens is extremely high. The battle can cost us a great deal: coronary heart disease associated with high levels of unmanaged stress; burn-out from unresolved, chronic job stress; the unpleasant feelings of an occasional fruitless encounter with a hopeless situation or an impossible person. The most frequent emotional response is anger or its more prevalent forms, disappointment and annoyance. Whenever we refuse to acknowledge the realities of a situation and blindly attack the givens, we choose to do battle against phenomenal odds, an effort that requires a great expenditure of energy. The major casualty, however, is not our ability to change the realities, but rather our self-control.

In the battle against the givens you can also expect constant excitation of your autonomic nervous system, a state usually manifested as anxiety. In fact, any of the various stress-related symptoms discussed in Chapter 1 can occur because you choose to take up arms against nursing reality.

One of the highest prices we pay for fighting the givens is our omnipresent despair and overwhelming powerlessness. "After all," we tell ourselves, "look at all the energy I've spent on this problem and how upset it makes me feel. Yet no matter how hard I try, nothing seems to change! So why bother? I've been beaten!"

Once the process becomes a daily experience, resignation and apathy aren't far behind. The givens have defeated you. In fact, there is no way of winning when you fight against the givens. Your energy and time are no longer available for projects or people with which or whom you could have a significant impact.

Some people turn this defeat around; they use the givens as an excuse for their personal failures or, indeed, for not even trying. A 69-year-old psychiatric patient with whom I worked kept trying to convince me that the reason he had become an alcoholic and never amounted to anything was his father. His father had abandoned him and his mother when he was quite young. So what could anyone expect from him? His whole life had been "ruined" by his father. This man had spent his entire life blaming the givens. Certainly a father could have improved his childhood; but did this unfortunate lack really account for his wasted life? Many people face unpleasant realities, some much worse than not having a father, but what they do with their lives is largely a matter of their choice and their responsibility.

Some nurses respond to the givens by becoming embittered cynics whose job "script" reads something like this: It's all hopeless. Nursing is a dying profession made up of impotent women who cannot unite to solve any problems. Look at all these problems! These nurses resist suggestions that might lead to solutions. Their struggle with the givens leads to a premature death of spirit; it leaves them in a continual state of emptiness and disappointment. The "ain't it awful" game sucks them in: ain't it awful that we don't have enough staff, that we have budget cuts, that families interfere with the patient's care, and on, and on. Ain't it awful?

Other embittered nurses adopt an active rather than a passive style, which I like to call the dragon-slayer approach. Nurses who operate in this fashion engage in headlong attacks on every negative reality they perceive. In their crusades, they seem to fight one unsuccessful battle after another, as if trying to slay dragons. Of course, there's nothing wrong with tackling reality and attempting to beat it into a more livable shape. However, the dragon-slayer's blind, scattered assaults usually result in failure. Rather

than controlling their emotional responses to the givens and taking a problem-solving approach, they react at once to everything. They may also become disappointed with their co-workers because the latter refuse to join
these crusades; co-workers in turn may even avoid these dragon-slayers
because dragon-slayers are always upset and angry about something. Such
an approach costs these nurses the satisfaction of being constructive
change agents and the respect and support of their fellow nurses. On rare
occasions, they may succeed in making some changes, but the odds resem-
ble those faced by David against Goliath. And if they do win, they will
probably have fought so hard, employing any means to win, that they will
have alienated friend and foe alike in the struggle. Making changes in the
health care system may sometimes feel like a battle against evil forces; in
fact, the change process is a mutual struggle among various professionals
who are all attempting to work together in providing optimal patient care.
Improving patient care is not a crusade against dragons.

UNHOOKING FROM FUTILE BATTLES

Now that you appreciate how expensive fighting against the givens can
be, how can you avoid these confrontations? How can you choose to unhook from these futile battles?

William Glasser (1975), in his book *Reality Therapy*, offers some advice
on the subject. He believes "Reality may be painful, it may be harsh, it may
be dangerous, but it changes slowly. All any man can hope to do is to struggle with it in a responsible way by doing right and enjoying the pleasures
or suffering the pain that may follow." He also thinks that all emotionally
ill people have one common trait: "They all deny the reality of the world
around them, and hence are unable to fulfill their needs."

Learning to unhook from emotional traps always involves a change in
perspective. Unless you begin to see things differently, to question your
expectations of reality, you can never hope to stop beating your head
against the wall. Edelwich and Brodsky, in their book *Burnout: Stages of
Disillusionment in the Helping Professions* (1980), suggest: "Accept the
givens: understand them; live with them; work with them. . . . Living with
the givens means accepting reality as the basis of one's actions, the starting
point of whatever one decides to do."

Some people never choose to stop fighting the givens. For example,
I've seen couples in conjoint therapy who conducted raging battles with
each other for decades. Each attempts to change the other into what would
be the ideal spouse. Despite all forms of therapeutic intervention, they te-
naciously cling to their position that the other person needs to change.
They end up never resolving the conflict, both dissatisfied with each other
and resenting their life situation. They choose never to accept the givens—
in this case, to accept the other person as he or she is.

It may be difficult to let go of fighting the givens because we feel righteously justified in our battle. We believe the givens to be wrong, bad, or not the way things *should* be, and our attack on them is thus justified. I think that life is not a simple choice between resignation to reality and a head-on attack of it; instead, we should recognize when we have personal power and when we don't and prevent ourselves from becoming emotional yo-yos everytime unpleasant realities arise. This is not to imply that you are passive; it means that you understand your limitations and work with your potential. Or, to quote the prayer of Alcoholics Anonymous (adapted from a statement by the German philosopher Reinhold Niebuhr):

God grant me the serenity to accept the things I cannot change,
Courage to change the things I can, and wisdom to know the difference.

The question is not whether givens should exist but rather how to handle your responses to these realities. Do you choose to stop wasting your energy attacking situations that can't change? Are you going to allow circumstances you dislike to control your sense of well-being and job satisfaction? It seems absurd to allow something or someone you dislike to control your life; yet, in fact, that's exactly what happens when you fight the givens. The choice is yours. You can spend your professional life attacking "the system," complaining about how bad "things" are, being furious at the shortcomings of health care or outraged at co-workers' insensitivity, or resenting your lack of professional freedom and autonomy. The other option you have is to acknowledge these unpleasant realities, learn to control your emotional responses to them, and do some problem-solving and assertive limit-setting to cope with them.

Once you realize that you can't necessarily change other people or many of the daily realities of nursing practice, you are faced with the issue of self-responsibility. Blaming the givens may be your way of avoiding personal responsibility for your emotions and your possible impact on the profession. After all, there is an advantage to deluding yourself and to believing that people and events are controlling you and making it impossible to do your job. In this way, you don't have to acknowledge your own power and your personal responsibility for self-control and well-being. (For further discussion of this topic, see Chapter 12, "Cognitive Approach to Stress Management.")

At times our awareness of reality may also be distorted. In *Value Clarification*, Simons and co-authors (1972) have described the tendency to focus exclusively on occasional mistakes while neglecting to notice all the things that go right as a "red pencil mentality." It's easy to lose our perspective and see only the problems. When this red pencil mentality is operating, we selectively attend only to the problems that exist in nursing. Certainly there are many real problems in nursing, but there are also numerous positive features Improvements have occurred in the profession and in working conditions in most hospitals. It isn't all bad. Sometimes, however, we're just seeing the problems, and our "reality" becomes a bit distorted, which leads to a pessimistic view of nursing.

At the same time that I caution you not to become unrealistically pessimistic, I also suggest that you not distort reality into a Pollyannist form of optimism. Voltaire, in his satire on optimism, *Candide* (1962), addresses the folly of blind optimism in the ironic tale of a young man who blithely maintains that "this is the best of all possible worlds"; however, over and over again, he faces the evils of humankind and nature. His optimistic naiveté finally gives way to the realization that reason is a unique human weapon in surviving the harshness of life. Far from being defeated by all his scuffles with villains, disasters, and the ravages of time, the hero ultimately accepts evil as an inescapable reality of life. He refuses to be totally consumed, but he also stops blindly holding false expectations that lead only to disaster. He discovers that "we must cultivate our gardens . . . let us work then without disputing . . . . It is the only way to render life supportable." Once he finally accepts the good and the bad he can then enjoy life as it is. Nursing isn't all good or all bad. It simply is whatever it is. You might check to see if you're falling into the common trap of "things shouldn't be this way."

HANDLING WORK GIVENS

For example, you arrive at work one morning only to discover that someone has called in sick and the unit is short-staffed. You say to yourself, "This isn't right. We *shouldn't have* to work with so few people." Whether it's right or wrong to work short-staffed is irrelevant. The reality is that you are down one person. You may now experience anger welling up—anger toward the system, the head nurse, or whomever called in sick. Or you could decide to calm down by using one of the temporary stress reduction techniques (described in Part 6, "Stress Reduction Techniques") and then use a problem-solving approach to handle the crisis (see Chapter 7). If the crisis of short-staffing occurs frequently, again you have some options. You can sit around complaining or you can do some long-range problem-solving to handle these chronic crises. For example, some hospitals have developed staff-patient ratio criteria for patient care that allow nursing administration to close admissions to units that are critically short of staff. Other hospitals have established float pools of extra nurses who are oriented to hospital policies and procedures; they are assigned to general service areas such as medicine, surgery, or pediatrics and are available to cover when the need arises. Still other facilities have call-back services for staff who wish to work extra hours at time-and-a-half pay and have signed up for available shifts.

The problem is not in the lack of solutions; indeed, there are *many* solutions I haven't mentioned in the previous example. The problem is in getting stuck in what we feel is a justifiably angry position—the "things shouldn't be" position, which makes it impossible to come up with solutions. One author suggests that "While [you] may come to recognize the impossible quality of certain goals and wishes, and be willing to relinquish their demands on [your] behavior, [you] may at the same time discover uncharted possibilities for productive work and pleasure" (Zaleynik, 1967). Again, we can unhook from the position of raging against the givens when we acknowledge what reality is. We can then use this awareness as our starting point. We need to be willing to take positive steps toward identifying a solution rather than simply reacting to problems. Unfortunately, in many instances you may need to go to great lengths to get reasonable needs met; or you may have to reevaluate the importance of these needs.

For many of us, the insight we gain from recognizing a situation and/or person as a given is enough to allow us to unhook from the futile battle against the givens. The next time you experience the fight-or-flight response ask yourself:

1.   Is this situation a given?
2.   Is there anything I can do that will immediately change it for the better?

This insight allows you to recognize the source of upset as a given. When, for example, you notice that you are upset because it's raining or snowing, a grumpy doctor is being predictably grumpy, you are in a slow lunch line, or you are in one of hundreds of other possibly irritating situations, the recognition that this is a given may allow you to say to yourself, "Hey, why are you getting upset over this? There's nothing you can do about it. Relax. Let it go."

I like to think of this type of insight as the kind of helpful advice I might get from a good friend who loves me enough to tell me what I need to know but may have been too blind to notice myself. We can all develop this internalized helpful friend by learning to become self-supporting. (See Chapter 15, "Developing Social Support: We're All in This Together.")

You might be saying, "What do I do with my gut reaction? How do I calm down when my body says run or fight and I can't do either? Sure, I recognize it as a given, *but* I'm still upset."

If insight isn't enough, there are several possible techniques you can employ to decrease your fight-or-flight response and bring your stress response down to a tolerable level. Visualizing the absurd or centering and focusing techniques (discussed in the following sections and in Chapter 17) are immediately useful in any nursing setting. Although many other stress reduction techniques also decrease stress by controlling the fight-or-flight response of the autonomic nervous system, they are not easily applied to typical work situations. For example, transcendental meditation, guided imagery, and desensitization work extremely well; however, they are difficult to use while performing patient care. You probably don't have the necessary 15 minutes right then to relax. You do, however, have the less than one minute necessary to use centering or visualization to calm down, and no one even notices what you're doing.

Visualizing the Absurd

Visualizing the absurd is especially useful when you are confronted with a person whose behavior is upsetting you. Focus your attention on the quality or characteristics of the behavior that is disturbing you (for example, a *loud, shrill voice* or a person *pointing a finger* at you or *glaring* at you). Take these qualities and exaggerate them while creating a visual picture—a cartoon or caricature of the person (a glare becomes the glassy stare of a rat's eyes or a loud, shrill voice becomes a buzzy saw). The more ridiculous your mental picture, the more effective it will probably be. Don't listen to what the person is saying; focus your awareness on the person's mannerisms, facial features, or qualities of behavior.

Whenever you use this technique, you are literally using the person's behavior to provide you with a calmer state; you are using humor to alter your perception. Indeed, humor can make the same statement as can complete seriousness, but the perspective provided by humor somehow allows you to bypass your intellectual defensiveness.

The chief psychiatrist of one psychiatric unit on which I worked provides an example of this technique. He was constantly focusing attention toward minor details while totally missing the more relevant major issues. It became infuriating to sit in departmental meetings; discussions revolved around how many pots of coffee should be given to the patients each day while the issues of philosophy of patient care and treatment planning were ignored. He also had an annoying habit of glaring at you through his glasses with a cold stare whenever you tried to refocus conversation on anything but the mundane. I reached the point of wanting to scream at him whenever he opened his mouth. Nothing that anyone had tried would budge him from his obsessive stance. Clearly his behavior was a given! Recognizing this, however, didn't help in the slightest.

One day I began to visualize him as a man with a severe visual impairment who could only see small objects directly in front of his nose. If you imagine looking around a room with a magnifying glass before your eyes you can begin to appreciate how it must have been for him to see any more than an object 6 inches away from his eyes. While sitting in meetings listening to him drone on and on, I allowed my mind to play with the idea of how distorted everything must appear to him. Once I began to see him as an infirm, blind man, I could easily tolerate sitting in the mandatory meetings without experiencing violent rage attacks. Whenever I raised a point and he peered out at me over his glasses, I calmed myself with the fact that "he has to stare because he can't see too well—poor dear!" No longer could I be intimidated by these looks.

An interesting strategy that developed from this visualization was that whenever we had to deal with big issues, I'd make a point of breaking them down into minute details—just the right size to place in front of his nose. Sure enough, he seemed more responsive to discussing them.

Centering/Focusing

Centering/focusing can provide immediate relief in any nursing setting. Whenever you notice yourself becoming upset and off-balance, no matter what the cause, you will have difficulty handling the situation until you gain self-control. Centering/focusing allows you to calm yourself without anyone even noticing.

CENTERING/FOCUSING

Directions:
  1. With your eyes open, stop whatever you're doing and focus all your attention onto your breathing.
  2. Take five slow, deep, diaphragmatic breaths. Concentrate on your breathing. Each time your mind wanders off your breathing pull it back and force your mind to empty itself of all other thoughts.
  3. As you're breathing in, say to yourself, "I'm breathing in warm, soothing air that will cleanse me." (Try to visualize this.)
  4. As you breathe out, say to yourself, "I'm exhaling tension and stress, thereby calming myself." (Try to visualize this.)

The first time I presented a lecture to an audience of 350 people I thought I was going to die. I approached the speaker's podium; it looked like the control panel of a 747 jumbo jet. There were hundreds of switches, dials, and monitors. Some of the switches were to raise or lower the three screens on the wall behind the stage. There were ten or more light controls as well as switches to record responses from the audience. I wanted to run off the stage and cry. I was so scared I knew I couldn't even read the notes I'd prepared.

I stopped looking at the control panel and focused my gaze on my notes. I didn't attempt to read the notes, although, to the audience, it probably looked like I was taking a last glance before beginning. I began my slow, diaphragmatic breathing. Each time I began to think something like, "What if you hit the wrong switch?" I would say, "You are breathing in warm, refreshing air that will calm you." I'll admit that in this situation it took about ten breaths, (that isn't much more than 30 seconds), to calm down. When I began the lecture, I felt calm, alert, and mentally sharp.

When the time arrived for questions from the audience, I again panicked: "What if they ask me something I don't know?" I was flooded with many of those good scare thoughts we all know only too well. Again, I stopped and took a few deep breaths before I acknowledged each person in the audience.

A word of caution: I'm not suggesting that if you don't know your material you can bluff your way through it just by breathing. I am saying, however, that you have a much better chance of communicating your ideas effectively when you are calm; this is true whether you're in a test-taking situation or giving a lecture. In fact, I always use this centering/focusing technique before I interact with clients or handle any emotionally charged interaction.

Once you have used one of these techniques to calm your acute fight-or-flight response, you can begin to evaluate other coping strategies for handling chronic problems with the givens.

CONCLUSION

I'm not saying that by accepting things as they are you resign yourself to thinking that nothing can be done to correct a situation. On the contrary, the opposite is true. Once you accept circumstances as they are, and only then, can you start to see what is possible and function within these realities. Nursing won't change by our wishing it were different or by getting angry over how "things shouldn't be this way." It will improve by our acknowledging the current givens in nursing and by our taking individual and united action to correct these unpleasant problems. It is not enough to want to see things in nursing change; we will have to take some action to initiate the changes.

History offers a myriad of people who lament what their lives might have been. I call these individuals the "if only" people. "If only things had been different, then I would have . . . ." "If only I'd been given . . . then I'd . . . ." But things are not likely to be different without our making a conscious choice to expend the energy required to produce change. There is an old Pennsylvania Dutch saying that accurately sums up the need to take personal responsibility for making our lives what we want them to be: "If wishes were horses, then beggars would ride." Everyone wants to ride, but if you don't want to work toward making changes, then acknowledge your choice. It's a perfectly legitimate position to consciously decide, for whatever personal reason, that you are not willing to expend the energy necessary to make a change. But at least by making this choice with awareness, you are acknowledging your self-control and rejecting the notion that you are a helpless victim.

As a nurse you have probably worked with patients who were paralyzed or deformed but who refused to be defeated and miserable as a result of their givens. While acknowledging the givens of their medical conditions, these patients may have overcome their limitations, adapting in unforeseeable ways. Most importantly, instead of being bitter about their "fate," they experience joy in their lives. It is amazing what we all are capable of accomplishing once we stop seeing ourselves as helpless victims of a cruel, unjust world. Nursing may not currently be the way we'd like it to be, but we can still experience a great deal of personal satisfaction from our profession; furthermore, we can still greatly contribute to our patients' well-being. The goal, then, in unhooking from futile battles with the givens is to maintain self-control while striking a balance between what is real and what is possible.

REFERENCES

Edelwich, J., and Brodsky, A. 1980. *Burn-out: stages of disillusionment in the helping professions.* New York: Human Sciences Press.

Glasser, W. 1975. *Reality therapy.* New York: Harper Colophon Books.

Kramer, M. 1974. *Reality shock: why nurses leave nursing.* St. Louis: The C. V. Mosby Co.

Simons, S., Howe, L., and Kirschen G. 1972. *Value clarification.* New York: Hart.

Voltaire, F. M. A. de. 1962. *Candide.* New York: Washington Square Press Inc.

Zaleynik, A. 1967. Management of disappointment. *Harvard Business Rev.* 67612:59–70.

5

Making Interpersonal Relationships Work for, Not Against, You

The social support received from family, friends, and co-workers can buffer against the destructive effects of job stressors as well as contribute to an overall sense of well-being. Although social support is a critical variable in developing or preventing distress, it is not a panacea for job stress.

Unfortunately, all too often instead of using our interpersonal relations to decrease job stress we in nursing have experienced these relations as one of our biggest job stressors. Many nursing articles and several research studies have identified interpersonal relations as one of the largest contributing factors to job dissatisfaction. Instead of feeling supported by co-workers, we may feel attacked or sabotaged by them; indeed, the result may be an increased sense of collective powerlessness. Rather than collectively problem-solving, we sometimes collectively complain ourselves into a position of despair and resignation.

The chapters in Part 5 discuss the positive and negative relationships between social support and stress. They concern ways in which nurses can develop and utilize interpersonal relationships more effectively in their work environment. Collective approaches to stress management, such as conflict resolution or collective bargaining, are not addressed. These approaches are difficult to employ until we accept personal responsibility for our own individual sense of well-being and stop seeing ourselves as helpless victims. Our numbers alone present great potential for change if we can begin to see our job satisfaction as our responsibility and not dependent upon what others—doctors, hospital administrators, patients, or nursing supervisors, *do to* us.

CHAPTER 14

Controlling Contagion: Disturbing the Stagnant Quo

EMILY E. M. SMYTHE

THE STAGNANT QUO—WHAT IT IS

A high level of stress can be much like an infectious disease. It saps an individual nurse's morale and contributes to his or her job dissatisfaction; in addition, it can have disastrous effects upon the whole nursing care system. As with any system, the dysfunction of one part (the stressed nurse) affects every other part (every other nurse) as well as the total system (Morrison, 1980). When a system has experienced excessive stress for a prolonged period of time, any change may be perceived as threatening. I call this condition the "stagnant quo."

The stagnant quo is a negative variation of the status quo. Stagnation can occur whenever corrective input and change are absent. It can also occur when the group norm of the staff becomes one of maintaining whatever is familiar—even if the familiar happens to be disruptive, malfunctional, or purposeless. After all, human beings are creatures of habit, and even bad habits can feel safe and familiar. Changes that might alleviate some of the problems causing the stress may be resisted because the nurses feel they don't have enough energy to adapt to the change. Any change requires an expenditure of adaptive energy and thus can be experienced as an additional stressor (Rahe and Holmes, 1967).

What then begins is the process of dying from within—entropy. Entropy literally means the "diminished capacity for spontaneous change." The energy of the system is not available for performing work (*Dorland's Illustrated Medical Dictionary*, 1974). During the process of entropy, energy is used in various nonproductive ways: complaining, acting without purpose, procrastinating, or functioning below one's level of competence, for example. The system dies after losing its ability to change. Change, of course, is inevitable; but the staff is no longer able to devise creative solutions or responses to the new demands associated with the changes. Everyone seems to get locked into doing things by the book, blindly following guidelines or unit policies, long after the rationale has been forgotten or has become outdated. The professional growth of the nursing staff stops.

If a stagnant quo exists in a patient care environment, outsiders can sense it when they enter the facility. They can see the lifeless faces of the nursing staff, who just seem to be going through the motions. There may not be any feeling of conflict present; instead, it may appear as if everyone has already given in. The individuals no longer care to notice what is happening around them, let alone fight for what they believe. It may also seem as if staff are walking around wearing blinders and saying, "If we don't see the problems, then they don't exist, and we won't need to get involved in correcting them." Avoidance becomes so ingrained as the staff response to problems that the unit motto might read: Let sleeping dogs lie.

If conflict does exist, you may notice that it occurs over issues that the unit personnel deem to be acceptable. These issues have been griped about continuously over the years; all that one needs to say is a key word and the complaint is automatically recalled. For example, when a nurse starts complaining about a daily occurrence, the listener already has a pretty good idea of what the problem will be. These are safe problems that everyone has recounted hundreds of times but no one seems sufficiently energized to tackle. Everyone complains about them and everyone receives an occasional nod of acknowledgment.

Of course, every now and then a new "live" issue comes up, and members of the staff become excited over it. Soon, however, the negative attitudes so ingrained in most of the staff squelch any positive move to deal with the problem. Someone will say, "You remember what happened the last time we tried to get anything changed around here? Nothing ever changes. No one will listen to us. They'll just say we're complaining again. Why bother? Sure it upsets me, but it's a hopeless cause." At this point, the ward's past history gets dredged up to suppress any possibility of exploration or problem-solving. The energy expended seems to be aimed at keeping everything the way it currently is while rechanting the continuous, lifeless litany of complaints.

In a nursing care setting where stagnation has set in, the environment usually looks sterile and institutionalized. Outsiders are struck by the feeling that no one really lives there or feels like a part of the place. Staff just pass through as though they are passing through a hotel room; the environment is occupied for periods of time, but no one really lives in it. The bulletin boards are covered with memos or work schedules. You won't find any personal touches—no pictures, announcements of parties, cartoons, professional articles of interest, or letters from former patients. None of the nursing staff seem to have any personal investment in what happens with the environment. They just put in their time and don't get involved.

You may be wondering why any environment as unpleasant as this would continue to exist. Why doesn't someone come along and change the stagnant quo? Several mechanisms help to spread the stress and maintain the stagnation by establishing resistance to positive, corrective changes while fostering pessimism. We all learned in our fundamentals of nursing classes how contamination occurs. There must be a vehicle or means of transmitting the pathogen from the infected carrier to a susceptible host who is vulnerable to the disease (Wolfe et al., 1979). Bitching and splitting are two of the most common vehicles for transmitting stress and for resisting its handling; these mechanisms can lead to the development of a stagnant quo.

BITCHING: THE PROCESS OF SPREADING STAGNATION

When bitching becomes prevalent, complaining is no longer a temporary way of releasing pressure; instead, the recital of gripes becomes a major feature in daily interaction with co-workers. The bitcher just can't wait to get together with someone else to play what Eric Berne calls the ain't it awful game (Berne, 1964).

You probably know someone who is constantly griping about everything and who never has anything positive to say but always has an abundance of complaints about what wasn't done or what ought to be done. You automatically begin to avoid this person to avoid getting helplessly cornered and being forced to listen to the current gripe.

For these individuals complaining is a way of life. Seeing themselves as helpless victims, they are reduced to feeble complaining as a way of mustering up support or making contact. I've found it useful to tell acquaintances who are always complaining that this behavior bothers me and that instead, I'd like to hear what's going well for them. (Of course, it's usually easier just to avoid a direct confrontation with the person. But I personally would appreciate it if friends were to give me honest feedback about my obnoxious behavior rather than simply avoiding me.) No one wants a relationship in which complaints are the common ground. This is particularly true when you're already stressed and one more person's negativity becomes an additional drain on your already depleted psychic energy.

A negative result of bitching is that frequently the complainer, conten simply to sit on the sidelines commenting on the game, stops looking for solutions to its problems. Naturally, everyone has to discuss problems before solutions can be found. But all too frequently what happens in unit meetings, nursing care plan meetings, or milieu meetings is that people get stuck bringing up one problem after another and producing only a random list of problems. It becomes a game of "Can you top this?" "Well, if you think that's bad, let me tell you about." Or "Guess what happened to me!" At the end of the meeting, everyone leaves feeling they have ventilated their concerns but that the problems still exist; participants realize that they are just as unequipped to manage the problems as they were before the meeting. This continual ventilation leads nowhere; it tends only to support the nursing staff's sense of frustration and resentment.

It's important to clearly state the purpose of any meeting. If the meeting's purpose is to voice complaints, that's fine, but if it's supposed to be a planning meeting, the group discussion needs to shift into exploring options once the concerns have been shared. If a lengthy discussion is necessary to allow all present the opportunity to air their grievances, a second meeting should be planned for problem-solving.

Another dysfunctional result of bitching is that some people feel their responsibility for the problem ends once they've voiced their negative concerns. It's as if they say, "Well, I've told you what's the matter here; now it's up to you to solve the problem." The saying, "If you're not part of the solution, you're part of the problem," always applies. All of us influence and are influenced by the systems in which we work. No staff member is merely a passive observer, absolved of responsibility. Identifying problems is only the first step in problem-solving. It is not the end point. (See Chapter 7, "Focusing on the Possible: A Problem-Solving Approach.")

If an issue has been discussed over a long period of time and no solutions are found, bitching can lead to a sense of helpless frustration. You'll hear people say, We've discussed this problem for months! Nothing happened. It's certainly not getting any better. Why bother? It's always going to be like that. At this point, complaining about issues has clearly evolved into a stagnant quo. The disruptive situation is now the status quo and staff no longer have any hope of resolving issues or instituting constructive changes. The bitching has become a way of spreading the disease of dissatisfaction and stress.

It isn't always bad to complain. In fact, at times it may be healthy. Blowing off steam by complaining to someone can be a valuable safety valve. All of us have experienced a bad day at work when we came home needing to tell someone how awful it was. This ventilating lets us get the frustration off our chests and provides catharsis for the pent-up emotions. The process of catharsis allows us to voice our concerns and feelings; it is an essential part of working through issues. It is, however, not an end in itself (Yalon, 1970).

We can all recognize the occasional need to blow off steam to someone. But when you're in this mood, you don't want your listener to offer solutions to the problems you're describing. If she does you may feel frustrated, as if the individual wasn't really listening to you. What could be happening is that you haven't made your needs clear. The other person was probably also frustrated by your response. After all, she'd given excellent advice and all you did was continue to gripe. Again, the clearer we can be about our needs, the more likely these needs are going to be met. If you say, I've had an awful day at work and just need to bitch about it for awhile, then your listener has been cued to settle back for your recounting the day's atrocities. The listener's energy can be focused on listening to you and offering condolence rather than advice.

Another positive aspect of ventilating feelings is that when you gripe about work problems you may be able to see the situation from a new perspective. Just saying out loud what you have on your mind often clarifies thoughts about which you've been ruminating. The person listening to you may be able to offer alternative ways of analyzing the situation, challenge assumptions you've made about what happened, or suggest workable solutions you hadn't considered.

Complaining to another person also offers you the opportunity to validate your reactions to a situation. Other people may endorse your feelings by saying, "Yeah, in that situation I'd have done the same thing" or "I certainly understand why that upset you. There's nothing wrong with your feeling angry!" Their comments let you know that your reactions are acceptable and not a sign of your own "craziness." Ventilating your complaints also offers others the chance to vocalize their support of you by letting you know that you're not alone. Whenever you've got troubles, you know you have a friend who cares and is willing to listen.

But be careful. Although there are positive aspects, griping, complaining, "blowing off steam," or whatever you want to call it can also be overdone and become a negative process, or bitching. And bitching is contagious! It may even be possible, as with other infectious processes, that carriers aren't aware of what they're doing and don't realize that their bitching is spreading dissatisfaction and stress to others.

Have you ever ended up upset and anxious after receiving nursing reports from the previous shift? The nurse giving the reports might have said: "Boy are you all in for it today! I've had a horrible time! It's been a madhouse here. Never get enough help to do the job. Some of these patients are really difficult cases." You may have come to work feeling great, well rested, and looking forward to work, but suddenly, you notice you're beginning to feel stressed and anxious and wish that you were anywhere but at work! What happened? You've allowed the nurse giving the report to contaminate your day by accepting her negative evaluation and by reacting to her anxiety and frustration. Her bitching has spread her upset to you.

This spreading of anxiety, dissatisfaction, and frustration by bitching can

occur at lunch, during coffee breaks, while socializing with co-workers after work, or whenever nurses get together and blow off steam. Usually,
after one of these sessions, instead of feeling better you notice you feel
upset and angry. It certainly wasn't a break! You're now left stewing about
all the awful things that were discussed. Most of us have difficulty not reacting to another person's emotional tales of woe. Remaining uninvolved
when someone complains about problems that they assure you are affecting your job requires special skills of centering and objectivity.

A word of caution. If you're going to take a break, then take a break.
Don't discuss work problems at lunch, coffee, or social gatherings with co-
workers. All of us need to be able to put aside work worries and to relax for
a few minutes before going back to face job stresses. Even if others are
unwilling or unable to stop their complaining, you at least have a choice of
whether or not you wish to be exposed to their illness. You always have
the option of placing a barrier of distance between yourself and their bitching, thus removing yourself as a "susceptible host."

The psychiatric consultation/liaison team I work with has a strongly enforced rule: *no* work problems are allowed to be discussed at lunch, coffee, or social gatherings! If there is a work problem that needs to be
discussed, it is discussed at our team meeting, a patient care conference, or
an emergency staff meeting, but not during our off-time. Of course, sometimes this rule is *very* hard to enforce, especially when there is some crisis
occurring. But it's even more necessary during a crisis to have a break from
the stress. We need to reenergize ourselves by talking about things outside
of work that give us pleasure and add a balanced perspective to the current
crisis.

Splitting

Another way of spreading or maintaining the stagnant quo is the process
of splitting. I like to describe it as the creation of two separate camps—us
and them. The us are, of course, the good guys who see things the way we
do. The them are the other ones—the archetypical bad guys, the Darth
Vaders of the organization. The them are all those other people who we
believe make our work miserable. Once you have an us and them split in
operation, it is extremely difficult to correct it; everyone is so embroiled in
fighting against the enemy that frequently the issues get lost. Furthermore,
no one is willing to compromise lest they lose ground to them. It can become like a feud, the cause of which no one even remembers: "But now
that it is a feud, we're going to fight to the finish!" "The problem isn't
mine, it's yours," they seem to say.

They become the scapegoat of the unit. A scapegoat can be a person, an
event, or a group of individuals. For example, the doctors, the hospital
administration, a particular nurse, or budget cuts can become the scape-
goats responsible for *all* the unit problems. When you polarize issues or

people, you have not only found someone or something to blame for your misery, but you also are no longer able to evaluate what is happening to you objectively. Now whenever anything bad occurs, it's the scapegoat's fault. If something happens to go right, it "certainly couldn't have anything to do with the (scapegoat) . . . in fact, it probably happened despite them!" you tell yourself. At this point, you are totally blind to available data that could correct or alter your view. Nothing can change your opinion, and you even start to amass data supporting your view; at the same time, you selectively ignore information that could threaten your opinion of the scapegoat's evil. You may even find that to maintain your hatred of the scapegoat and your view that the scapegoat is to blame for everything, you start avoiding any contact with "them." The more contact you have with people, the more difficult it is to see them as totally bad. Once you start to know them as real, complete people, you may start to see their point of view or notice that they too are human. For the splitting-scapegoating process to continue, you certainly must avoid resolving the differences you have; you must avoid any chance of collectively finding a solution to your mutual problem. For as long as you have a scapegoat, you can continue to disown any responsibility for what is happening. "It's all the scapegoat's fault, you assure yourself."

The natural tendency from the beginning of time was to look "on high" for the cause of human misery. In ancient times, the Greeks blamed the gods on Mount Olympus for problems here on earth. In modern times, at work, it's usually someone above us in the power hierarchy—the head nurse, the doctors, the hospital administration, or anyone else who happens to be above us. It must be someone who we believe has more power and control than we do. Essentially, you are saying, "Someone up there is dumping all these problems down on my head. I'm just a helpless victim."

Only in rare situations is there one person who alone is to blame for the state of affairs, good or bad. Especially with the complexity of health care, no one person is really totally responsible for operating the system or for providing patient care; all staff collectively contribute to both. In a way, the scapegoating of someone on high becomes a negative reenactment of a childlike fantasy. We believe that there is a fairy godmother protecting us by making the world safe and magical. But whenever we feel they aren't doing what they should, we become overwhelmed with disappointment and resentment. All our childlike faith turns into hatred.

The best approach to dealing with scapegoating and splitting is to establish an open dialogue that forces contact with the thems; this keeps the focus of discussion on the *shared* nursing care problem. Nature hates a vacuum; it fills it up. So it is with human beings. Whenever we are left not knowing—with an information vacuum—the natural tendency is to create information to fill the void. We create "perceptions" of what the other person is thinking, feeling, and believing from explanations manufactured in our own heads; we do this rather than checking our concoctions with the scapegoat. We invent personalized dialogues to explain what we don't know. More frequently than not our explanations of what the other person feels or believes are erroneous, or half-truths at best. Yet we tend to act on these false assumptions as long as there is no situation that forces us to confront the other person and hear his or her thoughts.

Meetings that compel both sides to sit down and share views and mutual problems help to correct these manufactured false beliefs. Once you have increased contact with them, you frequently realize that they have similar feelings and concerns; you discover that they are usually attempting to accomplish the same end—good patient care and personal job satisfaction. They're neither all good nor all bad, just human beings struggling with problems and experiencing stress. Also, once you begin a dialogue, you soon realize the need to accept some of the responsibility for working together toward a solution. When this happens, you've disturbed the stagnant quo.

Old-Timer–Newcomer

Dissatisfaction and anxiety that may be perceived as stress can also spread from the old-timers to the newcomers. The old-timers are staff who have worked in the setting for a long period of time. Many times, when a stagnant quo exists, even adding new personnel won't change the overall functioning of the system or the staff morale; this is because the old-timers manage to inflict their pessimism and defeatism on the new staff.

When the newer staff person makes suggestions to help eliminate the stagnant quo, older staff can frequently be heard advising them, "Hey, we've already tried all these ideas you're suggesting. Believe us, they won't work. Nothing works around here. Don't get so involved, just relax, go with the program, and forget it. You'll last a lot longer."

The new staff, with their enthusiasm and energy, actually become a threat to the stagnant quo, especially since the old-timers are probably so defeated they simply don't have the energy to undertake more change. The old-timers may have learned to survive in the system by detaching themselves from problems but continue to take pot shots from the sidelines in the form of complaints and bitching. Sometimes, when new staff sense the enormity of the problem and the lack of commitment by the old-timers to rectify the stagnant quo, they opt to leave the system; they would rather leave than become associated with the negative attitudes or poor quality of nursing care. Other new staff may simply attempt to battle it out single-handedly, ignoring the hopeless odds; they blindly and naively believe that if they just try hard enough, they'll succeed in the herculean task of changing everything. They usually end up frustrated and burned out.

Changing the stagnant quo requires united group effort. Staff will have to become sensitive to how the disease spreads and is maintained; they will need to devise an active plan to eradicate it (Storlie, 1979). In severe cases of stagnation staff turnover may be necessary to cure the unit's disease. On an individual level, any newcomer will have to guard against his or her vulnerability to group pessimism. One way to do this is by consciously avoiding debates with the hardened old-timers; instead, the newcomer must seek out a support group of other staff who share his or her concerns and enthusiasm.

Taking Problems Home

It is not uncommon to find that when we've been under intense job stress for an extended period of time, other areas of our lives suffer from that tension and conflict or from neglect. It is literally as if the job stress is carried home with us to contaminate our interpersonal relationships or leisure activities—introducing the stagnant quo even there. The usual demands at home become difficult to manage.

Of course, the reverse of this contamination process also occurs. Stresses at home can be taken to work; they can affect our work performance and job satisfaction. Many people who describe themselves as highly stressed can't separate out the stressors or causes for their discomfort because they are overwhelmed by every aspect of their lives (Appelbaum, 1981).

Naturally, it's hard to separate one facet of our lives from another. But during periods of high job stress, our outside interests and relationships can actually rejuvenate us and help us maintain a healthy perspective. People who have satisfying interpersonal relationships and a healthy sense of self-worth bolstered by meaningful interactions and personal accomplishments are far more resistant than others to the devastating affects of stress (Burke and Weir, 1977).

With prolonged, intense job stress, however, you may find that when you leave work you're exhausted and not at all interested in having an active evening. The idea of jogging, socializing, going to classes, or doing housework probably feels like much more of an expenditure of energy than you can manage. Even requests by your children or pets to play or overtures of affection by a loved one feel like just more demands. You might feel like screaming, "Leave me alone! All I want to do is relax! Don't bother me. I've had another bad day at work!"

As you begin to cut down on your contact with others and stop doing things you enjoy, you probably notice feeling that your upsetting job is the only thing happening in your life. Somehow you feel as if the job has taken over your entire life. In fact, that is exactly what has happened. You've allowed the job stresses to contaminate all the other aspects of your life (Cherniss, 1980).

It is vital to compartmentalize high-stress areas of our lives so that the rest of our personal lives don't suffer. (See Chapter 7, "Focusing on the Possible: A Problem-Solving Approach.") You'll find that if you force yourself to put aside the worries of work and attempt to continue doing things that you enjoy, you will be much less apt to allow the job stress to devastate your life.

CONCLUSION

If you are working in an environment dominated by the stagnant quo, you can take steps to relieve the stress this causes by separating yourself from the complainers, developing channels of communication with them, and protecting your personal life from work intrusions.

REFERENCES

Appelbaum, H. 1981. *Stress management for health care professionals.* Rockville, Md.: Aspen Publishers.

Berne, E. 1964. *Games people play.* New York: Ballantine Books.

Burke, R. J., and Weir, T. 1977. Marital helping relationships: the moderators between stress and well-being. *J. Psychol.* 95:121–130.

Cherniss, C. 1980. Individual factors in job stress. In *Staff burnout: job stress in the human services,* editor, C. Cherniss. Beverly Hills, Calif.: Sage Publications, pp. 137–141.

Dorland's Illustrated Medical Dictionary, 25th ed. 1974. Philadelphia: W. B. Saunders Co.

Morrison, E. 1980. Family therapy as prevention. In *Community mental health nursing: an ideological perspective.* St. Louis. The C. V. Mosby Co.

Raher, R. H., and Holmes, T. H. 1967. The Social Readjustment Rating Scale. *J. Psychosomatics Research* 11:213–218.

Storlie, F. J. 1979. Burnout: the elaboration of a concept. *Am. J. Nurs.* December:2108–2111.

Wolfe, L., Weitzel, M. H., and Fuerst, E. 1979. *Fundamentals of nursing,* 6th ed. Philadelphia: J. B. Lippincott Co.

Yalon, I. 1970. *The theory and practice of group psychotherapy.* New York: Basic Books, Inc., Publishers.

CHAPTER 15

Developing Social Support: We're All in This Together

EMILY E. M. SMYTHE

HOW SOCIAL SUPPORT CAN HELP

One day, on your way to work, you come upon a traveling medicine show, like those of yesteryear. You can't believe what you hear the medicine man say. "The miracle cure . . . this elixir is guaranteed to cure all your physical aches and pains caused by that everyday demon, stress! Believe me, ladies and gentlemen, there is nothing like this known to modern man. It can even help make you immune to those awful stress-related diseases of heart attack, arthritis, migraine headaches—to name only a few of the hundreds of ailments it is known to alleviate. It can even help to prevent cancer! Yes-sir-ee folks, you'll have to try it to believe it! What's more, research—yes, *research*—has validated my claims, enabling me to give you a money-back guarantee if you're not completely satisfied. So don't be nervous, don't hesitate, just step right up and buy a little bottle of this magical potion called 'social support'."

You, along with every other skeptic in the crowd who hears these wild claims, probably don't believe your eyes and ears. "How could 'social support', be so helpful in managing stress?'' you ask yourself. Yet the medicine man is able to back up his claims by hard, solid, objective evidence. He produces the type of evidence we've all learned to know and trust: scientific research conducted under rigorous standards by topnotch, high-powered, well-respected researchers at the best, well-established academic institutions. How can you doubt this type of evidence?

As you start to examine the reports he hands you to support his claims, you ask yourself, "How can social support prevent stress-related illnesses? How does social support enhance my sense of well-being?"

I'm not sure that the experts would be as extreme as our traveling medicine show man in proclaiming the virtues of social support, but research findings on its positive effects in reducing stress are fairly impressive. For example, Caplan (1981) states, "Empirical researchers confirm that exposure to high stress by individuals receiving adequate support does not increase the risk of mental or physical illness." These findings have been confirmed by numerous other respected authorities (Burke and Weir, 1977; Caplan et al., 1975; Cobbs, 1976; Cassel, 1976). One study of the mediating effects of social support on stress was conducted by the National Aeronautics and Space Administration at the Goddard Space Flight Center. In this study, physiologic responses to stress were measured (for example, hormone levels, serum glucose, and blood pressure). Participants were subjected to known job stressors, such as role ambiguity and heavy work loads. Those who had scored high on social support scales did not have the typical physiologic changes associated with the stress response and threatened health (Kiritz and Moos, 1974). The implication then was that adequate social support had made them "immune" to many job stressors.

After reviewing the available literature in 1976, Cobbs found that social support protects people in crisis from such varied pathologic states as arthritis, tuberculosis, and alcoholism, as well as from bearing infants with low birth weight, social breakdown, and even death. Social support also contributed to accelerated recovery from illness while reducing the need for pain medication (Cobbs, 1976).

In citing numerous research studies, House (1981) identified three ways that social support can decrease stress and enhance the individual's health:

> First, social support can directly enhance health and well-being because it meets important human needs for security, social contact and approval, belonging and affection. That is, positive effects of support on health can offset or counter-balance negative effects of stress.

> Second, support, at least from people at work, can directly reduce levels of occupational stress in a variety of ways and hence indirectly improve health.

> A third type of effect is the potential of social support to mitigate or buffer the impact of occupational stress on health. Here social support has no direct effect

on either stress or health but rather modifies the relation between them, much as a chemical catalyst modifies the effect that one chemical has on another.

It seems that modern-day research is beginning to "prove" what was known in Biblical times: "A faithful friend is the medicine of life" (*Apocrypha, Wisdom of Solomon*).

If, as we have seen, stress can be associated with the development of numerous physical and psychologic illnesses such as cardiovascular disease, depression, cancer, infectious diseases, gastrointestinal disorders, and a host of others, you can begin to appreciate the beneficial effects of social support in buffering illness and promoting health. Perhaps, then, the medicine show man wasn't totally falsifying his claims after all!

You must remember, though, that stress is a complex phenomenon. Being "stressed" and experiencing distress as a result involve the interaction of numerous interrelated variables that impinge upon us. If the demands made upon us by one or more stressors exceed our ability to cope with them, we will experience distress. If the stress is excessive and continues uncorrected over a period of time, cellular damage may occur; the net result is then physical or mental illness. So, unfortunately, although social support can buffer the effects of stress and can contribute to our resources and sense of well-being, it alone cannot prevent the wear and tear of uncontrolled stressors. As House (1981) puts it: "Social support is not now, nor will it ever be, a panacea for all problems of occupational stress and health. But it can be an important and effective component of a comprehensive effort to reduce work stress and improve health, both physical and mental."

I like to think of social support as a safety net. As I go through my hectic work day trying to balance job stresses, I can look down and see it there— my protection from too dangerous a fall. I may suffer a few minor bruises when I make a mistake, but the social support net will save me from falling into a hopeless pit of despair or depression. The security of knowing that the safety net is there gives me the confidence I need to take risks—for example, to assert my potentially controversial beliefs about patient care or to face an "angry mob" of dissatisfied family members. Sometimes I go through a whole day unaware of my social support; other days, when everything seems to be going wrong, I know it's there when I reach out to a friend for support and understanding or when I simply realize that I have a lot of great people behind me who believe in me and care about me.

Social support won't cure illness, but it can significantly protect you from the deleterious effects of occupational stress, particularly if these job stressors are givens over which you have little control. If you sincerely want to manage your job stress you will need to develop a healthy life-style that enhances your sense of well-being. (Chapter 6, "Balance: A Way of Developing a Healthy Life-Style," discusses this issue further.) Maintaining adequate social support is certainly one of the essential elements of such a life-style.

TYPES OF SOCIAL SUPPORT

There are four broad categories of social support (House, 1981). *Emotional support* is demonstrated by a person showing concern, listening, providing affection and love, and being trustworthy. *Appraisal support* is characterized by activities that are relevant to one's self-evaluation; included are such processes as affirmation and feedback. *Informational support* consists of receiving advice, information, and help with problem-solving. *Instrumental support* is derived from being given goods and services. Of these four types of social support, emotional support seems to be the most influential in enhancing one's sense of well-being and buffering the physical and psychologic disorders of stress.

All of us need emotional nurturing, yet frequently we fail to get the social support we so desperately need. Probably one of the most profound examples of how essential emotional support is was observed in the nineteenth century. Infants in foundling homes and orphanages were dying at a high rate. Some authorities estimate that as many as 95% of the infants died despite having their dietary, environmental, medical needs completely satisfied. Naturally, everyone was perplexed about why these infants would waste away and die for no apparent reason. This condition was, in fact, called *marasmus* (the Greek word for *wasting away*). The miraculous "medical" cure for this devastating condition was found to be "TLC" (tender loving care), which is simply a form of emotional support. Due to the concern for providing a clean, aseptic environment, the infants were not touched or caressed the way infants (and, I believe, adults) must be to thrive (Sehnert, 1981).

BLOCKS TO GETTING SOCIAL SUPPORT

If social support is so necessary for survival, what stops us from getting it? We, as nurses, have been taught how to give TLC to our patients; why can't we give the same degree of care to ourselves and our fellow nurses? There are many personal and professional reasons why nurses do not get or give the support we all need.

Personal Blocks

One reason is that we are afraid. We think that needing help from someone else is a sign of weakness—a personal failure. After all, we tell ourselves, "What's wrong with me that I can't cope with this job? No one else seems to be falling apart like I am." There has long been a conspiracy of silence in nursing, which has encouraged the faulty notion that if you don't see or talk about a problem, it doesn't exist. So we all walk around miserably, suffering alone. Recently this conspiracy has been broken; pick up any nursing journal and you will find articles acknowledging that nursing is a stressful profession with many unsolved problems that need to be addressed.

Some hospital administrators still identify nurses who verbalize their concerns as troublemakers and malcontents and insist that nursing supervisory staff weed them out or keep them in line. Many nursing students and practicing nurses have discovered too that if they ask questions or share their personal reactions to patients, these actions become identified as their problem areas on future performance evaluations. One may then begin to think, for example, "If I mention to my supervisor that I'm having difficulty handling dying patients, she'll think I'm incompetent and then watch everything I do." Raising concerns appropriately in this situation is not seen as a necessary step in the nurse's professional growth; instead it is taken as proof of her existing personality problems or her total failure. Frequently, beginning nursing students quickly get the message: Whatever you do, don't admit that something upsets you or that you don't know something. Fake it! Or you'll never hear the end of it. They'll label you as a problem student. Unfortunately, this negative reinforcement deprives the student and practicing nurse of valuable resources and much needed emotional support. Acknowledging weakness, they learn, only makes you vulnerable to attack.

Instead of each nurse smugly clutching her knowledge as a well-guarded secret, why can't we willingly share our expertise with each other? It seems ridiculous to expect any of us, no matter how brilliant, to know everything about everything given the complexity of modern health care. Instead of attacking another nurse who doesn't know something—as we've been attacked by physicians for years—why don't we encourage free exchange of knowledge while accepting ignorance as temporary? Being supportive is recognizing the potential for growth in each person. Where we are now is only the beginning of where we can be. Nurses have always criticized physicians for feeling and acting omnipotent and omniscient; so why are we now expecting the same of ourselves? We each have a great deal to give. We each have a great deal to learn. (One of the things that I love most about teaching is how much I can learn from my students.)

Another reason we may not seek social support at work is that we've concluded that "the only person you can count on is yourself." This attitude of going it alone probably developed from repeated disappointments and frustrations whenever we sought help from other nurses and supervisors. If you've been working short-staffed, with every nurse pushed past her limit and feeling unable to offer help to co-workers, it's not surprising that you finally decide that there's no one available to help, so why bother wasting the time and energy asking?

At times in our lives it may have been appropriate, perhaps even necessary, not to count on help from others who were unable or unwilling to give it. However, all of us need support in one form or another. Developing the personality style of "trust only thyself" in our work (discussed in Chapter 9) leads to not seeking help that is available; we face all situations as if no one is available or willing to help us. Rarely is this the case. In most instances, if we're suffering, several other co-workers are equally miserable. Collectively, the cry for help has a greater impact. Collectively, solutions for what seemed like hopeless situations can be found. The old axiom, two heads are better than one, definitely applies. At the very least, it is foolhardy to become like Atlas—carrying your world around on your shoulders all alone. A rather stressful notion! If in reality there is no social support available in your job, you might question whether the job is worth the stress you are experiencing. If your answer is yes or if you feel that you don't have the option to leave the job, look around for support that may be available outside the work environment.

You might also ask yourself, "Have I really made my needs known to other people? Have I asked for what I want?" Often we act as if other people ought to be mind-readers. We give all the nonverbal clues that we are upset and then expect the other person to know what the problem is, how we feel, and what we want them to do. When they fail to help us, we feel disappointed. "Why didn't you help me?" we ask. "Help you with what?" they reply. The more you can explicitly tell someone what you need, the better your chance is of having your needs met.

Those of us who are really stressed—especially to the severe, terminal degree of "burn-out"—tend to become socially isolated and emotionally withdrawn; again our needs for support are not met. We reason to ourselves, "I'm too exhausted from this job. I need peace and quiet—to be left alone! I don't have the energy to be with people, and anyway I'm so depressed I'm no fun to be around." We become like wounded animals that crawl into the bushes to nurse our wounds alone. Often this social withdrawal is not due to a lack of energy so much as it is to shame and embarrassment. This is especially true if many of our friends are co-workers who seem to be coping well with the same work problems.

We can also miss out on needed social support because we spend all of our time and energy complaining to others rather than truly communicating. The complaining, if done over and over again, leaves the other person drained of energy and uninterested in our problems. Complaining really doesn't promote closeness. It may, in fact, have the opposite effect. It may widen the distance between people once it becomes the exclusive mode of social interaction.

If we already have a damaged self-image and feel insecure in our interpersonal relations, we may not seek social support for fear of being rejected. We start to withdraw from social contact under stress because we feel that others will be uninterested or bored with our problems; we may believe that they'll see us as a burden. "Who wants to listen to all my problems? They're too depressing. I don't blame people for not wanting to be around me these days." Naturally our withdrawal behavior stems from our diminished sense of self-worth; but it also tends only to reinforce our faulty belief system: "If anyone really knew me, they'd reject me." So we leave the other person first or avoid the interpersonal contact before being rejected or abandoned. We never test our faulty premise that we're no good and so no one will care about us. We end up feeling abandoned in our hour of need because we can't risk asking for help that we fear won't be given.

Professional Blocks

In addition to personal reasons for not getting needed social support, there are reasons related to splits within the nursing profession that contribute to nurses' feeling alienated from and unsupported by other nurses. "United we stand, divided we fall." Perhaps this should become a primary motto of the nursing profession. Some of the splits center on issues like whether one is a "professional" or a "technical" nurse (or a degree rather than a diploma nurse); the use of temporary staff; the fragmentation of patient care; and the dynamics of "victimization." All these issues contribute to our lack of mutual support, increased perception of stress, and inability to solve professional problems.

The debate over the existence of two separate levels of nursing functions has raged for well over a decade. Proponents of the notion that there are and should be two distinctly separate levels of nursing education and practice advocate that the technical nurse (typically a nurse with an associate degree earned in a two-year college program) is prepared to perform the more mechanical and concrete tasks of nursing but does not have the broader theoretical knowledge base necessary for the complex functions of the "professional" nurse. Professional nurses, on the other hand, with a minimal baccalaureate degree in nursing (BSN) following four or more years in a university or college, are thought, for example, to assume greater responsibility for health care delivery. Such responsibility includes doing advanced problem-solving and setting priorities that include delegating tasks to their subordinates (the technical nurses, licensed vocational nurses, and nurse's aides) (Sehnert, 1981; Rogers, 1972; American Nursing Association, 1978). However valid and possibly necessary this movement toward two separate levels of nursing may be, it tends to increase our view of ourselves as separate entities rather than as a collective, collaborating group. Many nurses who do not have the BSN degree now endorsed by the American Nursing Association for professional training feel that their skills, education, and professional competence are being belittled. This is causing resentment and an ever-widening split between technical and professional nurses. It's hard to give support to or ask for understanding from someone you believe feels superior to you!

Rather than devaluing of technical nurse's skill and training or attacking professional nurses because they lack technical skills and have their "heads in the clouds," we need to develop career-ladder programs that offer anyone in the nursing community the opportunity to move, as desired, to various levels of nursing. Each level is not only clearly needed but also offers distinctly valuable services. Unfortunately, we seem to be acting like members of other underprivileged, low-status minorities who engage in horizontal violence against one of their own who advances beyond the group's status and power through pursuit of more education. Instead of both levels of nurses helping each other advance by sharing knowledge and skills, we attack each other mercilessly. I believe that those who have to make themselves look good by attacking others must have extremely low opinions of themselves. If you truly value what you have to offer, you need not belittle others for what they offer.

> The further apart we are, the smaller our relative numbers and the less chance of being able to have a successful impact on the health care system and to make the changes necessary for quality patient care and satisfying professional lives. The further apart we are, the more controlled and powerless we are as a group. (Dean, 1982).

It may be wise for us to pay close attention to Ben Franklin's sage advice on this matter: "Speak ill of no man but speak all the good you know about everyone."

Another factor tending to divide rather than unite nurses is the fact that many hospitals attempt to deal with severe personnel shortages by utilizing nursing registries and/or "float pools" composed of per diem staff. Temporary staff may feel no identity with the hospital; thus, they may not feel at all responsible for resolving hospital problems or patient care issues beyond the immediate and direct concerns of the shift to which they are assigned. There is nothing inherently wrong with the use of registries or staff pools; in fact, this type of "fee-for-service" approach to nursing care provides a creative solution to staffing shortages. However, on the negative side, temporary nurses who do not view themselves as part of the regular staff are less apt to give corrective feedback to the system, address the long-range issues of patient care and hospital policies, or to give collegial support to co-workers. Of course, this is only natural since in many instances nurses seek this type of temporary employment after experiences in health care systems that were unresponsive to their needs or concerns. Another source of friction is the difficulty of assuring the competence of registry nurses, who may not have been adequately screened or required to meet the standards of minimal competency required of permanent staff.

In any event, the existence of temporary staff certainly doesn't lead to a sense of shared concern or group cohesion. Frequently, temporary and permanent staff feel alienated from each other and may even sabotage or "dump on" each other. The permanent staff may say something like, "Give her all the tough patients. She's getting paid more; let her work more!" Or, "Who cares what she thinks about our unit? We don't need her criticism.

She doesn't know what's going on around here." The temporary staff person may think, "Why kill myself? I won't be here tomorrow. No point making waves by questioning the care of the patient. I'm just getting paid to do eight hours." The temporary staff may function like horses with blinders, plodding along, not seeing any of the peripheral issues. Although this may be a somewhat exaggerated picture of the way temporary and permanent staff view each other, such dynamics are usually operating to some degree, leaving both sides feeling unsupported and alienated. This situation simply adds to each individual's feeling of isolation and contributes to stress and frustration.

In many in-patient settings nurses also feel separated from each other as a result of the "team" concept of nursing care, which fragments patient care into specific tasks and responsibilities that are assigned to different nurses. One staff member, typically a practical or technical nurse or nursing attendant who is seen as lower in status than other members of the team, is assigned the less pleasant tasks. We all know these well—emptying bed pans, giving bed baths, assisting patients in ambulating, answering call lights. The nurse with higher status (BSN, team leader, or more experienced RN) performs the tasks that supposedly require more expertise and knowledge: passing medications, countersigning orders, performing specific procedures, communicating with the physicians. Sometimes there is an additional nurse with even higher status who coordinates a team of patients and staff; this individual would be the assistant head nurse, team leader, or charge nurse. No one staff member knows the patient completely because each one only focuses on a part of the patient's care. I met one patient who said, "I've met five nurses today and I still don't know who's taking care of me. When I ask one of the nurses for a pain pill, she says she'll have to get 'the nurse.' If I ask 'the nurse' for the bed pan, she tells me to wait a minute and she'll get 'my nurse.' Each time I want something I have to wait for the right nurse." Another patient put it this way: "To one nurse I'm a pill taker, to another I'm a bed pan sitter, to another I'm a body with a dressing that needs to be changed." This type of task orientation to patient care has tended to not only fragment the patient's care but has also tended to split the nursing staff into warring factions based on status. (I, for one, am hopeful about and pleased with the move toward primary nursing, which is aimed at decreasing fragmentation of patient care.)

The dynamics of "victim psychology" also operate in the nursing profession. When it occurs, the "horizontal violence" that characterizes victim psychology adds to the existing stresses in nursing and significantly hampers our ability to get support from one another.

Victim psychology is characterized by the concept that individuals in lower-status positions often tend to feel alienated from their peers. Rather than offering support and collectively defending their rights, they may pull against each other in backbiting or in open competition. Brooten and co-authors note: "As a group (nurses) are competitive, but unlike other groups that compete in the outside world for money, status and power, we compete with each other and tend to withhold support from those within our ranks who show signs of succeeding" (Brooten et al., 1978). Nurses, as low-status participants in the health care system, may not value acceptance by their low-status peers and may openly avoid being identified as nurses. Our concern with acceptance by the higher-status groups—physicians and hospital administrators—may deter us from supporting our low-status peers or even encourage us to openly attack fellow nurses. This kind of horizontal violence is typical of low-status groups who identify with the aggressor; members of the low-status group are, at times, more critical and harsh toward peers than are members of a high-status group. Many nursing authors believe that nurses' devaluation of themselves—as a profession and as individuals—stems from the fact that 98% of the nursing profession is female; we have been socialized, as women, to question our self-worth and to see ourselves as second-class citizens (Hughes, 1982; Dean, 1978; Heide, 1973). As novelist Erica Jong (1977) points out, "Every woman who has ever excelled in her field also knows that the bitterest experience of all is the lack of support, the envy, the bitterness we frequently get from our female colleagues. We are hard on ourselves and hard on each other, and women not only hold support from women, they openly attack. We have too little charity for each other's work and are too apt to let the male establishment pit us against each other."

An example of this phenomenon occurred in a series of stress management workshops that I presented. Staff from various levels of nursing felt abused and insulted by their fellow nurses. LPNs claimed that the RNs thought they were better than the LPNs and that the RNs were only interested in giving orders, not in listening to the LPNs' feedback. The RNs said that the assistant head nurses were removed from patient care and were more interested in minor administrative duties than in the needs of patients. The assistant head nurses felt that the head nurses and unit coordinators were solely interested in getting enough bodies to work the shifts, in adhering to policies, and in completing reports, rather than in staff or patient needs. The representatives of each nursing level felt that what they were doing was for the patient and that they alone were concerned most about patient care. Someone must be wrong. How could these nurses see the same situation from such different perspectives, leaving everyone feeling attacked and unsupported? What keeps each nurse from respecting the contributions of every other nurse? Certainly this devaluation of co-workers does little to improve the image of the nursing profession. The job of nursing is sufficiently difficult without our feeling attacked by our peers; they, if anyone, should understand and be sympathetic to the job stresses in nursing.

All too frequently we feel attacked from all sides with little or no support from within our own nursing ranks. Besides our colleagues' hostility, we often bear the brunt of patients' and their families' frustration, sense of powerlessness, and unending demands generated out of fear. Despite these attacks, we are expected to respond with sympathy and understanding while somehow single-handedly controlling our own reactions to our patients' and their families' sometimes cruel behavior. At times we may also be the target of physicians' displaced anger and frustration. Many physicians have unreasonable expectations of our ability to handle overwhelmingly complex situations; they may become enraged when their orders are not followed to the letter, regardless of the reasons for failure. After a day of being attacked from all sides, we may simply not have any remaining energy to support our fellow nurses. Giving much needed support to co-workers should be as high a priority as meeting patient needs!

Unfortunately, in many work settings it is far easier to be the object of criticism and self-belittlement than it is to receive support and help. Nurses operating under high-stress situations may be too survival-oriented to consider the needs of colleagues. Instead of having a reciprocal, supportive network of peers, we develop pecking orders that only dole out stress to those lower in the hierarchy. This displacement of anger does much to fan the flames and maintain a high level of job dissatisfaction and frustration; it keeps us at each other's throats instead of engaging in collective problem-solving or providing needed emotional support.

ASSESSING THE SOCIAL SUPPORT SYSTEM

How do we go about obtaining this much needed social support from our peers despite all the obstacles just discussed? Caplan (1974) has stated that social support systems are enduring interpersonal ties with people upon whom we can rely to provide us with emotional sustenance, feedback, resources, and assistance when we are in need. Typically, these supportive people share our values and beliefs; they allow us to expose our concerns and fears without worrying about ridicule or condemnation.

Naturally, there are many types and various degrees of social support. Ideally our social support comes from a number of people who make up a complex social network. We need support not only from friends and family outside of our work environment but also from co-workers and supervisory personnel on the job. Support may come from extremely intimate and close significant others, or it may come from mere acquaintances who provide assistance but with whom we wouldn't feel comfortable sharing our innermost feelings or concerns.

Support can be informational, such as that provided by supervisors, knowledgeable co-workers, or various, identified, resource personnel. Part of this informational support may also be in the form of relevant, corrective feedback about our job performance. Those who give us this type of support help to provide educational growth, validate our sense of mastery and competence, and stimulate our excitement and creativity in our work.

When we think of support, however, we more frequently think of emotional support rather than informational support. When we look for support, most of us think of having other people who will "be there" for us, unconditionally caring about our well-being—a spouse, lover, or intimate friend who gives us emotional support. Both informational and emotional support are essential parts of a social support network that will protect us from work stress while enhancing our sense of well-being. Expecting one or two people alone to meet all of our needs for support is a drastic mistake, similar to putting all of one's eggs in one basket.

At times, we have less need for someone to provide emotional support than for an expert nurse who can be a critical observer, providing valuable corrective feedback of our nursing practice. "In effect, a supportive social network complements and supplements those specific aspects of [our] functioning which are weakened by the effects of the stressful experience" (Caplan, 1981). To provide maximum protection from stress, social support should come from the work environment and from our friends and family outside of work. At this point it might be helpful to evaluate your social support systems both on the job and outside of work.

SOCIAL SUPPORT INVENTORY

The following questions are designed to help you identify your social supports. After completing the inventory, you should be able to determine if you have adequate support. The inventory will also help you identify the types of support you might need and who in your life might provide this support.

Outside Your Work Environment

1. Who in your life provides you with support by meeting your emotional needs (giving love, listening to your concerns, offering a shoulder to cry on, giving praise)?
2. Do you feel supported by your relatives?
3. Are your close personal friends nurturing, understanding, *and* available?
4. Are there people who meet your informational needs (give moral, ethical, or spiritual advice, for example, a religious leader, teacher, therapist, guru; give financial or legal advice; give health care advice)?
5. Are there people who meet your service needs (child care, house/apartment sitting, transportation, repair people you trust)?

SOCIAL SUPPORT INVENTORY (continued)

6. Do you know your neighbors and feel that you're a part of your neighborhood?
7. Do you belong to social clubs/organizations in your community (church, civic groups, PTA)?
8. Do you support political, ecological, or social groups that endorse your beliefs?
9. How frequently do you get together with friends by phone or for visits?
10. Are there people whom you care about and enjoy being with but whom you haven't seen recently? If so, what's stopping you from getting together with them?

In Your Work Environment

1. Are there co-workers with whom you can talk about job and/or personal concerns?
2. Are co-workers willing to provide help with patient care?
3. Are there nursing experts in your work setting who provide needed expertise and advice (in-service personnel, supervisors, experienced co-workers)? Are they available?
4. Is your supervisor emotionally supportive and understanding? Does your supervisor seem competent? Is your supervisor available?
5. Are there people at work whose criticism and feedback you value and find useful?
6. Do co-workers encourage your professional advancement/ growth?
7. Are there adequate ancillary services (pharmacy, transportation, social service) and equipment in your job?
8. Are you active in your professional organizations?
9. Are there organized staff group meetings where you work (regular nursing care plan meetings, staff meetings, support groups, team meetings, interdisciplinary meetings)?
10. Do you belong to any committees at your place of work?
11. Do you seek out educational opportunities for furthering your professional growth?

In our personal lives and our work environments there are numerous people who could potentially provide us with emotional support. Frequently, the problem isn't that potentially supportive people don't exist but that we are trapped into feeling alone and alienated because we are afraid to risk closeness with other people. Freudenberger (1980), in discussing closeness as a cure for burn-out, states: "Our A-No. 1 barrier to closeness is not *talking;* the second is not listening." If you think for a moment, I'm sure you can remember a situation when you wanted to get to know someone or share something with him or her but remained silently isolated while the moment slipped away! Of course, whenever you venture close to another person, you take a chance. There is absolutely *no* guarantee that the person will be delighted, or even mildly pleased, with the opportunity to become your friend. But I believe the chance of being rejected is worth the potential reward of reaching out to another person.

Friendship redoubleth joys and cutteth griefs in halves.

Bacon

One of the main goals in crisis intervention therapy is reopening the social network of the client in crisis. People under stress are more suggestible and potentially open to reaching out. Rather than waiting until work stress reaches a crisis level, however, it is better to establish a supportive social network by risking closeness.

The question, then, is how willing are you to become close to other people?

QUESTIONS TO EVALUATE YOUR WILLINGNESS FOR CLOSENESS

1. Do you express what you really want or feel? Or do you stop yourself by evaluating your feelings or worrying about how you will be judged by other people?
2. Are you able to listen to other people rather than forming an opinion about them based upon your preconceptions?
3. Do you feel comfortable sharing your fears and dreams with someone once you've gotten to know him or her?
4. Do you feel that most people who know you have a fairly accurate picture of who you are? Or do you hide your "real" self from everyone?

DEVELOPING AND MAINTAINING SOCIAL SUPPORT

In addition to being open to closeness, there are a number of ways by which you can increase your social support.

Outside of Work

We all need to become aware of the ways we can support each other informally on a daily basis, as well as through more formal approaches to establishing group support. Sometimes, the support we get from people outside work is just as important in reducing work-related stress as that produced by using stress-reduction techniques. The following suggestions are aimed at establishing and maintaining social support outside of the work setting.

1. Build support "rituals." Think for a moment about your favorite holiday season. What is it about this holiday that makes it so special? Probably one of the factors is that you renew friendships by getting together with people who are important to you. You also have rituals that you reenact. These rituals provide a continuity with your past while affirming a bond with your present loved ones. But why wait for those celebrations once or twice a year? Make support rituals a part of your life on a much more frequent basis. Plan celebrations for each holiday at home and at work; include decorations, music, and special foods. You'll feel a part of the holiday spirit and a sense of belonging with others.

2. Make a "family" celebration. If you are isolated in a distant place away from your family and old friends, create an "orphan" celebration. Get together with other unattached friends and co-workers. Each person can share his or her special childhood ritual or food. After spending one depressing Thanksgiving Day alone, I swore I'd never go through that agony again. For Christmas that year I decided to have a get-together of all the "orphans" I knew. It was such a delightful success that we all got together for nearly every holiday over the next three years. We'd even celebrate minor holidays like Ground Hog Day or create our own. None of us ever had to feel alone or unwanted.

3. Don't forget your birthday. Some of us hide our birthdays, but birthdays are special days for everyone, even those who resent aging. Make a fuss over your own as well as those of your friends, family members, and co-workers. Create a party. The guest of honor will feel special and well supported. Also don't forget to plan something for your own birthday if others haven't. Tell friends that you'd like to have them over to share your birthday celebration. Tell them that no gifts are necessary, just the gift of friendship.

4. Schedule regular get-togethers. If you live a hectic, stressed life, you may find that months somehow go by when you never get together with special people. Your best bet is to have a regular, monthly get-together (for example, the first Tuesday of each month). Force yourself to socialize by purchasing season tickets to a theater group or concerts.

5. Extend your circle of friends. When you have get-togethers, ask your friends to bring along other friends whom you don't know. It can be difficult to meet people in large, unfriendly cities. If you extend your circle of friends, you literally multiply your chances of meeting interesting people. You also avoid the hassles of trying to sort out strangers in singles' bars where you can end up feeling like a piece of merchandise being sized up.

6. Seek people through your interests. Rather than looking for available people by going to bars or singles' clubs, meet people through your existing interests, such as sports, politics, community action groups, child play groups, PTA. You will be supporting yourself by participating in the activity; in addition, you will be providing yourself the opportunity to meet congenial people.

7. *Join organizations.* Actively participate in groups that support your beliefs. If you feel strongly that the air ought to be cleaner, for example, seek out a group that endorses this belief; become involved in their activities. Do not allow yourself to develop anomie. Anomie is a subjective sense of purposelessness that develops when we do not have values that give our lives meaning and direction (Powell, 1958). The more we can do to build in a sense of belonging to society at large, as well as a sense of direction and meaning in our lives, the less apt we are to feel like overwhelmed victims of social stressors.

8. *Reach out and touch someone.* The telephone advertisement to "reach out, reach out and touch someone" makes a significant social statement. Decrease the physical distance between yourself and those you care about by using your phone. If you have moved away from supportive others, maintain your connection with them.

9. *Special little touches mean a lot.* When you care for someone who is suffering or overstressed, you can sometimes do more by sending a card or flowers or by taking him or her out to a play than you can by discussing problems ad infinitum. An old sage I knew once said, "A gift should be something the person would love to have but feels he really shouldn't get." A frivolous special treat that creates a special moment can go a long way toward cheering up a stressed-out friend.

10. *Turn drudgery into a party.* There is nothing worse than having to move! Wrong. Moving can become one big party with friends getting together to share the work and celebration at the end of the day. Any unbearable chore seems less miserable if it's shared with friends. At least you have someone to complain to and at best you can enjoy the experience by making the most of it. Look for the silver lining in each cloud. For example, when my husband and I lived in an apartment, we both hated to do laundry. Doing the laundry became a "Mexican standoff" with neither side willing to give an inch. Our solution, which became a cherished ritual, was to save up our laundry for as long as we could (sometimes three weeks). Then we would go together to a neighborhood laundry located several doors from a Chinese restaurant. After putting the laundry into the washers, we'd order our dinner and then alternate return trips to the laundry to load the dryers and put in extra change. It was a pleasant dinner out; and it seemed to halve the time required to do the miserable laundry.

At Work

Now that we've discussed support outside of work, I offer the following suggestions for giving support to peers and supervisors within the work setting and for getting the same in return. These, of course, are only a few of the possibilities. Ideally, once you recognize the need for support in your work environment, you will begin actively to seek out opportunities to give and get support in all of your interactions with co-workers.

1. Welcome the newcomer. Because of the high turnover in nursing staff in many facilities, existing staff may withhold support from new staff because it seems like wasted energy. Ideally, all staff should contribute to the orientation of new staff. Showing new staff members around the unit and introducing them to others requires no formal education! The more involved all staff are in welcoming new personnel, the more responsible they will feel for protecting newcomers and integrating them into the social structure of the unit. New nursing staff should also be introduced to nonnursing personnel with whom they will be expected to work—physicians, social workers, and pharmacists. This process conveys the message that we're all working together to provide patient care and that we feel that each nurse is an important contributor.

A buddy-system, in which one staff member coordinates the orientation of a newcomer, can be helpful. This arrangement allows the new person an opportunity to develop a trusting relationship with at least one other person. It also allows the orienting staff person the opportunity to carefully assess the newcomer's strengths and needs for further learning. Orientation shouldn't just be restricted to the first few weeks. Integrating new personnel into the system may continue for several months, especially if the orientee is a new graduate or a nurse returning to work after being inactive for many years. It is helpful to have a checklist for orientation that identifies the skills and tasks the newcomer must know how to perform. With a checklist as a guide, the newcomer can learn and demonstrate skills under the supervision of a previously certified staff member. This insures that the orientee has been adequately supervised in all areas of care, allows the supervising staff to share their knowledge, and provides the orientee an opportunity to assimilate new information at a comfortable pace. Having the checklist also indicates to orientees that we expect them to have questions and to need to learn some things, and that their lack of knowledge isn't seen as a failure, but as a normal condition to be remedied by the orientation process. This attitude toward learning encourages the orientee to ask questions. We have to indicate to all nurses that it's acceptable not to know everything as long as you're willing to ask for help and to learn.

2. Spread the learning. Learning shouldn't be something we do only in school. It is a life process—a process that enriches through sharing. Unfortunately, in nursing we fail to support each other by sharing openly and freely what we know or by acknowledging our expertise. An individual's growth to professional status can be fostered by mentors—guides who are accomplished nursing practitioners. Mentors in nursing can be colleagues who are willing to help other nurses learn and grow. They share wisdom from their own experience, which in many cases has been painfully learned. When I first graduated, there was a dynamic leader who helped in my transition from graduate to professional. Sometimes I think I would never have continued in nursing if it hadn't been for her help. Her role as my mentor was a combination of teacher and big sister. She was willing to question my brash assumptions and suggest alternate approaches to problems, and she always provided an excellent role model. Is there someone in your work setting who is or could be your mentor? Is there someone for whom you can be a mentor? Being a mentor is much more supportive than being a Monday-morning-quarterback who sits on the sidelines criticizing co-workers. It can also be a very rewarding role!

We must also remember that nursing supervisors are nurses, too. Once a nurse becomes a supervisor, she may no longer be seen by staff as "one of us." Instead she becomes "one of them," or management. It is true that many nursing supervisory staff sever their ties with staff nurses. Ideally, however, "supervision in the human services is intended to serve and support the staff. . . . Supervision serves a 'professional development' function as well as an administrative control function. . . . At its best, supervision becomes a mentor relationship. . . . In many settings, there also is a strong expectation that supervisors will help the worker to understand and constructively manage his or her own emotional response to the work" (Cherniss, 1980). The supervisor can become a staff advocate.

The supervisor also needs the support of the staff nurses. Sometimes, as a result of the perplexing problems in nursing, the supervisor becomes identified as the person who should be able to solve all our problems. I've heard unit staff complain about being overworked and short-staffed; they insist that the real problem is that the nursing supervisor won't give them more help. Do we really think that out of spite supervisors refuse to give us the several nurses that they have stashed away somewhere? They are experiencing the same stress! Rather than displacing our anger and frustration onto supervisors, and risking alienating them, why not try a collective approach? We're all in this together! Until we *really* buy this notion, we are only going to continue to divide ourselves.

If you are a supervisor in this situation, you too must acknowledge your impotence to solve the problem immediately. However, if you are willing to listen, to be responsive to your staff's concerns, you will at least be giving the staff much needed support. You will also then able to be a spokesperson for your staff in administrative deliberations. The time has come for nursing supervision to stop being a process of "keeping the girls in line." Nursing has progressed well beyond the point of being a "calling" or "mission." Nursing supervisors also need to stop protecting staff as though they were little children who can't survive the ugly truths of budget cuts, conflicting priorities, or in-house politics. It's not necessary for supervisors dealing with various frustrations and stresses to come crying to staff. It would be helpful, however, for the staff to have a realistic understanding of the administrative position on various issues and also of what steps are being taken to correct problems. An open dialogue between management and staff is essential (perhaps similar to what has successfully been practiced in many growing Japanese companies). Sharing yearly reports from administration give the nursing staff, as well as stockholders, a sense of being a part of the organization's concerns and growth. A good rule of thumb is to avoid alienating any of your supports. Don't foster splits between staff and management. Increase the dialogue and appreciation for each other's concerns and problems. Nursing needs to support its leaders as well as to get support from them.

3. *Develop peer support groups.* One of the best ways to establish formal support is through peer support groups. Peer support groups can be developed for any peer group—from staff nurses to nurse administrators. Peer groups can be developed for nurses within the organization of a particular unit or by nurses from different work environments. These groups also increase members' empathy for each other by allowing nurses to give to other nurses what we know how to give so well to our patients—time to listen and a willingness to show concern. By openly sharing work concerns, members can reduce some of the emotional tension while validating or altering their perceptions of work events. Once an open dialogue is established with co-workers, it becomes more difficult to project concerns or displace frustration onto them. The knowledge gained from "walking a mile in someone else's shoes" can alter what appears to be a hopeless standoff. In addition to improving communication and producing empathy, peer support groups provide an excellent opportunity for collective problem-solving, for stimulating new ideas, and for sharing professional expertise. Maslach's research on burn-out with health professionals indicates that staff members who are able to share their concerns with co-workers have a lower degree of work stress and lower rate of burn-out (Maslach, 1976). Members of peer support groups can also identify common concerns and then take active steps to learn new skills or techniques for handling work or professional problems. Some groups have concentrated on members' learning assertive skills, mastering relaxation techniques, or taking direct action to correct problems in the work setting.

A word of caution, however, is necessary. Peer support groups can become disastrous experiences if they are established as encounter groups in which members bare their souls and feel exposed and unsupported. Support groups are also not intended to become psychotherapy sessions. Staff who get caught up in rescuing a disturbed colleague usually are unable to work well together; they may develop a need to protect their co-worker rather than help him or her seek professional help.

Another potential pitfall of peer support groups is that they can unintentionally become a forum for confrontation in which personal conflicts are acted out in a vicious moblike attack upon one helpless victim. Peer support groups, in addition, are not intended to fulfill administrative responsibilities. If a staff member is not performing his or her job adequately, it is not the responsibility of peers to discipline the incompetent individual.

Finally, there needs to be an explicit rule that confidentiality is always respected. What is discussed in the group stays in the group. It doesn't become the latest material for gossip.

CONCLUSION

It has been demonstrated that when work group cohesiveness is high, there is a decrease in anxiety about work-related concerns and perceived work stress (Seashore and Barnowe, 1972). Social support is not a substitute for personal responsibility in your stress management, nor will it compensate for institutional stressors. It is, however, an essential ingredient in stress management.

REFERENCES

American Nursing Association. 1978. *Identification and titling of establishment of two categories of nursing practice.* ANA Conference Resolution 56.

Brooten, D. A., Hayman, L., and Naylor, M. 1978. *Leadership for change: a guide for the frustrated nurse.* Philadelphia: J. B. Lippincott Co.

Burke, R. J., and Weir, T. 1977. Marital helping relationships: the moderators between stress and well-being *J. Psychol.* 95:121–130.

Caplan, G. 1974. *Support systems and community mental health.* New York: Behavioral Publications.

Caplan, G. 1981. Mastery of stress: psychosocial aspects. *Am. J. Psychiatry* 138:413–420.

Caplan, R. D., Cobb, S., French, J. R., et al. 1975. *Job demands and worker health.* Washington, D.C.: National Institute of Occupational Safety and Health. (DHEW publication No. 75-160.)

Cassel, J. 1976. The contribution of the social environment to host resistance. *Am. J. Epidemiol.* 102:107–123.

Cherniss, C. 1980. The impact of supervision and social support from staff. In *Staff burnout.* Beverly Hills, Calif.: Sage Publications.

Cobbs, S. 1976. Social support as a moderator of life stress. *Psychosomatic Med.* 38:300–314.

Dean, P. G. 1978. Toward androgeny: victim psychology and the socialization of women. *Image* 10:10–14.

Dean, P. G. 1982. Go ahead, I'm behind you . . . way behind you. In *Socialization, sexism and stereotyping: women's issues in nursing,* editor J. Muff. St. Louis: The C. V. Mosby Co.

Freudenberger, H. J. 1980. *Burnout: how to beat the high cost of success.* Toronto: Bantam Books.

Heide, W. 1973. Nursing and women's liberation: a parallel. *Am. J. Nurs.* 73: 824.

House, J. S. 1981. *Work stress and social support.* Reading, Mass.: Addison-Wesley Pub. Co.

Hughes, L. 1982. Little girls grow up to be wives and mommies. In *Socialization, sexism and stereotyping: women's issues in nursing,* editor J. Muff. St. Louis: The C. V. Mosby Co.

Jong, E. 1977. Speaking of love. *Newsweek.* Feb. 21, p. 11.

Kiritz, S., and Moos, R. H. 1974. Review article: physiological effects of social environments. *Psychosomatic Med.* 36:96–114.

Maslach, C. 1976. Burn-out. *Human Behav.* 5:16–22.

Powell, E. H. 1958. Occupation, status and suicide: toward a redefinition of anomie. *Am. Sociolog. Rev.* 23:131–139.

Rogers, M. E. 1972. Nursing: to be or not to be. *Nurs. Outlook.* 20:42–46.

Seashore, S. E., and Barnowe, J. T. 1972. Collar color doesn't count. *Psychol. Today* 6:53–54.

Sehnert, K. W. 1981. *Stress/unstress.* Minneapolis: Augsburg Publishing House.

CHAPTER 16

Balancing Communication: Assertive Skills

JANET MUFF

Have you ever had difficulty expressing yourself in a staff meeting? Did you find yourself feeling hopeless, resentful, angry? Were you wishing you had the courage to speak up? Hoping someone else would?

Are you intimidated by the high-pressure tactics of supervisors, physicians, teachers? Do you have trouble standing up to these sacred cows? Do you remain silent but seething? Do you speak up but sound defensive? Do you say yes when you mean no?

Have you ever needed to give someone counseling? Did you avoid the problem, hoping things would change? Did you find yourself beating around the bush? Or did you find yourself being overly harsh when you finally gave the correction?

Most people have difficulty asserting themselves in some area of their lives or with some people in their lives. If you have this problem, your particular difficulty, as a nurse, may be with superiors, or subordinates, or even colleagues. The persons that give you trouble and your responses to them, whether nonassertive or aggressive, are determined by your basic personality characteristics and your upbringing. But whatever the reasons, difficulty being assertive often means that your needs are not being met, that you are unable to speak up or stand up for yourself, and that you may not feel good about yourself and your behavior. There is probably nothing more stressful than feeling that you have let yourself down.

NONASSERTIVENESS: A LEARNED RESPONSE

Naturally, the beginnings are important, and for most nurses the beginnings are in being raised female. This topic was discussed at length in Chapter 2, but briefly and most importantly, females learn to:

● Concentrate on home and family
● Emphasize nurturing and housekeeping attributes
● Live through and for others
● Rely on male providers for sustenance and status
● Focus on beauty and dress
● Avoid direct expressions of assertion, aggression, power strivings, and sexuality

The full development of their humanness is restricted.

Nursing, as a traditionally feminine occupation, is frought with traditional stereotypes and expectations. How can a nurse express anger when her role is to nurture and care for others? How can she say no to working a double shift when she has learned to live for others and place herself second? How can she express opinions in hospital committee meetings when she must live through and rely on male providers, in this case physicians? The stress, then, of being a woman in a "female" profession comes from the subjugation of oneself to males in authority and the denial of one's feelings, opinions, needs, and desires.

Many nurses, faced with societal and professional sanctions against assertiveness, *perceive* themselves as powerless to change their situations. Three factors—helplessness/powerlessness, lack of positive reinforcement, and nonrecognition, all of which have been described as stressors in nursing—lead to depression. People who are depressed are not motivated to assert themselves. The cycle is vicious and self-perpetuating. When, for example, a nurse needs something or dislikes something, she can be assertive, remain nonassertive, or become aggressive. Her behavior, to a great extent, depends upon how she *thinks* about herself and how she *perceives* her situation. The nurse who thinks of herself as relatively powerless and who perceives events as beyond her control will most often act nonassertively. She has, after all, been raised as a female to be nonassertive, and her work situation reinforces her upbringing. Certainly, some nurses are aggressive and others are assertive, but by and large, most nurses are nonassertive.

The Nonassertive Style: Thoughts, Words, Actions

How do you, as a nurse, signal your lack of assertiveness? By the way you think of yourself, by what you say to others (your verbal messages), and by how you say it (your nonverbal messages). Chapter 9 covered negative modes of thinking and unrealistic expectations both of which contribute to lack of assertiveness. This chapter concerns these stressors only in relation to nonassertiveness.

How you think about yourself contributes to and reflects your assertiveness. Consider the nurse who calls herself selfish when she refuses to come in to work on her day off, or the nurse who thinks it's unfeminine or bitchy or pushy to suggest that physicians retrieve their own charts from the chart rack, or the nurse who sees herself as a troublemaker when she defends her judgment to a nursing supervisor. In each of these cases, it is not simply what others might think or say about the nurse that is important but what she believes about herself. If you feel like a selfish, unfeminine, bitchy, pushy troublemaker, you will experience stress and you may be less assertive. Ultimately, your self-opinion will determine your assertiveness or lack of it. By the same token, your self-opinion will decrease or increase the stress you experience from being assertive.

Consider other ways of thinking that interfere with assertiveness. Do you, for example, restrict yourself to being assertive only when "an issue is of vital importance" or when "someone else will benefit" or when "you can be unemotional and in control" or if "others won't be hurt" by your behavior or when the time is "right"? Such qualifications effectively limit your assertiveness. Catastrophizing about all the terrible things that could happen if you act is another cognitive mode that inhibits assertion. How you think about yourself, the restrictions you place on self-expression, and your tendency to imagine negative consequences are the limiting factors.

The second way you signal assertiveness or nonassertiveness is by what you say to others. How *direct* are you? How *honest*? And how *spontaneous*? Directness means being able to state exactly what you think or feel to someone. Do you stud your comments with apologies and explanations? (I'm sorry about this, but would you mind moving?) Can you use "I" statements with confidence? (I do not want to work a double shift.) Do you find yourself clamming up when someone does something you don't like and then talking about it with others?

Honesty involves saying what you really mean rather than what you think you should be saying. Do you, for example, find yourself telling people what you think they want to hear? Are you reluctant to confront a peer whose actions are unprofessional? Can you speak your mind in meetings and make your opinions known?

Finally, spontaneity means expressing your honest feelings directly to the person involved at the time you are feeling them. Many of us lack spontaneity because we have learned to be indirect or dishonest. For example, a physician asks you to call another physician and request a consultation. You know that the policy of your hospital states that physicians should contact each other and not use nurses as go-betweens. Your gut says "no" but your mouth says "yes." You rationalize the yes as "not worth fighting over" or "keeping the peace" or "less hassle." You are being dishonest about your feelings and their validity. You may complain about the physician to a colleague, or you may snap at the next person who asks you for something, thus expressing your feelings indirectly. Assertiveness, then, involves recognizing your feelings (honesty) and expressing them at the time (spontaneity) to the person involved (directness).

A third way to signal your relative assertiveness is through nonverbal behaviors, including eye contact, facial expression, tone and volume of voice, and body stance. It is beyond the scope of this chapter to discuss these elements of communication except to say that nonverbal messages that are not congruent with verbal messages take precedence. For example, if you are asking for a raise and your body language connotes obsequiousness and insecurity, no matter how well thought out and assertive your words, your supervisor will attend to your behavior. The chances are you will undermine yourself.

Nonassertion: The Reasons Why

Now that we've looked at the general (social, developmental) reasons for women's nonassertiveness and can recognize nonassertive behaviors, we can begin to examine the individual dynamics that lead to nonassertion.

The first is fear—fear of displeasing others and fear of rejection. If, as we've said, women live for and through others, then women's self-esteem is tied to others. A nurse's self-esteem is tied to how much she gives to patients and to whether they and people in authority (physicians and supervisors) think she's doing a good job. Duty and self-sacrifice are the operative words, and both involve putting oneself last. The nurse is placed in a double-bind—to gain approval (and enhance her self-esteem) she must put herself last (which in turn diminishes her self-esteem). Self-esteem based on others' approval is precarious at best. The hidden lie is that others' disapproval makes one somehow bad. Asserting oneself means risking disapproval, which means loss of esteem (feeling like one is bad) which means *stress*. Many nurses choose not to take the risk and not to be assertive.

The second dynamic that leads to nonassertiveness is a mistaken sense of responsibility. If we say that the nurse feels bad about herself when others disapprove of her behavior, then we can also say the reverse: she will hold herself responsible for hurting other's feelings (she will have the power to *make* others feel bad) when she disapproves of their behavior. Again, we see the hidden lie that one person's thoughts have the power to make another person be. Again, we see the victim/narcissist connection (see Chapter 2). On the one hand, the nurse feels like the victim of others who control her; on the other, she feels responsible or guilty for controlling or hurting others. Implicit in this dynamic is a lack of separateness between self and other. Just as fear of others' disapproval inhibits the nurse's assertiveness, so does fear of the power and consequences of her own disapproval.

Believing that one does not have the right to be assertive is a third dynamic in nonassertiveness and comes in large measure from the traditional notion that women should be passive, dependent helpers. Women learn that they should rely on men for sustenance and reflected power, and female nurses do, in fact, rely on the males in their environments for these things. For example, as knights in shining armor rescued damsels in distress, so do physicians, imbued with benevolent paternalism, act as spokespersons in the media for overworked, underpaid nurses.

This brings us to the fourth dynamic leading to nonassertiveness: a reluctance to give up its benefits, namely the luxury of not being responsible and the security of not taking risks. Take the issue of questioning a doctor's order for example. Have you ever heard a nurse phrase her suggestions to a physician in a manner that suggests it was his idea? Do you know a nurse who will meekly accept a physician's wrath (at her temerity in questioning his orders) and who will complain to others about it but who won't speak up to him and "make waves"? This kind of nurse is not so different from a knight's lady, a kept woman, or a bird in a gilded cage, all of whom revoke freedom to gain luxury and security. Unfortunately, many soon find that a cage is a cage no matter how you gild the bars. A nurse who subscribes to peace-at-any-price thinking pays a high price in self-denial and stress.

AGGRESSION: A FEAR RESPONSE

Aggression and nonassertion are not so different as they seem. Both are responses to fear or anxiety, which are triggered almost automatically in certain situations.

Aggression: The Reasons Why

If we say that nonassertive behavior is in keeping with traditional female socialization, how is it that some nurses, albeit a minority, act aggressively? The connection lies in fear. Suppose an event occurs and you experience fear or anxiety. Your next response would often be anger. Then, depending upon the degree of threat and your sense of power, you would fight or flee. When our ancestors were engaged in primitive jungle combat, the choice of fight or flight was virtually automatic, as it still is in you when your life is threatened. In day-to-day anxiety-producing situations, however, fighting or fleeing are learned responses based on your perception of the situation, your role, and your relative power. The key point is that the response often *seems* so automatic that whichever emotion you experience—fear or anger—the other emotion is quickly buried. It is buried so quickly, in fact, that you may not recognize it.

For most women (and nurses) fighting is taboo. It is "unladylike." For them, an event occurs that triggers fear or anxiety, perhaps only unconsciously. They also experience anger, but this emotion is also frightening and gets buried. It may not even be recognized. A traditional woman learns to deny her anger, to squelch it, to cover it up. She may get a headache or an ulcer or be depressed. The fear generated by an event connects with other fears: her fear of what would happen if she asserted herself, her subconscious fears from previous similar situations, and her fear of being angry. Generally she is immobilized by fear and cannot assert herself.

For a minority of women, however, the anger is too strong, or they have not learned to control it well enough. They do not feel the fear as much as the anger, and they respond to the subconscious fear with aggression. The work involved in being aggressive is really a massive coverup for underlying fear, vulnerability, and powerlessness. Often the "work" is preferable to the pain of feeling anxious and helpless. It serves a defensive function.

Aggression and nonassertion, then, are flip sides of the same coin. The bravado of the aggressor masks a fearful, nonassertive person. Often when nonassertive people have "taken as much as they can stand," they blow up and become aggressive. People who go through assertiveness training often find that their first attempts at assertion are really aggressions. As with any new skill, assertiveness takes practice. Fear and anger are parts of all of us. The interaction, however, between ourselves and society ultimately determines the nature of our responses. We develop styles: nonassertive, aggressive, and assertive.

The Aggressive Style: Thoughts, Words, Actions

Those who respond aggressively, like those who respond nonassertively, have characteristic ways of thinking, speaking, and behaving that signal and reinforce their style.

Aggression is enhanced by certain kinds of thinking. For example, aggressive people may tell themselves, "I must win to be OK. To compromise is to lose." They often believe that the world is a hostile place, that people are basically out for what they can get, and that nice guys finish last. Sometimes they see themselves as the only ones capable of doing certain jobs. They insist that "my way is the right way" and spend considerable time and energy bringing others around to their thinking. If there is only one truth, and their truth is the real truth, then the truths of others are wrong. Aggressive people engage in power struggles. They see things as black or white. Often, they deny or ignore the rights of others.

These beliefs tend to become a self-fulfilling prophecy. If, for example, you believe that you "must come on strong to be heard," you may come on strong as a style rather than selecting instances when this kind of approach may be necessary. You will undoubtedly turn people off in the process. They will shut you out or become angry. In either case, you will have reinforced your beliefs that people do not listen and that the world is a hostile place. Carrying a chip on your shoulder is hard work; it is stressful. Coming on strong, struggling to bring others around to your truth, and arguing every issue are behaviors that expend a lot of energy. The price of aggression, like the price of nonassertion, is high.

Why, then, would someone hang on to aggressive behaviors? What are the benefits? Aggression is enabling; it gives you a sense of power and control. Sometimes it intimidates people into giving you what you want. It helps you to deny your own problems by viewing others as the problem. Aggression, like nonassertion, involves choice. (Granted, the choice for adults may no longer be conscious if the reaction is so ingrained as to be virtually spontaneous.) There are trade-offs in both responses: the nonassertive person trades self-esteem and self-expression for peace and security; the aggressive person gives up peace and security for self-esteem and self-expression. Both experience stress.

ASSERTIVENESS—NOT *JUST* A RESPONSE

An old nursery rhyme tells us that little girls are made of sugar and spice. Media stereotypes convey the message that nurses are angels of mercy or battle ax/sex pots. Sugar and spice? Passive and aggressive? Is this what nurses are made of? No, it is not what nurses are made of, but it *is* often how they behave out of learning and out of fear.

Aggression and nonassertion are responses to fear. Often they are so automatic that they seem to be innate character traits. Sometimes we do not see the event that triggers the response; we see chronically angry or passive individuals. These people, however, are responding to a long history of internal fears and to skewed perceptions of the world and their role in it. Assertion, unlike aggression and nonassertion, is not just a response;

it is often an initiation. Assertive individuals do not wait for things to happen and then respond. They make things happen.

Unlearning feminine stereotypes and overcoming fear are two components of assertiveness training. For many nurses, this means unlearning old behaviors and relearning new ones. Being assertive does not mean being rid of stress. It means expressing yourself honestly, directly, and spontaneously in thought, words, and actions, all of which can be stressful indeed. The payoffs for such hard work and for taking assertive risks are that you can express yourself openly, thereby getting your needs met, and that you come to respect yourself. Before discussing the how-tos of becoming assertive and the importance of assertiveness in stress reduction, let's contrast assertion with nonassertion and aggression in a typical hospital situation.

Assertion Versus Nonassertion and Aggression: The Case of the Vanishing Charge Nurse

The Situation   You are busy preparing a pain medication for Mrs. Jones, who is in the terminal stages of lung cancer. It occurs to you that this is a good opportunity to spend some time talking to Mrs. Jones, and you begin to plan what you want to say. Clara, the charge nurse, pops her head in the door and tells you that she'll "be off the floor at a meeting for a few minutes and you are temporarily in charge." This is the third time in two weeks that Clara has interrupted your schedule, and you feel annoyed.

The Nonassertive Style   If you are generally nonassertive, you might not say anything. Maybe your face would reflect annoyance; maybe not. You might feel resentful as you quickly administer Mrs. Jones' medication and rush to answer the telephone; or you might rationalize to yourself that Clara's activities take priority, and you do not have the right to feel annoyed. If Clara is your friend, a whole host of conflicting emotions may increase your sense of responsibility and confusion. What you do say, when and if you say something, may be indirect or apologetic. Chances are you'll wind up mad at Clara and madder at yourself.

How is it that people trap themselves into being nonassertive? One way is to fool themselves into thinking their feelings aren't real. Another way is to be overly concerned about hurting the other person's feelings. This often happens when co-workers and friends are involved. Trying to manipulate the other person into withdrawing their request rather than having to refuse is another possibility. An example would be if you, the nurse in the sample situation, began to debate with Clara the importance of her activities compared with yours, hoping she would remain on the unit and you wouldn't have to say no or assert yourself.

The Aggressive Style   If your style were more aggressive, you might become visibly angry. You might refuse flat out to accept the charge, or you might begin arguing and bolstering your righteousness with reminders of

Clara's past "failures." You might exaggerate and say things like, "You're *never* on the unit! You *never* think about how anyone else feels!" Blaming and "you" statements are hallmarks of aggression. The situation might escalate.

An aggressive reaction is often fueled by distorted thinking. A nurse with an aggressive style might be telling herself, "I'm going to let her know who's in charge." "No one's going to make a fool out of me." "I'm mad as hell and I'm not going to take it anymore." "The only thing she understands is the sledgehammer approach."

The Assertive Style   As an assertive nurse in the situation, you would have two immediate choices. First you could refuse to take charge and explain to Clara that you would be spending the next 15 minutes with Mrs. Jones, or second, you might acquiesce silently but discuss the matter in full when Clara returned.

The assertive nurse has acquired the skills that enable her to express her needs, desires, and refusals matter-of-factly. Situations are not catastrophes. She is not overwhelmed with hopelessness or anger. She may be objective enough to see options for both persons in a situation. You, the assertive nurse, might have told Clara that if she could wait 15 minutes, you'd be free to cover for her. Or later, you might have problem-solved with Clara a way to plan her absences and schedule you to replace her. You might have recognized that your steady assertions of your own competence and your "take charge" behavior invited her actions. And, having recognized that, you might have encouraged others to share the responsibility.

The options in a situation are generally limited by an individual's narrowed perceptions or overwhelming feelings. The nurse who is feeling angry or abused cannot be objective, often does not see the options, and feels trapped. Angry, sad feelings and a sense of being trapped lead to hopelessness, depression, and burn-out. Assertiveness gives one options.

In summary, let's look at a brief comparison of the characteristics of these three styles: nonassertive, aggressive, and assertive (see Table 16-1).

Chances are if you are a nurse and you are reading this book about stress, you are looking for something, hoping to change something, or wanting suggestions and options. Chances are if you are reading this chapter on assertion, you have already targeted assertion skills as something you'd like to develop. Now that you have a basic understanding of the three styles, the first step for your personal growth is self-assessment. You have probably recognized certain familiar behaviors or attitudes as you have read this far. Maybe you've tentatively assigned yourself a style. Maybe you see yourself as having a combination of styles. Maybe you are satisfied with your style but have some traits you'd like to change. Take the following self-assessment inventory to give yourself a more complete understanding of your style and to target areas where you might want to concentrate.

TABLE 16-1. COMPARISON OF NONASSERTIVE, AGGRESSIVE, AND
ASSERTIVE BEHAVIORS

Nonassertive	Aggressive	Assertive
Denies anger/experiences fear	Denies fear/experiences anger	Recognizes both fear and anger
Does not respect self	Does not respect others	Respects both self and others
Destroys relationships as avoidance and resentment build	Destroys relationships through angry outbursts, self-aggrandizement, and need to control	Builds relationships
Wastes energy by repeating situations that were not adequately resolved	Wastes energy in bluster and argument	Uses energy constructively
Fails to achieve goals	Occasionally achieves goals through intimidation	Achieves goals
Is stressful (low self-esteem, helplessness, hopelessness, depression)	Is stressful (power struggles, painful arguments, need to be ever vigilant)	Is stressful (defying traditional stereotypes; pain of being conscious)

ASSERTIVENESS INVENTORY

Directions

Each of the statements described below are typical nursing situations
that require assertive skills. The statements are designed to help you
pinpoint the type of situation that caused you difficulty. Circle the word
that best describes how frequently you are able to do the behavior in
each statement.

1. Say no when you feel someone is making an unreasonable
   request.
   always   sometimes   never
2. Tell a co-worker when you disagree with his or her statement or
   decision.
   always   sometimes   never
3. Ask for clarification when you don't understand what the other
   person is saying.
   always   sometimes   never

ASSERTIVENESS INVENTORY (continued)

4. Refuse to work a double or switch your schedule if you had previous plans.
   always   sometimes   never
5. Refuse to do a procedure when you feel it is not in the patient's best interest or when you question the physician's rationale for it.
   always   sometimes   never
6. Stand up for a friend when you feel he or she is being falsely accused or gossiped about.
   always   sometimes   never
7. Give a compliment to someone for a job well done.
   always   sometimes   never
8. Ask for help when you are working with a difficult patient.
   always   sometimes   never
9. Give your opinion about patient care during a care plan meeting or during rounds.
   always   sometimes   never
10. Refuse to cover for someone when they make a mistake and ask you to do something "as a favor."
    always   sometimes   never
11. Apologize to someone when you have made a mistake.
    always   sometimes   never
12. Ask your supervisor to give examples or explain criticism.
    always   sometimes   never
13. Tell someone you need time to think over your decision before replying.
    always   sometimes   never
14. Stop a co-worker when you see that he or she is about to make a mistake.
    always   sometimes   never
15. Tell a patient directly that you don't appreciate or will not accept his or her behavior.
    always   sometimes   never

Interpreting Your Responses

The more frequently you circled "always," the more consistently assertive you are. The statements you have circled "never" indicate the behaviors you may want to strengthen. For the statements you circled "sometimes" ask yourself, "What factors influence my being or not being assertive?" Is it the person involved, the size of your audience, when the situation occurs, or the nature of the situation (setting limits, initiating activities, or expressing positive or negative feelings)?

BECOMING ASSERTIVE: FOUR TARGET AREAS

Assertion difficulties can be grouped into four broad areas: positive feelings, negative feelings, limit setting, and self-initiation. Now that you have completed the assessment inventory, you have probably identified your own areas of strength and weakness. No one is solely aggressive, nonassertive, or assertive. Typically, each of us is able to assert ourselves in certain areas and not in others.

The following discussion of assertiveness is not meant to be exhaustive. There are whole books and training programs for that. It is an overview of the four target areas and is intended to demonstrate basic principles and skills. Specific assertive communication techniques are listed at the end of the chapter (see Appendix).

Handling Positive Feelings

Are you able to show warmth, appreciation, and affection? Expressing positive feelings is the first area of assertion and ranges from thanking a stranger for some small courtesy to telling family and friends that you love them.

People are often surprised that assertiveness has to do with positive feelings. Generally, being assertive is connected with negative feelings or with doing something distasteful. Women, as a rule, find it easier to share positive feelings than do men. Traditional female upbringing encourages warmth, nurturance, love, and emotionality. Also, as a rule, women find it easier to share positive feelings than negative ones. Again, upbringing plays a decisive role. Being "ladylike" and "feminine" means eschewing "masculine" behaviors such as anger, aggressiveness, competitiveness, and power strivings. There are two notable exceptions to the rule that women are freer to express positive feelings: when initiating relationships with men and when saying good things about themselves.

Giving and receiving positive feedback are certainly related to stress. Nurses often complain that they do not get positive feedback. They say things such as, "We don't even know this place has an administration until something goes wrong. Then they're on our backs." Or, "She never says anything nice, never tells us we're doing a good job. We only hear about our shortcomings." Studies (see Chapter 2) have shown that stress and burn-out in nursing are related, not so much because negative factors are present (nurses *expect* those) but because positive factors are absent.

Nearly all people, it seems, want to hear that they are doing a good job. Often, they are not seeking praise so much as simple acknowledgment that they and their work are noticed. Positive feedback generates good feelings, reinforces behavior, and makes negative feedback more readily heard. For example, a nurse clinician who works closely with groups of nurses in stress management has ample opportunity to validate perceptions, to acknowledge feelings, and to give encouragement. By the same token, she can also point out less desirable attitudes and behaviors if she has already created a climate of acceptance. Again, it is not compliments and praise that are so valued, but recognition, acknowledgment, and acceptance.

How do you give positive feedback assertively? We have all learned that saying things sincerely (in our own words) and looking people in the eye are important. Be specific rather than global about what you like. It is better to say, "Peter, Mr. Smith moves about so much better since you've been helping him with his exercises," than "Hey, you're doing a good job!" Be timely; mention the little things you see on a daily basis, rather than saving them up for evaluation time.

Refrain from giving positive feedback with criticism. Many of us have been taught to tell people what we like about what they're doing and then point out what they need to improve. Combining positive and negative feedback, we are advised, cushions the criticism and people will accept it better. They won't. The positive messages will be buried under the pain and rejection of being criticized. People need to hear both kinds of feedback but at separate times.

Similarly, positive feedback and requests should not be linked together. Telling people you like what they're doing and then asking them to do an additional task often makes them feel manipulated. How many times have you heard someone say, "Oh, Sharon, you are always so good about helping out in a pinch. Whenever things get crazy around here, I know I can count on you. Would you mind doing a week of nights?" How do you feel when this happens?

Some of us are better at giving positive feedback than receiving it. Having our successes acknowledged, especially in public, feels embarrassing. We have all heard that we should accept compliments gracefully. We know it is not OK to say, "Oh, this old rag? I've had it for years," when someone admires a party dress. But even knowing this, many of us deny, reject, deflect, and joke when people are telling us good things about ourselves. We feel stress.

Handling compliments assertively takes practice. It is enough to look someone directly in the eye and simply say, "Thank you." Another assertive response is to tell the person what her or his compliment means to you; for example, "I'm glad you found my care plan on Davey Williams helpful. I've had a hard time trying to figure out what's going on with him. Now that I think I understand, it's nice to know someone else feels the same."

Handling Negative Feelings

Negative feelings, like positive ones, have a range—from discomfort to fury. Handling negative feelings is the second area of assertiveness. It involves giving and receiving negative feedback, both of which may be stressful.

Many people have difficulty telling others what they don't like, what bothers them, or what they would prefer the other not do. Depending upon your individual dynamics, giving negative feedback can be particularly stressful when authority figures, subordinates, colleagues, or patients are involved. Do you know your problems areas? How, for example, do you, the head nurse, tell your supervisor that it upsets you when she intervenes in staffing or patient problems without consulting you first? How do you, the team leader, counsel a nurse's aide whose skills are not up to par? How do you, a staff nurse, handle your anger when a co-worker's repeated sick calls increase your weekend work load? How do you, a pain control nurse, tell your demanding patients that they cannot have their medication until the designated time?

Assertiveness techniques for managing these and similar situations include using "I" statements, describing rather than interpreting behavior, being specific and spontaneous, and using appropriate clout. Let's say, for example, you are the head nurse mentioned previously. If you confront the supervisor aggressively, saying, "You don't know what's going on. You tell the staffing office it's OK to float someone, but you don't check to see if we're getting any admissions. That's pretty insensitive!," chances are you'll get nowhere (except into trouble). These are "you" statements. They *blame* the supervisor and probably provoke anger or defensiveness. Telling your boss you don't like what she's doing is stressful enough without setting yourself up for retaliation. If, on the other hand, you say nothing, your nonassertiveness will probably leave you doing a slow boil. Nothing will change.

A better way to handle the confrontation might be to say, "Rita, I'm upset that you've changed our staffing without consulting me. Floating a nurse now, when we're expecting two admissions, means that no one will be able to attend the case conference on Mrs. Snyder." How is this different from the previous confrontation? First, you've taken responsibility for your feelings by saying, "I'm upset. . . ." You've made an I statement rather than a you statement. Second, you described behavior rather than assuming she didn't check admissions or interpreting her behavior as insensitive. You were *specific* where before you were general. And you were *spontaneous,* meaning you discussed the matter immediately. You did not actually use clout in this example, but you did spell out the consequences of her actions—that no one could attend the conference.

As in this example, descriptions of specific behaviors connected to feeling statements are less likely to be interpreted as attacking or punitive. It's hard to argue with feelings. You might link the two by saying, "When you [describe person's behavior], I [describe your feelings]." For example; "Dr. X, when you shout at me in the nurse's station, I get angry and then I can't hear what you're saying or help you." "Carol, when you close your eyes and lean back like that, I think you're not listening to me." "Mr. Adams, when you expose yourself, I feel uncomfortable."

How do you know whether to use clout? It depends on the situation. Wielding your muscle isn't usually necessary the first time you give negative feedback. Often, just stating your feelings and the consequences of the person's behavior are enough. In addition, you may need to spell out clearly what you want the person to do or not do. If that doesn't work, you may need to use clout in addition to other assertive techniques like the broken record (see Appendix). Clout involves using whatever leverage you have: referring to rules, regulations, or laws; using your legitimate authority (if you're a manager); calling on higher authorities; documenting the problem and taking it through channels. Clout should be titrated. You don't use an elephant gun to kill an ant. Suit your tone and your words to the situation.

When you meet resistance, just asking a person his or her name may be sufficient to get cooperation. It's surprising how people respond to a simple, "Now, what did you say your name was?" Occasionally, you might need to ask, "Are you refusing to . . .?" Or, if that sounds too harsh, "Do I understand correctly? You are refusing . . .?" The word refuse is motivating. So is having to give your supervisor's name. For hardened cases, you may need to use threats or spell out consequences: "If you do not . . . , I will . . .."

Lastly, you must carry out your threats. The purpose of clout is to give muscle to your words. Don't make idle threats. Don't paint yourself into a corner. Don't give ultimatums unless you can follow through. It is better to back off early than to back down late. That destroys your credibility. A final word about clout: it is often most powerful delivered matter-of-factly.

Now, put yourself on the receiving end. How do you handle negative feedback that is coming your way? Hearing that someone does not like what you are doing can be very stressful. Criticism is criticism even when it's "constructive." And criticism often hurts. It also surprises, annoys, enrages, or evokes any of a number of conflicting emotions that may catch you off guard or immobilize you. You may want to run or to fight. You may be so stunned you don't know what to do. The best initial response is to do just that: nothing. Stay put and listen. Don't talk. Don't interrupt. Don't explain. Listen.

Once you think you understand the problem, you must determine whether the criticism is realistic. This is not the same as legitimate. Realistic criticism is an accurate description of your behavior, usually accompanied by a statement of the other person's feelings or a request for change. Whether criticism is legitimate or not involves the concept of rights. Do other persons have the right to criticize you? Are their feelings right? Appropriate? Legitimate? The fact is that all feelings are legitimate. People do have the right to any feelings they might have about your behavior. (What you think about the logic of their feelings is another matter.) People also have the right to criticize, at least in this country. Freedom of speech mandates that people can say what they think. The only caveat to that rule is they must describe your behavior accurately, that is, realistically, if they are talking about you to others.

Once you determine that the criticism is realistic, you have two choices:

to accept the criticism and alter your behavior or accept the criticism and refuse to alter your behavior. If, on the other hand, you do not think the criticism is realistic or you do not like the way it is given, you have several choices. You can point out discrepancies and exaggerations. Let's say, for example, that the operating room nurse calls you and says high-handedly, "You sent Mr. Black up without the proper consent. You never get it right with Dr. Boyce's patients and he's furious. Can't you people read?" And so on. First, are there any discrepancies? Did the patient come from your floor? Did he have the right consent? In other words, is the fact that Mr. Black came from your floor without the proper consent realistic? Is the next statement—that You never get it right—realistic? Never and ever are generally exaggerations and, therefore, inaccurate. When the operating room nurse has finished speaking, assert yourself by clarifying any discrepancies and perhaps pointing out her exaggerations. (Don't say, "You *always* exaggerate!")

Criticisms can also be unrealistic in that they are value judgments, interpretations, or labels rather than descriptions of your behavior. "Can't you people read?" is a perfect example. It is the same as saying, "Are you illiterate?" The value judgment is implied. *Value* judgments are just that: judgments by one person that another's actions are good/bad, right/wrong, moral/immoral, smart/stupid, and so on. Interpretations, on the other hand, are often judgments, not about values but about motives. (What you're *really* saying is . . . .) Labeling goes a step beyond value judgments and interpretations. It involves making a value judgment (bad) and attaching a label: junkie, manipulator, bitch, and so on. It also involves making an interpretation (You forgot our date. You must be mad at me.) and attaching a label (passive-aggressive). Criticisms involving value judgments, interpretations, or labels generally also involve aggression.

Being the focus of another's aggression is stressful. As we've said, aggression evokes our fear and anger in intensities ranging from discomfort through pain. How do you assert yourself when you want to flee or fight or when you are feeling paralyzed? In addition to using assertive techniques (see Appendix), concentrate on the following:

- Getting to the source of the problem. Ask for more information or clarification. Be specific.
- Sticking to the goal. Ignore the aggression and discuss the issue. "You may be upset that no one oriented you to the unit yesterday. I wasn't here, but I'll look into it. Meanwhile, how can I help you today? What kinds of things do you need to know?" If someone is being particularly aggressive, you can say, "my intelligence or my morals or my deep psychological dynamics are not important. The point is . . . ." In other words, dismiss and redirect.
- Making the person aware of his or her aggression and its effects. "I don't like it when you shout at me."
- Limiting the behavior.

Setting Limits

The third area of assertion involves setting limits. When you set limits, you are in fact saying, "This is who I am, and this is how I expect to be treated." Generally, you are restricting access to your person, time, money, or energy. You are saying, "I will go this far," or "You may go this far with me." Before you can set effective limits, however, you must know yourself and your limits. How much of you is available? Do you have the time? Are you willing to spend the money or energy? Do you care? What are your goals, priorities, restrictions? What kind of trade-offs will you make? Can you make?

People who have trouble setting limits are people who say yes when they mean no. There are as many reasons why this happens as there are people who do it. Some are caught by surprise. Others are afraid (of hurting feelings, of making someone angry, of rocking the boat). Others feel they should, that it's expected, that they'd feel guilty if they didn't. Most people who say yes to things they don't want to do also say, I didn't realize I didn't want to until later. Many people, however, *do* know at some level. They get that icky feeling, that sinking feeling, that gut-level feeling. Trust your gut. When you say yes and mean no, you're denying yourself, your reality. You're swallowing your feelings. Your gut is the repository. It knows. Listen to it.

The first step, then, in setting limits is becoming aware of yourself, your conscious limits, and your gut reactions that signal your unconscious limits. Be aware of how you behave when you're feeling overloaded, overworked, overwhelmed, manipulated, and generally unappreciated. Do you withdraw? Avoid people, places, meetings? Get sick? Feel tired? Become bored? Are you irritable? Short-tempered? Overreacting?

Once you have an inkling that something is wrong, you can begin to analyze what is bothering you. This step is important. If you are not clear concerning what specifically is bothering you about someone's behavior, the only limit you can set is to avoid the person or situation entirely. You may begin by simply recognizing that you avoid someone. You notice that when Mary is your co-worker, you spend a lot of time in the medication room. At first, you may think you just don't like Mary, and you may defend yourself by saying, "I don't have to like everyone." No, you're right, you don't! But if being around Mary is uncomfortable enough to change your behavior, you owe it to yourself to figure out why. If being around Mary interferes with your work (by restricting your movements, by making you grouchy), you owe it to your patients. What is it about Mary that you don't like?

You don't like her incessant chatter, her clingingness. Now that you know what the problem is, you have a choice: live with it or set limits. The idea of setting limits is not to cut Mary off but to make her aware of what she does, how it bothers you, and what you want her to do about it. Once again you use behavioral descriptions and "I" statements: "Mary, I'm charting now. When you interrupt me, I lose my train of thought. Please wait until I'm finished." Be specific about what she does, and be spontaneous. Tell her at the time. Also, be specific about what you want her to do. At first, you might need to give her a time: "I'll be with you in ten minutes."

Mary will probably understand if you are clear and if you are consistent over time. Many of us are not clear, meaning we are not assertive. We use nonverbal behavior (the "cold shoulder"), hoping our Marys will take the hint. Then we get mad when they don't. Small problems are magnified until we're avoiding these persons altogether. Lack of consistency, too, perpetuates the problem. If your Mary's behavior has become a problem, meaning it isn't something that happened just once, you will probably need to set limits more than once to change the pattern.

Finally, consider the pitfalls to limit setting. Are you reinforcing the behavior that bothers you? Inconsistency of response and nonassertiveness certainly perpetuate problems. So do mixed messages. Do you, for example, wish your team members, nursing staff, or employees, could be more independent at the same time you solve their problems for them? Certainly it's quicker and more efficient if you are more experienced, but you are reinforcing their dependency. Do you wish the same staff would confront each other with their grievances rather than coming to you? Do you thank them for making you aware of the problem and thus defeat your goal?

Another pitfall in limit setting is trying to be reasonable. Getting involved in debates, answering questions, and making excuses keep you side-tracked. Be clear. Be firm. Is it uncomfortable for you to be responsible for the limit? Do you pass the buck? "Administration says . . ., They want us to . . .." Is it hard to say "I"? That one word, perhaps, is the key to assertiveness: knowing yourself, acknowledging your rights, and being responsible for asserting them. Saying "I" means being responsible.

Self-Initiation

The last area of assertion is self-initiation: getting yourself moving; getting what you want for yourself, your career, your life; going where you want; being proactive rather than reactive. What are you waiting for? Who are you waiting for? Are you waiting for someone to do it for you? Are you waiting for someone to take you where you want to go? Are you, a contemporary Cinderella, waiting because "someday your prince will come"? Forget Walt Disney! In the words of a contemporary feminist, "You have to kiss a lot of frogs before you find the handsome prince." Get moving!

Women (and nurses) have traditionally waited while men who earned more money, had more power, had more brains, and could vote, made the decisions. Slowly that is changing. Women are becoming autonomous. Women's rights are emerging. Do you know your rights as a woman health professional?*

- You have the right to be treated with respect.
- You have the right to a reasonable workload.
- You have the right to an equitable wage.
- You have the right to determine your own priorities.
- You have the right to ask for what you want.
- You have the right to refuse without making excuses or feeling guilty.
- You have the right to make mistakes and be responsible for them.
- You have the right to give and receive information as a professional.
- You have the right to act in the best interest of the patient.
- You have the right to be human.

As with any rights, these bring responsibility and risk. You have the right, for example, to an equitable wage, but others will dictate your salary unless you assume responsibility. You have rights, but you must assert them. Asserting rights, especially if those rights are nontraditional, involves risk: risk that you will surprise, shock, antagonize, and alienate people; that you will be hurt; that you will lose something or someone; that you will fail; that you will succeed and create even greater expectations and more work for yourself; in short, that you will increase your stress.

As with any rights, these involve choice. You must choose where and when you will exercise them. You must decide when to assert yourself and when to let go. You must weigh the issues.

CONCLUSION

Assertiveness alone does not reduce stress; rather it reduces feelings of helplessness, impotence, and frustration that contribute to stress. Unlike passivity or aggression, which are responses, assertiveness is a skill that must be learned and practiced. Whatever your area of difficulty—handling positive or negative feelings, setting limits, initiating activities—becoming assertive should help you achieve your goals and conserve energy while feeling good about yourself and others.

*From Chenevert, M. 1983. *STAT: Special techniques in assertiveness training for women in the health professions*, ed. 2. St. Louis: The C. V. Mosby Co.

APPENDIX: ASSERTIVE COMMUNICATION TECHNIQUES*

1. Broken Record

A systematic assertive communication skill in which you are persistent and keep saying what you want over and over again without getting angry, irritated, or loud.

By practicing speaking like a broken record you learn to be persistent and to stick to the point of discussion and to continue to say what you want. This technique helps you to ignore all side issues brought up by the other party.

2. Workable Compromise

A technique to use with an equally assertive person to work out a compromise. A workable compromise is one in which your self-respect is not in question.

3. Free Information

A listening skill in which you evaluate and then use the free information that people offer about themselves. It accomplishes two things; it facilitates conversation and it prompts others to respond easily and freely.

4. Self-Disclosure

Assertively disclosing information about yourself—how you think, feel and react to the other person's free information—permits social communication to flow both ways. This technique should be used with free information, because to elicit more free information you must be willing to self-disclose.

5. Fogging

A technique to assertively cope with manipulative criticism. You neither deny any of the criticism, nor get defensive, nor attack with criticism of your own. Instead you send up a fogbank. It is persistent. It cannot be clearly seen through. And it offers no resistance to penetration. By fogging you offer no resistance or hard psychological striking surfaces to critical statements thrown at you.

6. Negative Assertion

A technique to cope with criticism or with your own errors and faults by openly acknowledging them. This technique is to be used only in social conflicts, not in physical or legal ones.

*Reprinted from Donnelly, G. F. 1979. *Topics in Clinical Nursing* 1:1. By permission of Aspen Systems Corporation, © 1979.

APPENDIX: ASSERTIVE COMMUNICATION TECHNIQUES (continued)

7. Negative Inquiry

An assertive, nondefensive response that is noncritical of the other person and prompts that person to examine his/her own structure of right and wrong. For example, "I don't understand. What makes you think nurses are stupid?"

Sources:
1. Alberti, R. E., and Emmons, M. 1975. *Stand Up, Speak Out, Talk Back!* New York: Pocket Books.
2. Bloom, L. Z., Coburn, K., and Pearlman, J. 1975. *The New Assertive Woman.* New York: Dell Publishing Co., Inc.
3. Smith, M. 1975. *When I Say No I Feel Guilty!* New York: Bantam Books.
4. Fensterheim, H., and Baer, J. 1975. *Don't Say Yes When You Want to Say No!* New York: Dell Publishing Co., Inc.

REFERENCES

Baer, J. 1976. *How to be an assertive (not aggressive) woman in life, in love, and on the job.* New York: Signet Books.

Bower, S. A., and Bower, G. H. 1976. *Asserting your self.* Reading, Mass.: Addison-Wesley Pub. Co., Inc.

Butler, P. E. 1976. *Self-assertion for women: a guide to becoming androgynous.* San Francisco, Calif.: Harper and Row, Publishers, Inc.

Chenevert, M. 1978. *Special techniques in assertiveness training for women in the health professions.* St. Louis: The C. V. Mosby Co.

Clark, C. C. 1978. *Assertive skills for nurses.* Wakefield, Mass.: Contemporary Publishing, Inc.

Jakubowski, P., and Lange, A. J. 1978. *The assertive option: your rights and responsibilities.* Champaign, Ill.: Research Press Co.

Phelps, S., and Austin, N. 1975. *The assertive woman.* San Luis Obispo, Calif.: Impact Publishers.

6

Stress Reduction Techniques

The stress reduction techniques presented in this section are systematic procedures that decrease the stress response. They can also be used to provide a generalized sense of calm and relaxation that alters your negative perception of stress in general, thus cutting off the experience of distress.

Each technique requires active practice until the skill has become a natural part of your stress response and your overall stress-management program. Experiment with the different stress reduction techniques presented to see which ones match your personality style and are most effective for you. Feel free to adapt the techniques to your own needs. Hopefully, the sample of stress reduction techniques presented will whet your appetite to explore additional techniques listed in the resource and reference sections. What is presented in this section is a sampling of techniques that have been found useful in managing job stress; they are easily adapted to the work setting or as part of your daily routine. There are also many additional, exciting approaches to stress reduction such as reflexology, acupuncture, or "touch for health"; these are not presented because of the space constraints of the book and because proficiency in their use requires supervised practice. Many nontraditional approaches to stress management have been used for centuries in the East and are now just beginning to become known to Westerners. I hope this book will be just the beginning of your journey to develop a healthier life-style while managing job stress.

For each of the stress reduction techniques presented in Part 6, the presentation of basic principles and supporting research is followed by explicit directions for utilizing the technique; in addition, examples are provided of how to generalize the technique to your work environment and daily living.

CHAPTER 17

Relaxation: An Active Process

JEFFREY STOLROW

You can learn to control stress through systematic physiologic relaxation, in addition to the stress-control techniques you have learned in previous chapters. Relaxation of the body will help to relax the mind. Psychophysiologists have named this action the psychophysiologic principle.

First you need to understand the process of relaxation in order to have a better idea of how it works. Then, to help you relax your body, you will learn simple and effective relaxation techniques, some of which have been practiced for thousands of years. Relaxation takes time and effort. Because your time is at a premium, I will give you some tips to help you relax faster and with more consistency, and I will discuss recommendations for exercises to control specific stress-related problems.

THE PROCESS OF RELAXATION

Before we begin with the relaxation techniques, give yourself permission to relax. At this moment some of you may be saying to yourself, she is crazy! If only I could relax! No, I am not crazy. After working with hundreds of adult patients, many of whom are professionals, I have concluded that one of the hardest choices you face is giving yourself permission to relax. Think about this idea for a moment. The beliefs of our Western society tell us to be thoroughly competent in all tasks. You are not reinforced for leisure time, but you do receive copious praise for maintaining a continuous work schedule without breaks. We are a rushed, frazzled, and harassed culture, and no one knows this fact more than you, the nurse! Because of the demands of your profession, you may have identified with these irrational beliefs without being aware of it. You must modify these beliefs if you want to relax successfully. If you do not change these attitudes about yourself, you have the potential to develop dangerous cardiovascular disease, like high blood pressure and coronary artery disease (Friedman and Rosenman, 1974).

To modify your belief system, remember that you have the following rights. Say them to yourself before you relax. Recalling these rights will help you to incorporate relaxation into your daily activities: Give yourself permission to take the time to relax.

- You have the right to decide what to do with your body.
- You have the right to decide what to do with your time.
- You have the right to choose to relax, and you deserve this time for relaxation (Jakubowski and Lange, 1978).

If you are a runner, tennis player, or musician, you know that being successful at these activities demands constant and repeated practice. To hit a good forehand in tennis takes time, proper instruction, and motivation. Learning to relax requires these things too. I recommend that you set aside 30 minutes each day for your relaxation. You may think this time will be impossible to find, but you will be rewarded if you decide to take it. Deep relaxation for 30 minutes can be more beneficial than taking a two-hour nap (Jacobson, 1938). Instead of giving you less time to do things, relaxation will give you more time to engage in your chosen activities. Also, you will have more energy! So take your calendar or work assignment sheet and write in an appointment for yourself to relax each day. It is a good idea to make your period of relaxation at the same time of day, because this regular practice will create a habit of relaxation.

After three or four weeks of repeated practice, you should notice beneficial physiologic and psychologic changes. However, do not be discouraged if you cannot relax quickly. Dr. Edmund Jacobson, who developed a relaxation technique called progressive relaxation, states that it can take one year of daily practice to master this exercise. As you practice, you will be aware of large increases in your motor performance, plateaus when there's little change, and other times when nothing seems to work. This pattern of learning is found in all types of motor skills, so give yourself permission to take your time and make mistakes—relax.

To learn relaxation successfully, I recommend using a four-step process of relaxation. The steps in this process are becoming aware of your body, discriminating between tension and relaxation, choosing to relax or remain tense, and selecting the appropriate relaxation technique.

The first step in learning effective relaxation is becoming aware of your body. Without this awareness, you will not be able to relax because you will not know when you are tense. The process of awareness will be challenging for you. In this culture every attempt is made to limit body awareness. If you find this statement difficult to believe, think about television advertisements. The most frequent advertisements are for medications that control headache pain, for minor tranquilizers, and for alcohol. We are an anesthetized culture. Instead of promoting awareness, the society fosters denial. So what if your head is pounding with a migraine headache or you have not slept for three days! The society demands that you deaden your senses so you can get to work on time and appear as if you are performing your duties effectively.

Society is not concerned with why these physical signals are occurring, but you should be! Your body is giving you warning signals that need to be observed. To help you get back in touch with your body, I will give you awareness tips for many of the relaxation exercises. Use these cues when you are relaxing quietly and when you are confronted with a crisis situation on the job. As your awareness increases, you will have greater self-knowledge, which fosters control and mitigates anxiety and fear.

Once your awareness of your body has increased, the next step is to learn the difference between tension and relaxation. It is just as important to know when you are tense as it is to know when you are relaxed. After all, if you are not aware of increasing levels of tension, you will never know when to use the relaxation techniques. The mastery of 100 techniques is ineffective if you do not know when to use them.

As you learn better discrimination, remember not to evaluate yourself. Tension and relaxation are normal physiologic states that simply exist; do not attach moral judgments and evaluations to these physiologic conditions. You are not bad or awful because your teeth are grinding or because you have a tension headache. Likewise you are not good or wonderful because you are not experiencing these signals. It is impossible to be aware of yourself and judge yourself simultaneously. So let go of the judgment, and I believe you will be pleasantly surprised with the serenity that will take the place of anxiety and inadequacy. Besides, you and I know there is always someone around who will be delighted to evaluate your performance!

Now, for the most difficult step of the process—choosing to relax. For the professionals I have worked with, including nurses and physicians, the choice to relax is both difficult and crucial. You may have awareness, be able to discriminate, and be an expert in relaxation, but the whole process has failed if you do not choose to use it. You are not learning these skills for fun. You are learning these techniques to survive in your profession and avoid stress-related disease like essential hypertension, ulcers, adult-onset diabetes, and heart attack. Choose to relax! It will seem impossible when you are faced with deadlines, patients to care for, progress notes to write, and staff meetings to attend. And it seems easier to continue with predictable and habitual behavior patterns that in fact may be damaging your body. Behavioral changes are difficult because they involve effort, risk, and unpredictability. However, your choice to relax is essential to your professional competency.

The fourth step is to determine what relaxation technique is appropriate for a specific stressful situation. (If you have physical symptoms and suspect an organic problem, always consult a doctor before beginning relaxation exercises.) Each one of us is an individual. We begin with a genetic potential that is influenced by a learned history and set of environmental factors that are different for each person. Therefore, each of you will respond somewhat differently to a stressor or a relaxation technique. Even though it is impossible to recommend specific relaxation techniques with certainty, clinical experience and a review of the literature have verified that some relaxation techniques can be more effective for specific situations and problems. Still, there are individual variations. If a relaxation technique works for you, use it. If it does not work, do not use it. Sample the various techniques for several weeks. Continue to use those exercises that feel comfortable and control stress.

PHYSIOLOGIC CUES ASSOCIATED WITH RELAXATION

Initially many people have difficulty knowing when they are in a relaxed state. To help you interpret your experience, the following list describes physical sensations associated with relaxation. You may be deeply relaxed and not experience all of these sensations. What you experience depends on your own unique physiologic profile (Erickson, et al., 1976).

1. *Breathing.* Your rate of breathing will decrease and your abdomen will move with each breath. Your breathing will feel light and easy.
2. *Swallowing.* You will rarely feel like swallowing.
3. *Heaviness.* Your body, especially your arms and legs, will typically feel heavy. Your muscles produce this sensation when they have achieved a low state of resting tension.
4. *Warmth.* Your body, especially your arms and legs, will feel warm. Deep relaxation enhances blood flow to the extremities.
5. *Reaction to external stimuli.* You will not be as aware of your surroundings.
6. *Eyelids.* Your eyelids will have a tendency to gently close, and they will rest easily, without fluttering.

7. *Time*. Your subjective experience of time will be altered. Sometimes time will seem to pass more quickly, and sometimes it will slow.
8. *Attention*. Even though your attention is focused, you may experience short periods of "drifting" from the relaxation exercise. Deep relaxation may produce spontaneous imagery, dream-like states, or fleeting thoughts.
9. *Orientation*. When you decide to come out of the deeply relaxed state, you will probably stretch, or shift your physical position. This natural adaptation process will prepare you to continue your daily activities.

All relaxation techniques have in common the use of centering—controlling the mind's tendency to wander, repetition of movement, and the cognitive awareness of distinguishing between tension and relaxation (Girdano and Everly, 1976). Experiencing tension and relaxation at the same moment is an impossibility. Tension and relaxation are mutually exclusive experiences. Learning to relax the body completely through any of the techniques presented in this chapter inhibits the fight-or-flight anxiety response associated with stress because relaxation elicits parasympathetic responses that inhibit the sympathetic anxiety response (Jacobson, 1938). Once you learn to use any of these techniques to elicit the relaxation response, you will be able to successfully inhibit anxiety and distress.

To this point, I have given you a framework for the relaxation process. I will now incorporate this framework in the discussion and demonstration of specific relaxation techniques. I hope you derive great benefit from their use. I will begin our discussion with breathing because of its prime importance in the relaxation process.

TECHNIQUES

Breathing

Diaphragmatic breathing is the most important and effective relaxation technique you will learn. It can be used exclusively or in combination with all other relaxation techniques to promote rapid and successful relaxation of the central and autonomic nervous system. Because the breathing centers of the brain are closely related to the reticular activating system, relaxed steady breathing promotes relaxation in general. Yoga philosophy states breathing is the master of the mind, and thus regulated breathing is the "elixir of life" (Girdano and Everly, 1976). Diaphragmatic breathing is relaxing because it promotes a balanced blood neutrality, helps to relax the striated and smooth muscles, saves mechanical energy, and ventilates the lower one-third of each lung. Improper, shallow breathing inhibits the oxygen–carbon dioxide exchange, leaving the body without the oxygen it needs while continuing to circulate contaminated waste products in the bloodstream.

In the classic book on homeostasis, *The Wisdom of the Body*, Walter Cannon (1967) stated that the body can store practically every substance except oxygen. Since it is impossible to store oxygen, you must breathe continuously and effectively to maintain a constant supply of oxygen for your tissues. If, like most Westerners, you take this process for granted, remember that a six-minute interruption in the supply of oxygen to the body can produce brain death. To put it differently, breathing is the most important need of the body, a fact recognized in the East, where breathing has developed into a fine art.

Awareness of Breathing   To learn breathing awareness, recall the four-step process of relaxation. The first step in learning to relax is awareness, so try to become aware of your breathing. In a quiet, dimly illuminated room, sit or lie down. Next, close your eyes and begin to focus on your breathing. Do not force your breathing; just observe it, as you would observe a beautiful landscape. As you focus on your breathing you may want to become aware of some of the following things:

- Do you breathe with your shoulders or back?
- Do you pause between inhalation and exhalation?
- What does it feel like when you breathe in, and what does it feel like when you breath out?
- As you breathe, do you feel relaxed or uncomfortable?

You may become aware of other valuable sensations. Use these sensations as well as the ones I have mentioned to help develop awareness of your breathing pattern. Also, become aware of your breathing when you are tense, anxious, or angry. Compare this pattern of breathing with relaxed breathing. As you make these comparisons, your discrimination between relaxed and tense breathing will become more refined.

Discrimination Between Tension and Relaxation in Stressful Breathing Patterns   Place one hand on your chest and one hand on your stomach. Next, tighten your stomach muscles hard and take four or five deep breaths through your chest. Notice by visual observation and touch that the hand on your stomach will not move, but the hand on your chest will rise and fall with each breath. This type of breathing may begin to make you feel uncomfortable; be aware of these sensations. If you stop breathing completely, neither hand will move. Try this maneuver for 20 or 30 seconds. You will probably find this activity very uncomfortable (Figure 17-1A).

If you are not engaged in vigorous physical exercise and you are aware of shallow chest breathing or you are not breathing, you are in a state of physiologic arousal. Hyperventilation and hypoventilation are associated with tension and anxiety. These breathing states upset the blood neutrality, which has an immediate and adverse effect on the brain and body tissues. Also, these patterns of breathing increase the tension in the striated and smooth muscles; this tension wastes energy. Furthermore the lower one-third of each lung is not adequately ventilated with either hyperventilation or hypoventilation. This is a serious problem because the lower one-third of each lung has the greatest ability to absorb oxygen molecules. Finally, chest breathing is inefficient because the lungs must expand against the ribs, which are relatively inflexible and prevent proper lung expansion. Hypoventilation is inefficient because oxygen is not being delivered to the tissues. This condition can have especially adverse effects on the brain, which needs a constant supply of oxygen to process neural information. If these patterns of breathing are associated with tension, how do you know if you are breathing inadequately? Second, how do you know if your breathing is relaxed?

Relaxed, Diaphragmatic Breathing   Relax your chest and stomach muscles, but do not remove your hands. Take an easy breath, and let the breath go down into your abdomen. When you are performing this diaphragmatic breathing correctly, the hand on your stomach will go out as you breathe in, and it will go back when you breath out. The hand on your chest should not move when you perform this exercise. When you breathe diaphragmatically, you are relaxing. This type of breathing is also called belly breathing, because the abdomen expands and contracts with each breath (see Figure 17-1B).

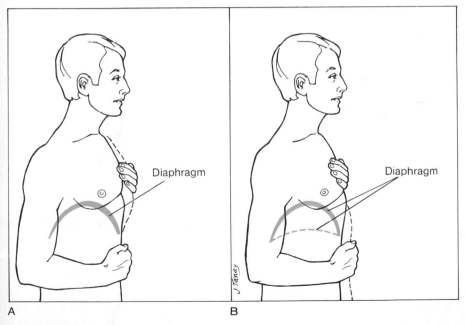

A   B

FIGURE 17-1.

A. Chest breathing.
B. Diaphragmatic breathing.

Babies and young children are excellent diaphragmatic breathers, as are professional musicians and broadcasters. If you have difficulty with this type of breathing, do not be discouraged. After all, since you were very young you have been told to suck in your stomach and stick your chest out. Society trains you to breathe anxiously! Please take your time. If you find this breathing is difficult, experiment by lying down and loosening any tight clothing around your abdomen and throat. Also, do not practice for long periods. Short, spaced periods of practice of five minutes are preferable to long and frustrating practice sessions.

I do not give my patients formulas for how many breaths to take within a period of time. The normal breathing rate for adults is 16 breaths per minute. If you are breathing faster than this number, slow your breathing rate. Spend approximately as much time breathing in as you do breathing out, and pause between breaths. As you become more proficient, the length of time it takes you to breathe in and out will increase, including the time span between breaths. Do not breathe too deeply. The diaphragm is a very efficient muscle, so just breathe lightly. Diaphragmatic breathing saves energy. It is preferable to breathe in through your nose, but you may breathe out through your nose or mouth.

Diaphragmatic breathing is an important physiologic activity because of its ability to relax you; in fact it is essential for all other relaxation techniques. Diaphragmatic breathing is unobtrusive; it can be used whenever you are aware of hyperventilation or hypoventilation. Practice diaphragmatic breathing for approximately five minutes, two times per day in a relaxed environment. Also, use diaphragmatic breathing when you are confronting any stressor, such as a belligerent patient or staff member. Diaphragmatic breathing will immediately prevent further arousal and in most situations will relax you as long as you continue it. Diaphragmatic breathing is your first line of defense against stressful situations so use it often and with confidence!

Progressive Relaxation

The technique called progressive relaxation was developed in the 1930s by Edmund Jacobson, M.D. It is designed to control muscle tension and anxiety by deeply relaxing the skeletal muscles, which are known as voluntary muscles because they are consciously controlled. Jacobson showed that anxiety and deep muscle relaxation are contradictory physiologic states; therefore, if you can succeed in relaxing some of your muscles, you can't be anxious at the same time. By monitoring muscles with physiologic instruments, Jacobson demonstrated that the repetitive practice of alternating tension and relaxation in a progressive series of voluntary muscle groups facilitated a state of deep muscle relaxation and low central nervous system arousal. Designed to be performed in a quiet atmosphere, this technique takes about 20–30 minutes to finish.

As you learn this basic relaxation technique, there are two things to keep in mind: a selective focus of attention and a repetition of movement.

Selective focus of attention refers to concentrating all of your attention on the muscle that is being tensed and relaxed at a given moment. Ignore all other distracting stimuli whether they are environmental, such as the noise of a telephone, or internal, such as thoughts about what you will be doing tomorrow. If you find yourself becoming distracted, say to yourself, "These distractions are occupying my attention and may be important, but I would like to gently come back to focusing on my muscles." Do not become angry or frustrated when distracted because these feelings will create more tension. Be patient. Learning selective focus of attention is a subtle process that is mastered in small steps. Through daily practice, you will eventually become skilled at directing your attention to a specific muscle.

The second fundamental principle of progressive relaxation is repetition. The alternating pattern of tensing and relaxing each muscle group is repeated according to a plan. This repetition is progressive because each major muscle group throughout the body is tensed and relaxed in a systematic manner. The repetition of movement is important because it limits distractions that may interfere with the technique. Also, repetition produces a quieting effect in the mind. By focusing away from the pressures and preoccupations of daily living, you will become more aware of subtle body sensations.

Discrimination Between Tension and Relaxation in Striated Muscles   Progressive relaxation is based on the ability to distinguish tension from relaxation. Surprisingly you may have little awareness of the sensation of muscular relaxation, so it is important to attend to the difference between these physiologic states. Learn to identify the specific physical sensations associated with each of these conditions.

Tension and relaxation feel different. Tense muscles usually feel tight. Extreme levels of tension will cause aching, twitching, or burning. Tight muscles may also inhibit movement in the adjacent joints. Most people say that relaxed muscles feel heavy, though I have had patients report lightness. Sometimes the feeling of heaviness is accompanied by warmth, an indicator that the smooth muscles in the arteries are relaxing.

As you compare tension and relaxation, spend three times as long studying the muscle in the relaxed state. For example, if you choose to tense a muscle group for 15 seconds, then remember to relax it for 45 seconds before continuing.

Use only a moderate level of tension when you contract a muscle. Do not perform isometric contractions! An isometric contraction will cause your muscle to shake involuntarily, and you will feel very sore after the exercise.

As you moderately tense and relax your muscles, you should develop the ability to tense only one muscle group at a time. For example, when tensing your right fist, do not tense your jaw. The term differential relaxation is used to denote this selective ability to tense and relax specific muscles at will. Differential relaxation is not an easy task, so do not be discouraged if you are not a professional in several sessions.

Guidelines for Progressive Relaxation   Find a comfortable surface and lie down on your back. Loosen any constricting clothing such as belts or collars, and remove your shoes and any jewelry that may distract you. Then close your eyes and take a moment to become aware of your breathing. Now take approximately one minute to become aware of your muscles. Scan your muscle groups, starting with your head and progressing to your toes. Do not attempt to relax a tense muscle. Experience the various states of tension throughout your body.

After completing this "body scan," focus your awareness on your right hand. Notice its resting state. Now begin to tense your right hand until you feel a moderate increase in tension. When a moderate level of tension is present, hold the tension for approximately 10–15 seconds. Study the contraction of the muscle. Now release the tension and let your hand relax, spreading your fingers. Do not let your fingers spring out as they relax. Let them relax smoothly. Once you have relaxed your right hand, study the relaxation for 30–45 seconds. Do not move your hand once it is relaxed! Notice how your muscles relax, and compare this sensation with the tension that was present when your hand was in a fist. Study the difference.

The process of progressive relaxation for your right hand will be the same for your other muscle groups. These are steps in progressively relaxing a muscle group:

1. Focus your awareness on the selected muscle group.
2. Moderately tense the muscle group for 10–15 seconds and study the tension.
3. Relax the muscle group for 30–45 seconds and study the relaxation.
4. Note the difference between tension and relaxation in the muscle group.
5. Progress to the next muscle group and repeat steps one to four.

Remember to continue breathing normally. You will have a tendency to hold your breath when you tense a muscle. Steady and easy breathing throughout the exercise will enhance the relaxation process.

PROGRESSIVE RELAXATION EXERCISE

Now you are ready to practice progressive relaxation. Close your eyes and then, using the five-step process just described, progress through this sequence.

1. Tense your right hand into a fist.

PROGRESSIVE RELAXATION EXERCISE (continued)

2. Tense your left hand into a fist.
3. Tense your right arm, contracting the biceps muscle.
4. Tense your left arm, contracting the biceps muscle.
5. Contract your forehead muscles by raising your brows.
6. Contract your eyelids and brows by closing your eyes tightly.
7. Clench your jaw.
8. Tense your tongue by pushing it up against the roof of your mouth.
9. Tense your neck by pushing it into the relaxation surface.
10. Contract your shoulders by shrugging them toward your ears.
11. Contract your chest muscles by taking a deep chest breath.
12. Tense your abdomen by tightening your stomach muscles.
13. Tense your lower back by arching it.
14. Tense your lower back by flattening it.
15. Tense your mid and upper back by pushing your shoulders into the relaxation surface.
16. Tense your buttocks muscles by pulling your buttocks together.
17. Tense your thighs by straightening your legs.
18. Tense your calf muscles by pushing your feet down or pulling them toward you.
19. Tense your feet by pulling your toes up.

When you have completed progressive relaxation, remain still and continue to focus on your muscles for about ten minutes. Enhance your relaxation and improve your awareness. Do not move or tense your muscles during this period! Then take several deep diaphragmatic breaths, stretch your arms and legs, and open your eyes. Get up slowly and resume your daily activities.

Cues Indicating Relaxation in Key Muscle Groups   Research and clinical experience have demonstrated the necessity of relaxing certain muscle groups in order to achieve deep relaxation. Therefore it is especially important for you to learn the difference between tension and relaxation in these five areas. Once you have tensed and relaxed each of these muscle groups, keep them relaxed for the remainder of the exercise.

The following cues indicate relaxation if you are lying on your back with your eyes closed:

1. *Legs.* When your legs are relaxed, each foot will angle out slightly. Your feet will appear to form the shape of a **V**. When your legs are tense, the feet will be parallel to each other, angle in, or angle out sharply. Look at your feet to check this angle.

2. *Abdomen.* When your abdomen is relaxed, it will gently rise and fall as you breathe in and out. When your abdomen is tense, you will not detect the movement. You may place a hand on your abdomen to check this activity.

3. *Lower back.* When your lower back is relaxed, it will make complete contact with the surface you are lying on (if you are sway backed, place a pillow under your knees to flatten your lower back). When the lower back is tense, there will be a space between the lower back and the relaxation surface. To check tension in your lower back, place a hand between your lower back and the floor or bed. Notice the amount of pressure on your hand. Then gently tense your lower back by arching it until you feel that the pressure on your hand is easing. Now see if you can become aware of the corresponding rise in tension. It is not necessary to produce greater tension. Now relax your lower back. Next, gently push your lower back into the surface until you feel a moderate increase in pressure on your hand. Once more, be aware of the tension in your lower back. Then release the pressure and relax. This two-step process should relax your lower back effectively without causing discomfort.

4. *Neck.* When your neck is relaxed, your head will angle slightly to the right or left, so that the side of your head makes contact with the floor or bed. When tense, your neck may seem comfortable and relaxed, but the back of your head, not the side, will be touching the surface. You may check neck tension by opening your eyes. If your neck is tense, you will be looking at the ceiling. If your neck is relaxed, you will see a wall.

5. *Jaw.* When your jaw is relaxed, your lips and teeth will part, and your mouth will hang open slightly. Your face will feel like it is elongating. When your jaw is tense, your mouth is closed. You can check jaw tension by looking at your mouth in a mirror. Make sure your mouth is hanging open!

Recommendations for Progressive Relaxation   When you have the time and privacy it requires, progressive relaxation is excellent for the control of anxiety. As a general purpose exercise, it may also be used to control overall levels of tension, give you more energy to perform your work, and keep you calm. This technique is effective too in controlling musculoskeletal disorders such as muscle tension, headache, bruxism, insomnia, and muscle spasms and in improving concentration (Jacobson, 1938). Its role in the process of desensitization is discussed in Chapter 11, "Perception: Believing Is Seeing."

Yoga

Yoga is a philosophical method for unifying the mind and body. A discipline that has been practiced for thousands of years in the East, its various schools emphasize selfless service, love and devotion to God, mind control, and wisdom. I will discuss a variation called Hatha yoga, which focuses on assuming body postures called asanas. The asanas facilitate deep relaxation when they are performed with proper breathing, known as pranayama. The diaphragmatic breathing discussed previously is an essential ingredient in all Yoga methods. The asanas also help to replenish body energy and vitality. Research in the East and West has documented the effectiveness of Hatha yoga in reducing adrenocortical activity, increasing the efficiency of the cardiovascular system, relaxing the peripheral circulatory system, reducing blood pressure, and decreasing serum cholesterol. Clearly, Hatha yoga is an excellent technique for stress management. It is also a proven technique for increasing the flexibility of the muscles, joints, and connective tissue.

In this section, I will describe asanas for reducing high states of muscle tension in the neck, shoulders, back, and legs because these are the areas associated most frequently with the stress response in our culture.

Guidelines for Hatha Yoga   Observe these guidelines in practicing Hatha yoga to insure an enjoyable and relaxing experience and to avoid injury.

1. Stretch to a comfortable position. You should feel a gentle pull in the stretched area, but never pain.
2. When you have stretched as far as you can without pain, hold the position for a minimum of ten seconds. Do not rock back and forth. You may practice the same stretch more than once within a session.
3. Breathe diaphragmatically, and remember to keep your jaw and abdomen relaxed while you stretch.
4. Do not practice the Hatha yoga sequence after a meal or you may become nauseated. Wait at least 30 minutes.

The asanas are capable of physically manipulating the internal organs including the stomach and intestines.

The Asanas   Each of the following asanas is beneficial for relaxation. Practice them in a quiet environment on a flat surface with carpeting, a towel, or a mat. You may practice these asanas individually or as a sequence. If you do them in a sequence, I recommend that you follow the sequence suggested here, but this may be varied according to your preference and need. See illustrations for each exercise.

HEAD TWIST

This exercise relaxes the neck and upper back. The asana may be performed lying down, seated, or standing (see Figure 17–2).

Exercise:

A. Clasp your hands around the back of your head so that your

HEAD TWIST (continued)

elbows are parallel. Gently begin to pull your head down, moving your chin toward your chest. When you feel the stretch, hold the asana for ten seconds. Then release your hands, relax your neck, and let your head rise.

B. Put your right hand on the right side of your chin and your left hand on the back of your head. Be sure to note the position of the fingers in the picture. Now, twist your head gently to the right and hold this position for ten seconds. Then, bring your head back to the forward position.

C. Put your left hand on the left side of your chin and your right hand on the back of your head. Now, twist to the left and hold for ten seconds. Then, relax your neck.

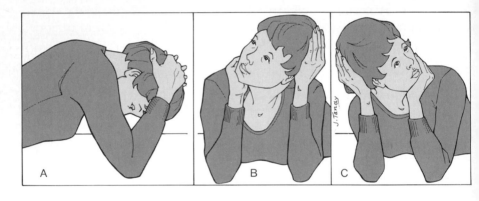

FIGURE 17-2.

Head twist.

CHEST EXPANSION (ARDHA CHAKRASANA)

This asana helps you to develop better breathing by relaxing your chest and shoulders (see Figure 17-3).

Exercise:

A. Stand in a comfortable posture with a straight back. Your feet should be slightly apart. Then bring your hands to your chest with palms facing away from you.

B. Straighten your arms in front of your chest.

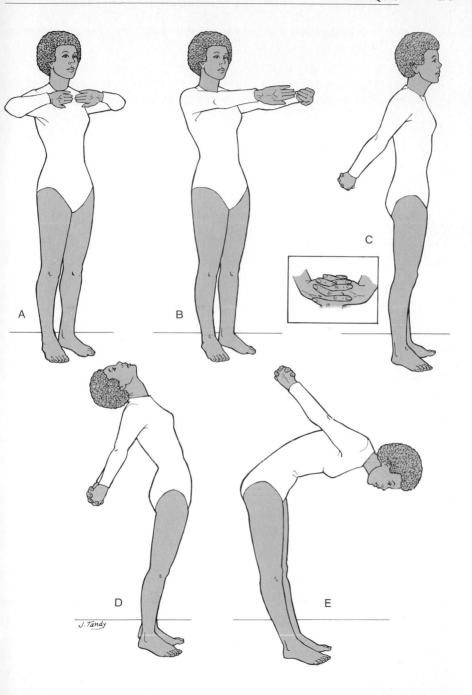

A   B   C

D   E

J. Tandy

FIGURE 17-3.

Chest expansion.

CHEST EXPANSION (ARDHA CHAKRASANA) (continued)

C. Slowly bring your arms behind you, clasping your hands in the manner shown in the picture. Keep your arms as high as possible and notice the stretch in your shoulders. Keep your elbows locked and do not bend at the waist or neck.

D. Now, bend backward and feel the stretch in your lower back. Do not bend back too far. Keep your head up and maintain the upward stretching in your shoulders. Hold this position for ten seconds.

E. From this position, bend forward at the waist and let your arms come over your head, elbows still locked. Your forehead should be pointing toward your knees, and the knees are locked. Hold this position for ten seconds. Then straighten up, unclasp your hands, and breathe easily. Make sure to bend your knees slightly as you assume the upright position.

LEG CLASP (PADAHASTASANA)

This posture stretches the back and hamstrings (see Figure 17-4).

Exercise:

Stand in a relaxed upright position with your hands at your sides. Now begin to bend forward, clasping your hands behind your knees (A). With your hands firmly against the back of your knees, begin to pull your trunk toward the floor (B). Hold this position for ten seconds. [As you develop better flexibility, you may move from the knee clasp to the back of the calves, and finally to your ankles (C).]

Unclasp your hands and straighten up, remembering to bend your knees slightly as you assume your upright posture.

BACK STRETCH (PASCHIMOTTANASANA)

This is an excellent posture for stretching the spine and lower back (see Figure 17-5).

Exercise:

A. Sit on the floor with your legs straight and directly in front of you (if your hamstrings are tight, it will be difficult to straighten your legs; just straighten them as much as you can without pain). Take your hands and clasp your legs, just above your knees.

B. Now lift your arms over your head and then bring them to your knees.

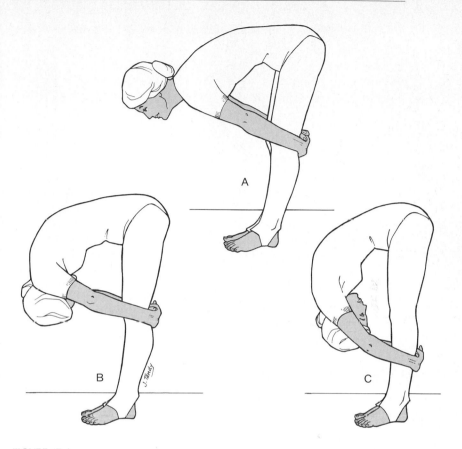

FIGURE 17-4.

Leg clasp.

BACK STRETCH (PASCHIMOTTANASANA) (continued)

C. While gripping your knees, bend forward at the waist. As you move forward, your elbows will angle out. Make sure to keep your head down. Hold this position for ten seconds. (As you develop better flexibility, you can clasp your legs below the knees. In the extreme position, the hands clasp the ankles and the head touches the legs.)

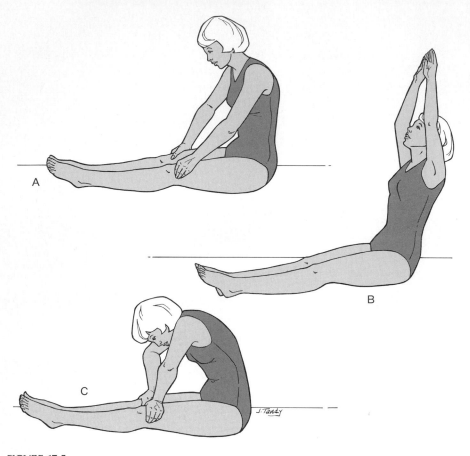

FIGURE 17-5.

Back stretch.

SHOULDER STAND (SARVANGASANA)

This posture stimulates the thyroid gland and aides the return of venous blood from the legs (see Figure 17-6).

Exercise:

A. Assume a relaxed supine posture.
B. Press against the floor with your palms while contracting the leg and abdominal muscles. Slowly begin to raise your legs.
C. Swing your legs back over your head and move palms to your hips to support your weight.

SHOULDER STAND (SARVANGASANA) (continued)

D. Now bring your legs up as far as you can without pain. Note that
your chin is against your chest and your legs are straight. You
may hold this position for up to a minute.

E. When you decide to relax, bend your knees and bring them
toward your head. As they drop place your hands back to the
floor.

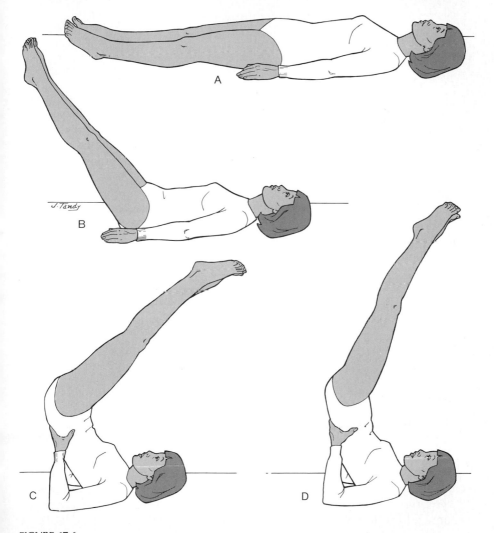

FIGURE 17-6.

Shoulder stand.

DEEP RELAXATION (SAVASANA)

This important posture facilitates a state of deep relaxation and has been shown to reduce blood pressure significantly.

Exercise:

Lie on the floor in a supine position with your arms at your side, palms down. Make sure your legs are relaxed (look for the slight outward angle in your feet). Let your jaw relax, parting your lips and teeth, and allow your neck to angle slightly to one side. Now, focus on diaphragmatic breathing for about one minute with your eyes closed. Then, open your eyes and continue with your daily activities.

Recommendations for Hatha Yoga   When you become aware of rising muscle tension in your body, perform a single asana. The standing postures are useful at work when you cannot lie down to perform the whole sequence. If you feel embarrassed doing an asana around others, you can always make a quick exit to an empty corridor or the privacy of a bathroom.

I have found the neck twist helpful when I have jaw, neck, or shoulder tension. This exercise is also helpful if you feel the beginnings of a tension or migraine headache. Many of these headaches begin with increased neck tension and may be forestalled by this exercise. For aching shoulders and stiffness in the middle or lower back, use the chest expansion. If the chest expansion does not relieve your tension, try the leg clasp, which accentuates the stretch in your spine and hamstrings. When an empty room is available, the shoulder stand is an excellent posture to perform after standing for long periods. If you have tension in your lower back, try the back stretch. Finally, the deep relaxation posture is great whenever you can take one minute to lie down. By focusing on your breathing, the posture will quickly calm you and center your concentration.

Centering

My clinical and personal experiences make it clear that tension and anxiety inhibit *centering,* which is the ability to hold focused attention on an object or thought. High levels of tension and anxiety make people feel as though they are out of balance. Thoughts become scattered; it is difficult to attend; there is a sense of not being grounded in the environment; there are feelings of dread. Extreme states of anxiety can result in paralysis of thought and action. I am sure you have experienced some of these feelings as a nurse, and some of you may have these feelings most of the time.

Centering is an integral part of other relaxation techniques. Recall the principle of selective attention that is so important in progressive relaxation. We are treating it specifically here because when further developed and paired with other techniques, centering can provide rapid and prolonged relaxation.

To center, you must choose a centering object or thought on which to concentrate awareness. Your attention should not be forced or even particularly active. Rather it is a form of passive concentration. If you should become aware of thoughts or images that are not associated with the centering object, just let go of these perceptions and come back to the focus of attention. Make sure not to evaluate yourself for not attending as well as you would like. This attitude will only create more tension.

As a center object, you can choose something external, such as a favorite picture of a loved one, a pastoral scene, or a favorite ring. Place these items in your work area so they can be easily observed. When you are tense, seek out the object and attend to it for several seconds. Perhaps you may take a diaphragmatic breath too. Several seconds of centering in this manner will lower your tension dramatically.

I especially recommend the use of adhesive colored dots as centering cues. They are inexpensive and can be purchased in large quantities at the drug store. Place the dots on objects like your watch, the rear view mirror of your car, or in various places at work. When you see the dot, say a coping statement to yourself and follow it by taking a diaphragmatic breath or relaxing a tense muscle group. For example, when you are rushed for time and look at the dot on your watch, you might say, "Wow, what am I doing being so tense and burning up all this energy? I have a right to decide what to do with my time and I am going to relax!" Next, take a diaphragmatic breath or relax your jaw. Now you are centered and it only took five seconds!

One problem with these external cues is brain tendency to seek out novel stimulation and ignore stimuli that are repetitive. Unfortunately, your brain will habituate to your external cues after a period of four to six weeks, causing you to look right through them. To prevent this problem, make sure you change the color, shape, or location of your cues periodically to maintain their novelty and effectiveness.

Centering cues may also be internal. Images of favorite scenes, numbers, or words can elicit rapid relaxation in any environment.

Centering is easier to perform in a relaxed setting, but in the midst of a crisis when you cannot take 20 minutes, you need to pair centering with relaxation that can help you center quickly. They need to be techniques that will keep you functioning at an optimal level of effectiveness without making you so relaxed that your performance suffers.

Guidelines for Centering   Use the following steps to link your centering cues to a state of deep relaxation:

1. Choose an appropriate cue that is relaxing.
2. Next employ a relaxation technique that will place you in a state of deep relaxation.

3. When you are deeply relaxed, allow the internal cue to form in your mind and focus on that cue for several minutes. In our example, I would focus on the word "meadow."
4. Whenever you relax deeply, focus on your internal cue. Do this for 15–20 relaxation sessions.
5. Then when engaged in your daily activities, allow the internal centering cue to come into your awareness. You will be surprised by the immediate relaxation a cue word such as meadow will produce.

This effect is not the result of magic but is the consequence of a simple and eloquent learning paradigm known as classical conditioning. By pairing deep relaxation with the centering cue meadow, you elicit the relaxation reponse without spending 15 minutes to do it. This five-step procedure can be used to facilitate relaxation for any cue you choose.

Autogenic Training

Developed in the 1920s by Johannes Schultz, M.D., and Wolfgang Luthe, M.D., autogenic training is designed to help you learn to control autonomic processes such as peripheral blood flow, breathing, heart rate, solar plexus activity, and blood flow to the head as well as to relax the striated muscles. You achieve this through reducing environmental and internal stimulation, mentally repeating psychophysiologically adapted verbal formulas, and passive concentration. Six standard exercises focused on a different organ or physiologic system employ training formulas to facilitate the desired physiologic response. Used extensively in Europe and Asia, this relaxation exercise is gaining acceptance in the United States, where a number of institutes have been established to teach autogenic training to professionals (Schultz and Luthe, 1969).

Guidelines for Autogenic Training When practicing this relaxation technique, it is important to maintain a state of passive concentration. Autogenic training is effective only when you center on the part of the body indicated by the formula. For example, when you say the formula, "My right arm is heavy," you must simultaneously be aware of your right arm. I suggest trying to make a mental picture of your right arm, but if you find this difficult you may focus on awareness of the proprioceptive and kinesthetic cues given by your arm. During the exercises any goal-directed behavior, active interest, or apprehension must be put aside! Do not try to make anything happen, but be aware of any physical sensations you experience.

Before beginning this technique, lie down on a comfortable surface and make sure your limbs and trunk are supported. If you have low back pain a pillow under your knees will help to take pressure off it. A firm pillow under the head can be helpful. Perform this technique in a quiet room of moderate temperature and reduced illumination.

When you are comfortable, close your eyes and become aware of your breathing. Use diaphragmatic breathing, as you have already learned, in a steady rhythm for about one minute. Next, relax your neck and jaw. Then spend about one minute performing a body scan. Scan your voluntary muscles for tension that might distract you. If you find tense muscles, increase the tension momentarily; then let them relax. Relaxed breathing and lower muscle tension will facilitate the effects of the exercises. Be sure to begin each exercise session with these steps.

Now that you are relaxing, begin to focus on the autogenic training formulas. Combined with the relaxation techniques already described, they will produce beneficial physiologic changes. More elaborate sequences than the one that follows are possible, but they require longer periods of practice. Practice the exercises and formulas regularly. Say the formulas to yourself, repeating each formula the number of times indicated. Make sure you do not alter the content of the formula in any way! Be sure to allow a three to five second pause after each formula.

There are several ways to perform the standard exercises. You can memorize the formulas, which is not as difficult as you may think, or you may make a tape by repeating the formulas in a quiet room. Whether you memorize the sequence or make a tape, say the phrases slowly and rhythmically. If you are good at visualization and do not like to repeat the formulas mentally, try flashing each formula across your visual field like a film strip. Keep your eyes closed. Let the formula continue to flash for the three to five second period. Then, go on to the next formula. I believe you will find saying the formulas easier (Schultz and Luthe, 1969).

AUTOGENIC TRAINING STANDARD EXERCISES*

First Standard Exercise

My right arm is heavy. (three times)
My left arm is heavy. (three times)
Both arms are heavy. (three times)
My right leg is heavy. (three times)
My left leg is heavy. (three times)
Both legs are heavy. (three times)
My arms and legs are heavy. (three times)

Second Standard Exercise

My right arm is warm. (three times)
My left arm is warm. (three times)
Both arms are warm. (three times)
My right leg is warm. (three times)

---

*The sequence for the heaviness and warmth formulas is for right-handed and right-footed individuals. If you are left-handed or left-footed, begin with the left arm or leg. Then focus on the right side.

AUTOGENIC TRAINING STANDARD EXERCISES (continued)
My left leg is warm. (three times)
Both legs are warm. (three times)
My arms and legs are heavy and warm. (three times)

Third Standard Exercise
My heart beat is calm and regular. (five times)

Fourth Standard Exercise
It breathes me. (five times)

Fifth Standard Exercise
My solar plexus is warm. (five times)

Sixth Standard Exercise
My forehead is cool. (five times)

Ending:
After you have completed the exercises, always end the autogenic training session with the following three-step procedure:
1. Flex your arms energetically.
2. Breathe deeply three times.
3. Open your eyes.

Autogenic training can produce a very low state of arousal. If you still feel sleepy or groggy after doing this procedure, continue to repeat it until you feel alert. Low arousal decreases motor performance, so do not jump right up and run to your car. Take time to let your body readjust to a normal level of alertness. Enjoy your feelings of relaxation.

Discrimination between Tension and Relaxation in Autogenic Training   The autonomic nervous system controls the smooth muscles and glands and innervates the heart. Awareness of the following physical sensations will verify that you are relaxing a specific organ or physiologic system controlled by the autonomic nervous system. However, it is not necessary to feel anything for the exercise to be effective.

The First Standard Exercise. The aim of this exercise is voluntary muscular relaxation. Most people experience heaviness in the limbs as the muscles relax, although some report feelings of lightness. Refer to the section on progressive relaxation for further discussion of tension and relaxation of muscles.

The Second Standard Exercise. The aim of this standard exercise is peripheral vasodilation. Most people feel warmth in the arms and legs as the vasomotor system relaxes.

You can check vasomotor relaxation by feeling your fingertips or toes before and after the relaxation session, or you can use an inexpensive alcohol thermometer to monitor your peripheral temperature. Place the bulb of the thermometer on the tip of your middle finger and attach the thermometer snugly with porous tape, such as micropore tape. It should not be so tight that you experience throbbing. Note your temperature before you begin and when you finish. Hand temperatures of 70–85 degrees are in the range of vasomotor tension, whereas temperatures of 88–97 are in the relaxed range. If your palms and fingers are sweaty, this indicates tension even if your hands are warm. When you finish the exercises, feel your hands again. If your palms and fingers are dry, then your autonomic nervous system is relaxed.

Third Standard Exercise. The aim of this exercise is the voluntary regulation of heart rate. As you relax, your heart rate will slow and become more rhythmic. You can check your pulse or place your hand over your heart. As you know, there is great variation in heart rates, especially if you exercise aerobically. Monitor your heart rate briefly before you begin autogenic training and use this reading as a baseline level.

Fourth Standard Exercise. This exercise will help you control breathing. As you become more relaxed your breathing rate will slow and become more rhythmic.

Fifth Standard Exercise. This exercise affects the solar plexus, a nerve center for the abdomen. (Imagine a circle approximately 3 inches in diameter below the xiphoid process.) Tension may manifest itself here as heartburn, stomach pain, or bowel sounds, although of course a recent meal can also produce these symptoms. When the solar plexus is relaxed, the abdominal region will feel warm, and there will be no bowel sounds or pain.

Sixth Standard Exercise. The forehead is cooled by the action of this exercise. It may be difficult to notice the difference, since the maximum decline in temperature is only several degrees.

As you practice autogenic training, you may be aware of other sensations like sinking or loss of awareness in the limbs, or imagine movement in your arms or legs. Do not be apprehensive about these sensations—they are signs of relaxation.

Recommendations for Autogenic Training Autogenic training, like progressive relaxation, is capable of producing a profound state of relaxation. You may use this technique for the long-term control of tension. Once you develop the ability to do the technique lying down, you can begin to perform the standard exercises in a supported, seated position. Being able to perform the exercises in a chair is advantageous when a bed or floor cannot be used. Unfortunately, this technique is not recommended when you only have a few minutes to relax, or when you are confronted with a stressor that must be controlled quickly.

Make sure to allow yourself 15–20 minutes each time you practice autogenic training. This time interval is necessary to lower your arousal level and increase your energy.

In addition to its value in controlling tension, autogenic training has been proven effective in the control of high blood pressure, migraine headache, Raynaud's syndrome, and gastrointestinal disorders (Schultz and Luthe, 1969).

Meditation

Meditation is a term that covers a broad spectrum of disciplines. All of the techniques in this chapter are meditative techniques. Meditation can be a simple act like diaphragmatic breathing, or it may take the form of religious contemplation like the Jesus Prayer. I believe that each of you will find some meditative techniques to be compatible with your temperament and life-style. Although the other exercises may seem useless, practice the ones that are comfortable for you, but do not give up on the exercises that may be initially uncomfortable or annoying.

You will discover that most of the exercises involve a selective focus of attention (centering) and a repetition of action. If you practice autogenic training, it is important to focus on that part of your body represented by the formula. If you practice transcendental meditation, you need to center on your mantra. When you perform Hatha yoga, you focus on physical movement and repeat actions. In progressive relaxation, you repeat the process of tensing and relaxing each of your muscles. If you enjoy religious devotion, you may repeat the phrases of the rosary. For those of you who have practiced Benson's relaxation response, you will repeat the word one.

Here are different types of meditative practice that facilitate relaxation.

Concentration   Concentration, centering, or focusing are words describing the essence of meditation. A beautiful and simple technique to develop this state is the passive awareness of a candle flame. To perform this meditation, take a candle and place it on a simple stand approximately 1 foot away from you. Next sit down so that the candle is in your line of sight. Make sure that the background behind the candle is neutral; complex backgrounds are distracting. Now begin to gaze at the candle flame in a state of passive concentration. Focus your awareness on the flame, and if you are distracted by thoughts or sensations, let these distractions pass and return gently but firmly to the flame.

Begin your practice by gazing at the candle for one minute intervals. Though one minute does not seem like much time it may be difficult for you to focus your awareness any longer in the beginning. As you practice, you will be able to focus on the flame for longer periods. Ten to 15 minutes of focused attention should be enough time to achieve a state of alert but physically relaxed awareness.

Mantra   A mantra is a word or phrase that is repeated in a rhythmic pattern. Mantras have spiritual connotations and are found in all of the world's major religions. I shall present several mantras from different religions. If you choose to use a mantra, you might select one that is compatible with your religious background.

Begin your mantra by sitting in a comfortable position and closing your eyes. You may repeat the mantra silently or aloud. Always focus on the mantra with passive awareness. As you gain familiarity with your mantra, you may repeat it at any time. The following mantras have been used for thousands of years and have facilitated a deep sense of spiritual awareness.

1. Aum (pronounced AH-OWM). This word, which is a fundamental sound or the blending of all sounds, has its roots in Eastern religions.
2. Lord Jesus Christ, Son of God, have mercy on me, a sinner. This phrase is a classic Christian mantra from the Gospel of Luke. It is also known as the Jesus Prayer.
3. It is in pronouncing thy name that I must die and live. Widely used in Islam, this mantra is a quotation from Muhammad.
4. Blessed is the person who utterly surrenders his soul for the name of Yahweh to dwell therein and to establish therein its throne of glory. This mantra, whose author is Zohar, summarizes the beliefs of the Jewish mystics.

Two popular relaxation techniques use the repetition of a word to produce relaxation: transcendental meditation (TM) and Benson's relaxation response. In TM you are given a secret mantra word designed to fit your unique personality. Many feel that the crucial element of this technique is matching the right word to the right person. By repeating this mantra, you are able to relax and achieve an altered state of consciousness. Research studies have demonstrated the effectiveness of TM in facilitating a relaxed state. Findings have reported decreases in heart rate, oxygen consumption, blood pressure, and muscle tension (Bloomfield et al., 1975).

Herbert Benson, a Harvard University professor who was very much interested in the physiologic effects of TM, designed an experiment to analyze the effects of the mantra on the relaxation process. His results showed that the repetition of the word one was just as effective in producing relaxation as was using a secret TM mantra (Benson, 1975). He concluded that the repetition of the mantra was the critical variable in facilitating the relaxed state, not the word used. From this research, he developed Benson's relaxation response, which uses the mantra one to produce relaxation. The advantage of Benson's technique is that it costs little to learn to meditate and relax. In contrast, TM costs considerably more money.

Movement   Meditation may be performed through movement as well as by centering while sitting quietly. Hatha yoga, which I have already discussed, is an example of centering on body movement to promote relaxation and peace. T'ai chi is an Oriental martial art that is a form of movement meditation. You may think that karate or jujitsu are strenuous and stressful forms of exercise, but they are actually relaxed and focused forms of meditation. If you are a person who is oriented toward movement and action, the martial arts are excellent forms of meditation, as well as self-defense.

Mindfulness The last form of meditation I will discuss is mindfulness. When you are mindful of your environment, you are acutely aware of your internal and/or external actions. Individuals who practice mindfulness are aware of a flowing, dynamic reality in which the mind observes the person's own thoughts, feelings, or physical sensations. To describe mindfulness, I shall use the example of mindful walking from *Journey of Awakening* by Ram Dass (1978).

In mindful walking you focus on the movement of your legs and body to develop a passive awareness of the action of walking. Focus on the sensations of contraction and relaxation in the muscles, as well as on the various angles of the joints. Walk with your arms and hands quietly at your sides or clasped behind your back. As you take your steps, be aware of the rising and falling of each foot. Notice the rhythm of your walking. Also, become aware of how your various moods affect your pattern of walking. Try not to look at your legs or feet while you meditate on mindful walking, but be aware of the physical sensation.

Mindfulness can be directed to many activities, including thinking, eating, breathing, or playing. Note how you have already developed mindful breathing from studying the breathing exercises. The key elements in mindfulness are passive awareness and alertness. Remember not to judge or evaluate your thoughts, feelings, or actions as you attempt this.

Recommendations Although meditation is an excellent way to relax, I believe the essential purpose of the meditative disciplines is to develop a systematic understanding of reality. Meditative disciplines provide a process through which this reality may be perceived. You may wish to look beyond meditation as a relaxation technique and explore the various paths of the meaning of the cosmos.

Biofeedback

Although the use of biofeedback depends on the use of equipment I will mention it because of its popularity and its usefulness. Biofeedback is used in conjunction with relaxation techniques to enhance awareness, promote discrimination between tension and relaxation, and facilitate passive concentration and deep relaxation. Sensors placed on the surface of the body detect subtle changes in physiology and transmit the information as bioelectric signals to the biofeedback instruments (see Figure 17-7). The biofeedback instrument filters the signals, amplifies them, and symbolically displays these signals to you in the form of auditory, visual, or tactile information (Brown, 1977).

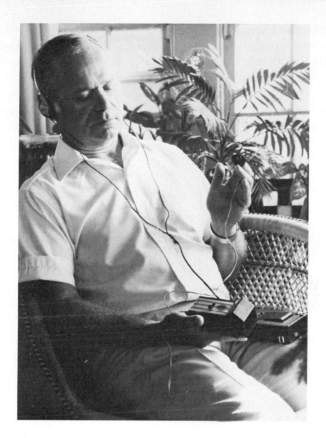

FIGURE 17-7.

Biofeedback is a popular alternative healing therapy that represents a shift toward independence and away from professional control. This man uses biofeedback to reduce job-related stress and to improve his racquetball game.

Biofeedback, then, is information that can be used to learn how to control physiologic systems. Using this feedback information in the form of signals you can begin to associate your conscious thoughts, feelings, and actions with the subconscious bodily processes being monitored. The important element of the learning process is to associate the external signal such as a light or tone with internal states of thinking, feeling, or bodily sensation. Once you have made the association between the moment-to-moment feedback signal and your internal activity, you can learn to reproduce the internal physiologic state at will.

For example, consider electromyographic biofeedback, or feedback from the voluntary muscles. Prior to muscle contraction, your muscles produce ionic electrical activity in the microvolt range (1 microvolt is about one million times as dim as a flashlight battery!). As your muscles tense, they produce more electrical activity, which is picked up by sensors placed on the surface of the skin. The increase in electrical energy drives the pitch of the auditory feedback tone higher. When your muscles relax, they produce less electrical activity, and this decrease in energy drives the pitch of the feedback tone lower. Suppose we place an electromyographic electrode on your forehead, an excellent site for monitoring facial muscle tension. When you clench your jaw, the feedback tone rises significantly. As you relax, the feedback tone drops dramatically. You can become aware of the position of your jaw and how your lips and teeth are parted during this relaxation. After you have tensed and relaxed your jaw several times and listened to the changes in the feedback tone, you will make the association that tensing the muscles of the jaw produces a significant increase in facial tension. Conversely, a relaxed, loose jaw will produce a significant decrease in facial tension. This is true, of course, whether you are being monitored by the biofeedback instrument or trying to get to work on time. The advantage of biofeedback is its ability to give you concise and objective information about what your body is doing at any given moment and thereby to accelerate the learning of complex motor skills such as those required to relax.

Types of Biofeedback and Their Clinical Applications   In clinical practice there are four basic types of biofeedback instruments: electromyographic biofeedback, electrodermal biofeedback, temperature biofeedback, and electroencephalographic biofeedback.

1. Electromyographic biofeedback. As we have just seen, this type of feedback instrument monitors muscle tension from voluntary muscles like the jaw.
2. Electrodermal biofeedback. This instrument monitors the electrical activity of the skin. Tiny sweat glands in the palms and fingers are innervated by the sympathetic nervous system. The sympathetic nervous system is a branch of the autonomic nervous system that helps to mobilize the body when it is confronted with a perceived threat. If the sympathetic activity is increasing, then the sweat glands secrete more sweat. Also, there are changes in the membranes of the sweat glands. Declining sympathetic nervous system activity causes the sweat glands to secrete less sweat. By learning how to control the electrodermal feedback, you are learning how to control your autonomic nervous system.
3. Temperature biofeedback. Temperature biofeedback, like electrodermal biofeedback, is a measure of sympathetic arousal. The sympathetic nervous system innervates the smaller arteries and arterioles of the peripheral circulatory system, especially in the fingers and toes. As your sympathetic nervous system becomes more tense, it constricts the muscles surrounding these blood vessels, causing less blood to flow through them. This response causes the surface temperature of the skin to cool. Lowered arousal in the sympathetic nervous system pro-

duces a relaxation of the smooth muscles in your arteries and arterioles with a corresponding increase in surface skin temperature.
4.   Electroencephalographic (EEG) biofeedback. These instruments measure the electrochemical activity of the brain cells, especially those oscillatory potentials at the surface of the cerebral cortex. The EEG wave forms change as states of consciousness change, and certain EEG wave forms have been identified with specific states of consciousness. For example, alpha waves are usually associated with a relaxed, passive attention, whereas beta waves correspond with active, focused attention. EEG feedback can help you to identify physiologic and mental cues associated with different EEG wave forms. Once you have made the associations between the feedback and your different patterns of awareness, you can learn to control consciousness.

Recommendations for Biofeedback   If you want to learn how to use biofeedback, or to obtain national certification, contact the Biofeedback Society of America (The Biofeedback Certification Institute of America, 4301 Owens Street, Wheat Ridge, CO 80033).

CONCLUSION

First, relaxation is a motor skill and must be practiced at regular intervals to maintain the benefits. When you have gone for a week or two without doing an exercise, note how your tension has been increasing. Then, make a note in your schedule to relax for 20 minutes, three times per week. As you begin to relax again, you will find that doing the exercises becomes easier as the habit is reestablished. Eventually, you will be back into your relaxation routine.

Second, you have been introduced to many relaxation techniques and may be confused about which ones are right for you. Breathing occupies the primary position in the hierarchy of relaxation and will be an essential component to any relaxation exercise. With that as a starting place remember the following guideline: the more tense you are, the more you need to use active, movement-oriented relaxation techniques to reduce high levels of muscular tension. Begin by walking around the block and then proceed from more active to more passive techniques until you experience relief. Perform several yoga asanas to release high levels of tonic muscle tension. Then perform progressive relaxation for about five minutes. Your mind and body may now be relaxed to the degree that focusing on the autogenic formulas or practicing meditation will be successful and rewarding.

As you continue relaxing, you will get a more consistent mental and physical response to lowered arousal, you will relax faster, and you will find that your relaxed state will generalize to your everyday activities. Relaxation will give you more energy to do the activities you enjoy, and it will lessen the negative impact of activities that create tension and anxiety. You have the right to decide what to do with your time and your body. So relax, because you deserve it!

REFERENCES

Benson, H. 1975. *The relaxation response.* New York: William Morrow.

Bloomfield, H., Cain, M., Jaffe, D. et al. 1975. *T.M.: discovering inner energy and overcoming stress.* New York: Delacorte Press.

Brown, B. 1977. *Stress and the art of biofeedback.* New York: Harper and Row.

Cannon, W. 1967. *The wisdom of the body.* New York: W. W. Norton.

Erickson, M. H., Rossi, E. L., and Rossi, S. I. 1976. *Hypnotic realities.* New York: Halsted Press.

Friedman, M., and Rosenman, R. H. 1974. *Type A behavior and your heart.* New York: Alfred A. Knopf.

Girdano, D., and Everly, G. 1976. *Controlling stress and tension: a holistic approach.* Englewood Cliffs, N.J.: Prentice-Hall, Inc.

Jacobson, E. J. 1938. *Progressive relaxation.* Chicago: University of Chicago Press.

Jakubowski, P., and Lange, A. 1978. *The assertive option: your rights and responsibilities.* Champaign, Ill.: Research Press.

Ram Dass. 1978. *Journey of awakening.* New York: Bantam Books.

Schultz, J. H., and Luthe, W. 1969. *Autogenic training,* Vol. 1. New York: Grune and Stratton.

CHAPTER 18

Creative Imagination

JESSICA G. SCHAIRER

Basic Principles
Imagination Exercises for Specific Situations
Imagery for Problem Solving
Conclusion

Imagination, daydreaming, imagery, visualization, self-hypnosis, meditation, prayer—these terms can all be considered to describe related phenomena. They are all states of mind in which attention and concentration are focused inward on subjective cues and images or sensations that are usually fleeting.

In these states of focused attention, you can get in touch with thoughts and feelings of which you might otherwise be unaware. You can become aware of underlying sources of stress, or the connection between otherwise seemingly disconnected events. And using this focused concentration, you can observe and even generate images and sensations leading to the creation of new solutions to seemingly intractable problems.

Daydreaming is commonly considered a rather passive and aimless activity. However, it appears to be an important part of the creative process for many artists and writers, and even entrepreneurs—people whose life work entails finding unique and creative solutions to a variety of problems.

I believe that bringing this kind of creativity into the everyday work of nursing deroutinizes it and thereby reduces its stressfulness. Krieger (1979) has demonstrated that nurses who focus concentration on conveying tender loving care through touch can have a remarkably positive effect on patients. This approach gives a creative and meditative aspect to the daily work of bedside nursing.

The techniques discussed here make explicit and direct methods that many people have used spontaneously and successfully for centuries. What is new is the greater scientific respect and understanding these processes have achieved.

Imagery techniques can be used to increase self-awareness of physical stress, to facilitate problem solving, and for health maintenance, future planning, and personal growth and self-development. In fact, it is no exaggeration to say imagery can help in almost any realm of endeavor, just as it is no exaggeration to say that logical thinking can help in almost any situation. This is because visualization is another kind of thinking; it appears to be associated with the right hemisphere of the brain in the same way logical thinking is associated with the left hemisphere. Although developing cognitive ability increases your options for dealing with life, you will be amazed at how you can enhance these powers by focusing your attention on your imagery and learning to use it actively. It's much like what happens when an individual who can play the piano by ear starts taking music lessons—the kind of music she or he can produce on the piano can become infinitely richer and more complex. But in the same way that almost everyone can sing and enjoy music, almost everyone can use imagery to improve and enrich daily life.

BASIC PRINCIPLES

The exercises in this chapter do not demand extraordinary psychic powers. They are systematizations of what many people do naturally and spontaneously. Research on coping styles suggests that they are actually most helpful to those individuals who are "ineffective copers" (Weisman and Worden, 1976) or "catastrophizers" (Brown et al., 1981); "effective copers" or "minimizers" are using these techniques already. For example, in a study of pain experimentally induced by immersing subjects' hands in ice water, a minimizer might spontaneously think of cupping his hands in a cool mountain spring to get a drink, while the catastrophizer imagines himself parachuting into the North Sea during World War II. The catastrophizer's image helps him be brave and withstand the pain. The minimizer's image recodes it into something much more pleasant. Both images contain the same reality element—the hand immersed in cold water.

When we think of imagery, we usually think of visualization, but visual imagery is not every person's preferred modality. Some people prefer auditory imagery—sound and music. And some people feel most comfortable with kinesthetic imagery—physical feelings and sensations (Bandler and Grinder, 1976). For example, think of a cat. What color is it? If you immediately have a cat of a specific color, you are probably a good visualizer. If you are more aware of thinking of the texture or warmth of a cat, you are more kinesthetically oriented. If you think of the cat's purr, you are more auditorily oriented. Of course, a person can use all three modalities, or even more, by including smell and taste. However, most people have a preferred modality.

Let's try another example. Imagine yourself lying on the beach. What are you aware of first? The warmth of the sun? Or the sound of the surf and the cry of the gulls? Or the brilliant blue sky? Or perhaps the smell of the salt air? Whichever comes to you first gives you an indication of which sensory modality is most comfortable for you. However, you can also begin to see in this example how a rich image is built up in as many sensory modalities as possible.

To develop your capacity to use imagery, it's usually best to start with the sensory modality you're comfortable with and then embellish your image with input from other modalities, as I just did with the image of the beach. In the exercises I give in this chapter, I try to include something to stimulate image production in every modality.

In recent years, a great deal of exciting research has been done on the use of imagery in various settings. A number of intriguing hypotheses that relate imagery to the functions of the right hemisphere of the brain are now just beginning to be understood. Imagery appears to be the language of the right hemisphere of the brain, in the same way that words are the language of the left hemisphere. If this is so, learning to consciously think in images is the equivalent of learning to consciously use the right hemisphere of the brain. It certainly seems to enhance creativity, which in many people seems to be powerfully assisted by the right hemisphere.

Most people find it easiest to do the exercises in this chapter if they are in a state of deep physical relaxation, as described in Chapter 17. However, these imagery exercises are not necessarily physically relaxing.

Psychophysiologic research has been done comparing transcendental meditation, which focuses passively on a mantra, and kundalini yoga, which focuses actively on becoming one with a higher power. Although passive meditation is physiologically relaxing, active meditation can be very physiologically arousing—in some cases similar to orgasm. In more passive meditations, brain waves are predominantly alpha. In more active meditations, brain waves are predominantly beta (Krieger, 1979).

Practically, what this means is that it is easier to enter a state of deeply focused concentration from a state of deep physical relaxation, but you may or may not remain deeply relaxed physically once imagery is introduced. How relaxed you are will depend on the imagery you're dealing with and the purpose for which you are doing it. Most people who are in a state of deep hypnosis report feeling deeply relaxed. Yet it has been my personal observation, using biofeedback monitors, that they are often physiologically aroused but unaware of it. This is the clearest example I have seen of the difference between psychologic and physiologic relaxation.

Once again, I want to refer you to Chapter 17 on physical relaxation techniques. Once you have mastered one of the techniques described there, you will be able to enter a relaxed and receptive state at will, ready to use the visualization techniques discussed here. After two or three weeks of practice, most people find all they have to do is take three deep diaphragmatic breaths and they are able to trigger their relaxation response (Benson and Klipper, 1976) and are ready to start using imagery. However, if you have not already mastered a relaxation technique, you would do well to start each exercise with at least three to five minutes of diaphragmatic breathing while sitting or lying quietly with your eyes closed.

The exercises that follow give you many opportunities to practice creating harmonious and positive images, even under difficult and stressful conditions. You may find it helpful to record each one on audio tape and then play it back in order to practice the exercise without the stress of trying to remember an unfamiliar sequence. Speak very slowly and gently to yourself. The dots (. . .) indicate pauses. They should be as natural as a breath.

EXERCISE 1: 20 STEPS TO YOUR SPECIAL PLACE*

Start by getting as comfortable as you can: loosen any tight clothing, and make sure you will be uninterrupted. Take the phone off the hook. Take three deep, diaphragmatic breaths . . . in and out . . . in and out . . . in and out. Let your eyes close and with every breath, begin to feel your body relax more and more.

Now imagine yourself at the top of a flight of 20 steps. They can be anywhere you like, any kind of steps. Just see yourself at the top. In a moment you will begin to descend.

You are on the first step . . . beginning to feel more and more comfortable and relaxed . . . . The second step . . . beginning to notice that parts of your body are more relaxed . . . . The third step . . . maybe your arms are more relaxed than your feet . . . . The fourth step . . . or maybe your feet are more relaxed than your arms . . . . The fifth step . . . it really doesn't matter, as your entire body becomes more and more comfortable and relaxed . . . . The sixth step . . . perhaps noticing a warm heavy feeling in your hands and feet . . . . The seventh step . . . noticing your breathing becoming slower and more even . . . . The eighth step . . . . The ninth step . . . . The tenth step, half-way down the steps . . . wondering what you will find at the bottom . . . . The eleventh step . . . feeling a pleasant feeling of relaxation flowing through your entire body . . . . The twelfth step . . . with nothing to bother you, nothing to disturb you . . . . The thirteenth step . . . the fourteenth step . . . the fifteenth step, almost at the bottom. The sixteenth step . . . feeling more and more comfortable and relaxed . . . . The seventeenth

*Adapted with permission. Barber, J. Rapid Induction Analgesia: A Clinical Report. *The American Journal of Clinical Hypnosis*, Vol. 19, No. 3, 1977.

EXERCISE 1: 20 STEPS TO YOUR SPECIAL PLACE (continued)

step . . . your entire body feeling heavy and warm . . . . The eighteenth step . . . perhaps feeling a pleasant tingling sensation in your hands and feet . . . . The nineteenth step . . . almost at the bottom of the steps . . . . The twentieth step, the bottom of the steps.

Now, while you continue in a state of deep physical relaxation, in your mind's eye, see yourself in your special place, where you feel most comfortable and secure . . . . Your own special place—maybe it's in the city or the country . . . . Maybe it's in the mountains or by the shore . . . . Wherever it is, it is your special place . . . . See its colors . . . hear its sounds . . . smell its special scent . . . . Take a moment to really enjoy the special feeling the image of it brings . . . that special feeling of comfort, peace and security.

Now, while you are in this state of deep physical and emotional peace and relaxation, you are best able to focus your attention on whatever you wish. In these moments of silence, focus on your inner images.

Leave at least five to ten minutes of silence here. If you wish, you can play some music during this section of your tape. Many people like organ music, especially fugues. Any of the exercises following this one could also be done here. Or if you like, you could just focus on your breathing or a single phrase, such as I am one, and the images it arouses.

In a moment, you will ascend the staircase, feeling more and more refreshed and alert. See yourself once again at the bottom of the staircase. See yourself on the twentieth step, beginning to walk back up the staircase . . . the nineteenth step . . . the eighteenth step . . . the seventeenth step, still comfortable and relaxed, but with every step beginning to feel more and more refreshed and alert . . . . The sixteenth step . . . the fifteenth step, with every step feeling refreshed and renewed . . . . The fourteenth step . . . the thirteenth step . . . the twelfth step . . . feeling more and more refreshed and alert . . . . The eleventh step . . . the tenth step, halfway up the steps. The ninth step . . . the eighth step . . . with every step feeling more and more alert, more and more refreshed . . . . The seventh step . . . the sixth step . . . slowly letting everyday thoughts come back to mind . . . . The fifth step, getting ready to open your eyes . . . . The fourth step, beginning to feel your eyelids flutter . . . . The third step, letting everyday thoughts come back to mind and your attention come back into the room. The second step, gently open your eyes. And the first step, feeling refreshed and alert, glad to have taken these moments to relax and pay attention to your inner self.

Just rest quietly now for a few moments with your eyes open; then stretch and return to your everyday activities.

IMAGINATION EXERCISES FOR SPECIFIC SITUATIONS

The exercise just given includes physical and mental relaxation through imagery. It also contains a section of silence in which any of the following exercises can be done. However, as discussed in the basic principles section, once you have a good conditioned relaxation response (Benson and Klipper, 1976), you will not need to do a full-scale physical and mental relaxation exercise in order to focus on your inner imagery. Instead, you can just take three deep breaths and focus on a personal code word of your own choosing, such as relax or one or even meadow or ocean—whatever works for you. In the following exercise I will refer to this warmup process as *relax deeply.* Take as little or as much time as you need to trigger your relaxation response.

EXERCISE 2: IMAGERY FOR PHYSICAL SELF-AWARENESS OF STRESS

You may be aware of general feelings of tension and stress but unaware of how these feelings affect you physically. This exercise focuses on the physical effects of stress and uses imagery to undo them.

Relax deeply. Attend to your entire body, becoming aware of areas that are still tense. Imagine you have x-ray vision. What do you see in those parts of your body? Imagine your vision is an electron microscope. What do you see now? You may get a strong sense of your body without any visualization at all. That's fine. What does it feel like?

Maintain this image or kinesthetic sense of the effect of tension in your body. Imagine the body's natural healing process at work. If you have become aware of muscle tension, focus on the lengthening of the muscle fibers with relaxation. If you have become aware of increased pulse or a subjective feeling of increased blood pressure, visualize the heart slowing and the blood vessels relaxing. Focus on the healthy functioning of your body. (This approach is especially suited to health professionals who understand physiology.)

Alternatively, you can give your tension or pain a color. Focus on the changes in the color as you become more and more deeply relaxed. You may also find it gets larger or smaller or becomes less and less attached to your image of your body as you focus on it in a relaxed and quiet way. You can learn a lot about your physical reaction to stress just by quietly observing.

Or you may identify a resonance, a hum. Hum with it, louder and louder, softer and softer, higher and higher, lower and lower, until it fades away.

IMAGERY FOR PROBLEM SOLVING

There are a number of different approaches to problem solving through imagery.

EXERCISE 3: WAITING FOR AN IMAGE

Simply relax deeply and pose the problem to yourself. Then just wait to see what images or thoughts come to mind. You will often be presented with an image or kinesthetic sensation that may suggest a novel solution.

EXERCISE 4: MOVIE SCREEN

A more linear approach than just waiting for an image is to relax deeply. Imagine a movie screen in your mind's eye. Project the current problem on the screen. Then run different possible solutions on the screen, as if you were viewing them in a theater. Try to be as detailed as you can. Carry each idea out to its full and logical conclusion. You can even split the screen and run two competing solutions side by side and see which works better. You may be surprised at what you see—details you weren't aware of may suddenly become clear and important.

This approach is especially useful if you are trying to deal with administrative problems or any problems with many details in a complex configuration, such as planning a nursing protocol in critical care or the emergency area. See yourself going through it. Even better, if you can, feel yourself going through it as if you are engaged in the action, rather than as an external observer. See it through your own eyes, rather than seeing an image of yourself performing on the movie screen. If you have trouble seeing yourself reaching your goal, visualize yourself there first and work backward, perhaps using the split screen, to imagine how you might get there.

This exercise has the advantage of breaking the task up into discrete, doable segments, rather than one massive, overwhelming whole. It also has the advantage of using a more right-hemisphere approach and calling on resources that otherwise might not be consciously available.

EXERCISE 5: IMAGINING SUCCESS: THE SELF-FULFILLING PROPHECY

The self-fulfilling prophecy is usually thought of in negative terms: believing an undesirable outcome will occur will in fact cause its occurrence. However, the same effect can be seen in positive directions as well.

Imagery can be used to enhance positive self-fulfilling prophecies. In the previous exercise you visualized yourself at your goal and then explored how you might get there. There are other times in life when you know exactly what to do but doubt your ability to do it. Losing weight, writing reports, and stopping smoking are behaviors in this category. I find that everybody can tell me all the steps they need to go through to accomplish these goals. If they are at all confused, I ask them to tell me what they would advise some third person to do. The trick is to phrase these behaviors in a positive and nonpunitive way to yourself.

For example, people who wish to lose weight typically view a diet as a horrible self-deprivation that can be endured for only a short period of time. However, a much more successful viewpoint is to see a healthful diet as the best way to nourish your body by feeding your body good food in the right amount. Here the image of nourishment replaces deprivation. This image is much easier to live with in the long run.

EXERCISE 6: CAREER PLANNING

Another good use of the self-fulfilling prophecy is in career planning. Relax deeply and try to see yourself next year and then five years from now. What are you doing? Do you like what you see? If you don't, what would you like to see instead? Don't discount your wish, no matter how unusual it seems to you now. Elaborate the image; really get into it. If you find you really like this image, start imagining how you might get there. Many highly successful people do this all the time, quite spontaneously. It enables them to be open to opportunities they otherwise might not notice, and these opportunities help them get where they want to go.

EXERCISE 7: THE INNER GUIDE*

Relax deeply. See yourself on a road. A glow of light is coming down the road. The light becomes a figure. Who or what is it? This is your inner guide. Ask the figure your questions. Listen closely for an answer. The answer may not be in words. Agree with your inner guide to meet again before you say goodbye.

This exercise is especially good for questions of inner development—questions that do not have an obvious answer.

*(This exercise is adapted from Carl Simonton et al., 1978.)

CONCLUSION

I have attempted to give you an overview of a process as old as human-kind and as richly creative as art or dreams. It is an attempt to make available to your conscious mind processes that occur in everyone, all the time, but usually unconsciously.

If this chapter has sparked your interest, I urge you to read further. Good starting points are Samuels and Samuels (1975) and LeShan (1974). These are two encyclopedic sources of visualizations and meditations. If music is your modality, you might wish to investigate Halpern's work (1976). And for a view of how active imagination can be integrated with psychotherapy in a profoundly meaningful way, Hannah's book (1981) is excellent.

Imagery is an intensely personal experience. Although some themes are universal, every individual's experience is unique. Being in touch with your own inner life, as expressed in your own images, can be a great source of strength and balance in withstanding the daily stresses of nursing with its constant exposure to human suffering and pain. I hope that through these exercises you find yourself more in touch with your own inner strength and more able to use it in your daily life.

REFERENCES

Bandler, R., and Grinder, J. 1975. *The structure of magic*, Vol. 1. Palo Alto, Calif.: Science and Behavior Books, Inc.

Bandler, R., and Grinder, J. 1976. *The structure of magic*, Vol. 2. Palo Alto, Calif.: Science and Behavior Books, Inc.

Barber, J. 1977. Rapid induction analgesia: a clinical report. *Am. J. Clin. Hypnosis*, Vol. 19, No. 3.

Benson, H., and Klipper, M. Z. 1976. *The relaxation response*. New York: Avon Books.

Brown, J. M., Chaves, J. F., and Leonoff, A. 1981. *Spontaneous hypnotic strategies in two groups of chronic pain patients*. Paper presented at the American Psychological Association Convention, Los Angeles, August 25.

Halpern, S. 1976. *Spectrum suite: soundscapes #1*. Palo Alto, Calif.: SRI Records and Tapes.

Hannah, B. 1981. *Encounters with the soul: active imagination as developed by C. G. Jung*. Santa Monica, Calif.: Sigo Press.

Krieger, D. 1979. *The therapeutic touch*. Englewood Cliffs, N.J.: Prentice Hall, Inc.

LeShan, L. 1974. *How to meditate*. New York: Random House.

Samuels, M., and Samuels, N. 1975. *Seeing with the mind's eye: the history, techniques and uses of visualization*. New York: Random House.

Simonton, O. C., Matthews-Simonton, S., and Creighton, J. 1978. *Getting well again*. Los Angeles: J. P. Tarcher, Inc.

Watzlawick, R. 1974. *Change: principles of problem formation and problem resolution*. New York: W. W. Norton & Co., Inc.

Weisman, A., and Worden, R. J. 1976. *Vulnerability and coping: a research report*. Cambridge, Mass.: Harvard University, Department of Psychiatry.

Annotated Bibliography

SHEILA K. BYRNE

For additional suggested reading on stress management see the references for each chapter. This is not a conclusive listing of relevant books but rather the ones I have found to be most useful for my nursing practice and personal knowledge. They are listed alphabetically for each part of the book.

PART 1: THE EFFECTS OF STRESS UPON THE NURSE'S WELL-BEING

Applebaum, H. 1982. *Stress management for health care professionals.* Rockville, Md.: An Aspen Publication.

> Explores the psychosocial and physiologic impact of stress on the health care "manager." Focuses solutions to the stress problem primarily upon systems interventions. Includes extensive amounts of stress literature, at times in almost an outlined form.

Edelwich, J., and Brodsky, A. 1980. *Burn-out: stages of disillusionment in the helping professions.* New York: Human Sciences Press.

> Concise account of what the author identifies as four stages leading to burn-out in human service occupations. Discusses each stage (enthusiasm, stagnation, frustration, and apathy) in detail. Symptoms and responses of each stage are elucidated by examples from human service workers' experiences. Discusses intervention, including short-term, long-term, institutional, and personal.

Freudenberger, H. J. 1980. *Burn-out: how to beat the high cost of success.* New York: Bantam Books.

> Gives numerous case studies of burned-out individuals and their experiences and attempts to handle the problem. Offers some useful suggestions for making work more tolerable.

Friedman, M., and Rosenman, R. H. 1974. *Type A behavior and your heart.* New York: Alfred A. Knopf.

Presents basis of type A and type B personality behavior, correlating type A to the coronary-prone individual.

Kramer, M. 1974. *Reality shock: why nurses leave nursing.* St. Louis: The C. V. Mosby Co.

Identifies the issues that lead to "reality shock" in new graduates and the unsuccessful ways nurses attempt to deal with the stresses/pressures of the nursing professions, and presents an approach, the anticipatory socialization program, for more effectively preparing nurses for their professional responsibilities. Essential reading for everyone in nursing (includes some nursing research studies).

Lazarus, R. S. 1966. *Psychological stress and the coping process.* New York: McGraw-Hill Book Co.

Research on stress and adaptation is presented in everyday language offering a conceptual framework to understand the relationship between psychologic events and the stress they produce. Emphasizes the perceptual and personality factors of stress appraisal.

McConnell, E. A. 1982. *Burnout in the nursing profession.* St. Louis: The C. V. Mosby Co.

An anthology, largely from journal articles, of current information on the burnout syndrome. Section headings: Coping Strategies for Preventing Burnout, The Burnout Syndrome, Potential Causes, The Cost of Burnout, and Historical Development of the Concept of Burnout in the Nursing Profession. Offers additional reading suggestions.

Muff, J., editor. 1982. *Socialization, sexism and stereotyping: feminist issues in nursing.* St. Louis: The C.V. Mosby Co.

Collection of primarily original articles that address the effects of various feminist issues upon the nurse and the nursing profession. A must for any nurse who wants to understand the personal and professional stressors of nursing.

Pelletier, K. R. 1977. *Mind as healer/mind as slayer: a holistic approach to preventing stress disorders.* New York: Delacorte Press.

Presents research and theory in a readable, understandable fashion. Provides an in-depth explanation of the mind-body connection and the stress-illness continuum. Discusses specific diseases of American culture such as cancer and heart disease. Useful description of various stress reduction techniques, including meditation, autogenic training, and visualization.

Selye, H. 1974. *Stress without distress.* New York: Signet.

Easy-to-read description of stress theory. Selye's philosophy of life as a prescription to manage stress. Focuses on positive use of stress.

Selye, H. 1976. *The stress of life*. New York: McGraw-Hill Book Co.

> Presents a "simplified summary of contemporary view on the scientific basis of the entire stress concept as it applies to any field." Describes the "discovery of stress," and the development of "stress-distress" theory.

PART 2: PHILOSOPHY OF SELF-CARE

A barefoot doctor's manual: a guide to traditional Chinese and modern medicine. 1972. Prepared by the Revolutionary Health Committee of Human Province. Mayne Isle & Seattle: Cloudburst Press.

> "This medical manual is an expression of modern China's intense effort to remember its past, to use what has been shown to be effective, and then build on this knowledge with modern Western and Chinese techniques." The concepts of health presented are based on the underlying theory of balance or disequilibrium of opposing forces. One-third of the manual is an illustrated guide to over 500 medicinal plants and their use. Curative practices are presented in diagrammed/illustrated step-by-step details. One of the *most* interesting books I've ever read!

Ardell, D. B. 1977. *High level wellness*. Emmaus, Pa.: Rodale Press and Bantam Books.

> Discusses the concept of five dimensions of high-level wellness: self-responsibility, nutritional awareness, stress management, physical fitness, and environmental sensitivity. Includes resource guide and annotated bibliography sections.

Baer, C. 1979. Effecting time management. In *TCN: Stress Management*, Rockville, Md.: Aspen Systems Corporation.

> An excellent article for the nurse who *never* has enough time. Exposes many myths related to time and offers hints for organizing and using time effectively.

Blattner, B. 1981. *Holistic nursing*. Englewood Cliffs, N.J.: Prentice-Hall, Inc.

> Presents holistic concepts and their application to nursing. Includes self-assessment tools and exercises. Focuses on a high-level wellness model of care instead of the traditional "illness" model of many nursing schools. The book grew out of an introductory course in holistic nursing.

Engel, G. L. 1977. The need for a new medical model: a challenge for biomedicine. *Science* 196(4286): 129–136.

> Critism of traditional medical model, which ignores the psychosocial influence of health care and illness. Offers model for medical care that shares responsibility and decision-making with a health team and the patient.

Ferner, J. D. 1980. *Successful time management.* New York: John Wiley and Sons, Inc.

A self-teaching guide for time management. Includes self-assessment tools and planning guides. Addresses issues such as controlling interruptions, effective delegation, and procrastination.

Flynn, R. A. P. 1980. *Holistic health: the art and science of care.* Bowie, Md.: Robert J. Brady Co.

Introduces concepts of health and high-level wellness and integrates humanistic nursing concepts with holistic health theory. Overview of "mind-body connection-disconnection" and neurophysiologic and psychosomatic research as they relate to holistic health practice. Contains a holistic wellness assessment section.

Hastings, A. C., Fademan, J., and Gordon, J. S., editors. 1981. *Health for the whole person: the complete guide to holistic medicine.* New York: Bantam Books.

Offers information from authorities in holistic health movement in a "survey" format. Extensive annotated bibliography section for each chapter. Presents both traditional and nontraditional approaches to health care and maintenance.

Knowles, J., editor. 1977. *Doing better and feeling worse: health in the United States.* New York: W. W. Norton.

Noted medical authorities address current problems in health care system as well as offer suggestions for future directions to improve health care. Reinforces need for personal responsibility in health maintenance

Lakin, A. 1973. *How to get control of your time and your life.* New York: Signet Books.

Helpful, practical suggestions for time management. Easy reading but very useful.

Veith, I., translator. 1972. *The yellow emperor's classic of internal medicine.* Berkeley, Calif.: University of California Press.

This translation covers some of ancient, traditional Chinese medicine as it was collected during the second century B.C. It is in dialogue form between the Yellow Emperor and his physician; addresses the relationship between human beings and nature and the causes and cures of illness. Amazing reading when you consider the advanced knowledge of anatomy and physiology known at that time.

Wiley, L. 1978. The ABC's of time management. *Nursing '78* 8(9):105–112.

Describes ways that staff nurses can effectively implement techniques of time management.

PART 3: SELF-AWARENESS TOOLS

Boston Womens' Health Collective. 1971. *Our bodies, ourselves: a book by and for women.* New York: Simon and Schuster.

> Self-care book designed for women to help them understand themselves and take responsibility for their wellness. Covers topics such as relationship, nutritional awareness, and physical fitness.

Ferguson, T., editor. 1980. *Medical self-care: access to health tools.* New York: Summit Books.

> Presents eight previously published issues of *Medical Self-Care* along with new articles. Extensive annotated bibliography and resource section for each chapter. Of interest for stress management are articles on eating, support groups, psychologic self-care, health workers, and self-care and stress/unstress.

James, M., and Jongeward, D. 1971. *Born to win.* Menlo Park, Calif.: Addison-Wesley Pub. Co.

> Combines transactional analysis and Gestalt therapy concepts to help people take responsibility for their lives and increase their basic sense of self-worth. Includes self-assessment questions. A classic.

Progoff, I. 1975. *At a journal workshop.* New York: Dialogue House Library.

> Introduces the *Intensive Journal* process with explicit directions that allow the reader to utilize this format without additional guidance or supervision. Extremely useful life-long process to increase self-awareness and personal growth.

Progoff, I. 1980. *The practice of process meditation.* New York: Dialogue House Library.

PART 4: THINKING YOUR WAY OUT OF DISTRESS

Beck, A. T. 1976. *Cognitive therapy and the emotional disorders.* New York: Meridian Books.

> Describes cognitive therapy as an approach to deal with various psychologic problems primarily through a problem-solving method. Discusses how we distort "reality" through faulty thinking. Emphasizes the patient's need to learn how to correct his or her thinking versus depending on the therapist to "cure" the problem.

Ellis, A. 1975. *A new guide to rational living.* Los Angeles, Wilshire Books.

> A guide to rational emotive therapy; identifies commonly held irrational beliefs and rational ideas to refute these with a step-by-step plan to develop rational thinking.

Glasser, W. 1965. *Reality therapy: a new approach to psychiatry*. New York: Harper and Row Publishers.

> Discusses the three Rs: 'reality,' responsibility, and right/wrong. First half of book presents theory of reality therapy; second half gives examples of how this can be applied to practice.

Glasser, W. 1976. *Positive addiction*. New York: Harper and Row Publishers.

> Addresses the negative aspects of addictive behavior such as drugs and alcohol and contrasts these with "positive addiction," being "hooked" on self-nurturing practices. A how-to book on turning a helpful activity into an addiction.

Gridano, D., and Everly, G. 1979. *Controlling stress and tension: a holistic approach*. Englewood Cliffs, N.J.: Prentice-Hall.

> Focuses on self-responsibility for health and illness and gives numerous self-assessment tools. Emphasizes the conceptual knowledge necessary to understand stress-reduction techniques. Stress management is generally presented from a life-style approach.

McKay, M., Davis, M., and Fanning, R. 1981. *Thoughts and feelings: the art of cognitive stress intervention*. Richmond, Ca: New Harbinger Publications.

> Workbook that provides "simple step-by-step directions for mastery" of various cognitive approaches to stress management. Introduction to such topics as problem-solving, covert assertion, and stress innoculation.

Morse, P. R., and Furst, M. L. 1979. *Stress for success*. New York: Van Nostrand Reinhold Co.

> Focuses on individual's ability to alter stress while criticizing the "invader-invaded" view of illness. Emphasizes the individual's responsibility to choose rewarding life-styles that minimize stress and disease.

Simoris, S. 1972. *Values clarification*. New York: Hart Publishers.

> Utilizes the assumption that one's values and beliefs determine how one interacts with others, perceives life events, and evaluates the sense of self-worth. Numerous experiential exercises to help clarify personal values that influence professional functioning.

PART 5: COLLECTIVE APPROACH FOR STRESS REDUCTION

Claus, K. E., and Bailey, J. T. 1977. *Power and influence in health care*. St. Louis: The C. V. Mosby Co.

> A great resource for nurses in leadership positions. Breaks down the negative attitudes that are assigned to the concept of *power*. Power is defined as a positive force commensurate with humanistic values of nursing. This book will help you

define personal, organizational, and social power and use it effectively in bringing about planned change.

Berne, E. 1964. *Games people play.* New York: Grove Press.

Introduction to transaction analysis that focuses on interactional styles in interpersonal relations. Useful in identifying personal patterns of interactions and "life-scripts" that help to influence current interpersonal dynamics.

Bower, S. A., and Bower, G. H. 1976. *Asserting your self: a practical guide for positive change.* Reading, Mass.: Addison-Wesley Pub. Co.

The book's goal is to provide an assertive training process for better self-management. An instructor's manual is also available. Step-by-step guide gives clear how-to information, exercises, and self-assessment tools. A good beginning book.

Brooten, D. A., Hayman, L., and Naylor, M. 1978. *Leadership for change: a guide for the frustrated nurse.* New York: J. B. Lippincott.

Excellent presentation of leadership skills that facilitate the development of optimal health care, with the nurse described as an equal participant in the health delivery system.

Butler, P. E. 1976. *Self assertion for women: a guide to becoming androgynous.* San Francisco: Harper and Row, Publisher.

Describes how being socialized as a woman contributes to nonassertive, victimized position. Many useful exercises and techniques to develop assertive skills.

Clark, C. C. 1978. *Assertive skills for nurses.* New York: Contemporary Publishing Co.

Essential for any nurse who wants to learn assertive skills as they apply to the nursing profession. Excellent examples; useful exercises and concrete suggestions for work environment. Can be used as part of a support group or for individual growth.

Cherniss, C. 1980. *Staff burnout: job stress in the human services.* Beverly Hills, Calif.: Sage Publications.

Series of monographs and edited collections of original articles that deal with issues and themes of current concern in community mental health and related fields. Addresses issues of social support and supervision.

House, J. S. 1981. *Work stress and social support.* In *Addison-Wesley Series on Stress.* Reading, Mass.: Addison-Wesley Pub. Co.

Extensive review of research related to the relationship between stress and social support.

Veniga, R. 1979. Administrator burn-out—causes and cures. *Hosp. Prog.* February:45–52.

> An excellent article that is a must for all administrators/managers. Describes symptoms of burn-out and delineates those life-styles/work-styles that are based upon unrealistic expectations and can contribute to eventual burn-out. Several organizational situations that place administrators in frustrating and defeating positions are identified and several unique measures for burn-out prevention or intervention are identified.

PART 6: STRESS REDUCTION TECHNIQUES AND COPING STRATEGIES

Basmajian, J. V., editor. 1978. *Biofeedback—principles and practice for clinicians.* Baltimore: Williams and Wilkins.

> Descriptions of the clinical application of biofeedback are presented by recognized authorities. Biofeedback principles and techniques are applied to such diverse areas as rehabilitation, pregnancy and labor, voluntary movement disorders, and cardiovascular diseases.

Benson, H. 1975. *The relaxation response.* New York: Avon.

> Explains physiologic nature of stress and simple meditative technique to cope with stress. Reviews research to support usefulness of techniques. Numerous quotes from ancient teachers: Buddha, St. Augustine, Lao-tse.

Berkeley Holistic Health Center, compiler. 1978. *The holistic health handbook.* Berkeley, Calif.: AND/OR Press.

> Offers a "variety of representative systems for healing the whole person," giving a "comprehensive and multidimensional view of the holistic movement." Presents diverse healing systems and techniques such as holistic nutrition, autogenic training, Native American healing, and reflexology. Mostly nontraditional approaches.

Crasilneck, H. B., and Hall, J. A. 1975. *Clinical hypnosis: principles and applications.* New York: Grune and Stratton.

> Overview of theoretical concepts and application of hypnosis, giving detailed induction techniques.

Davis, M., Eshelman, E. R., and McKay, M. 1980. *The relaxation and stress reduction workbook.* Richmond, Calif.: New Harbinger Publications.

> Workbook giving brief introduction of theory, assessment tools, and activities/exercises for stress management techniques. Gives good overview of such techniques as progressive relaxation, rational emotive therapy, and autogenic training.

Samuels, M., and Samuels, N. 1975. *Seeing with the mind's eye*. New York: Random House.

The "complete" book of visualization; numerous illustrations and exercises giving suggestions for the therapeutic use of visual imagery. Presents the physiologic, psychologic, and historic aspects of visualization.

Shapiro, D., and Walsh, R. 1979. *Meditation: self-regulation strategy and altered state of consciousness*. New York: Aldine Press.

Presents self-regulating strategies as well as research findings demonstrating the change that occurs during meditation and altered states of consciousness.

Simonton, O. C., Matthews-Simonton, S., and Creighton, J. 1978. *Getting well again*. Los Angeles: J. P. Tarcher.

Applies visual imagery to clinical treatment of cancer and endorses the view that positive imagery can stop or slow down the growth of cancer. Addresses the psychosomatic aspects of cancer. Further research is needed to validate the usefulness of their approach but at least their method is helpful in helping patients feel better.

Resources

This section is a sampling of available resources for continued growth; it focuses on stress management and personal development. The resources are listed alphabetically. In addition to the resources listed here, most colleges and universities offer classes or workshops on stress-management–related subjects; numerous schools of nursing and hospitals are beginning to implement holistic health practices into their services and education; and most communities offer recreational facilities or physical fitness programs. Look under telephone directory listings such as physical fitness, exercise programs, relaxation, and other specialized techniques (hypnosis, gestalt therapy, cognitive centers). You will also find that once you get on someone's mailing list, you will soon receive a tremendous number of unsolicited "self-help" announcements and advertisements, some of which are useful, others of which are pure junk!

ORGANIZATIONS/ASSOCIATIONS

Autogenics. International Center for Autogenic Therapy, Medical Center, 5300 Cotes des Neiges, Room 550, Montreal H3T IYE, Canada.

> Offers information about autogenic training and therapy.

Biofeedback. Biofeedback Society, University of Colorado Medical School, 4200 E. Ninth Ave., Denver, Colo.

> Research-oriented society offering information on the most recent practice and theory of biofeedback.

Chinese Medicine. Center for Chinese Medicine, 230 South Garfield Avenue, Suite 202, Monterey Park, Calif. 91754.

> Nonprofit, educational organization offers seminars and workshops on Chinese medicine for health care professionals. Presentations on acupressure, pain control, proper nutrition, and relaxation.

Holistic Approach to Aging. Association for Humanistic Gerontology, 1711 Solano Avenue, Berkeley, Calif. 94707.

> Publishes "comprehensive members catalogue" and list of national conferences and seminars.

Holistic Approach to Aging. The Gray Panthers, 3700 Chestnut Street, Philadelphia, Pa. 19104.

> "A national coalition of old, young, and middle-aged activists" who emphasize "the relationship between personal growth, self-development, holistic health and liberation from negative stereotyping."

Holistic Nursing. Holistic Nurses Association (A.H.N.A.), Box 116, Telluride, Colo. 81435.

> Excellent means to become part of a holistic nursing network. Offers newsletters, "Beginnings"; articles on holistic practice, and news of holistic educational opportunities throughout the United States.

Holistic Nursing. Nurse Consultants and Health Counselors: The Healing Center, 465 Brussels, San Francisco, Calif. 94134.

> Holistic healing is offered to groups and individuals by therapists. A contact for learning how to establish your own holistic counseling service.

Homeopathy. Nutritional Center for Homeopathy, 6231 Leesburg Pike, Falls Church, Va. 22044.

> Offers material and information on homeopathy.

Human Growth and Wellness. Institute for Advancement of Human Behavior (I.A.H.B.), Box 2288, Stanford, Calif. 94305.

> Presents national workshops and seminars on topics related to the human growth and wellness movement. Examples of recent presentations and speakers: "The Human Connection," Rollo May, Gerald Piaget, George Bach; "Wellness: Optimizing Health in Mind and Body," Hans Selye, Arnold A. Lazarus, and O. Carl Simonton; "Frontiers of Health," Muriel James, Albert Ellis, and Meyer Friedman.

Hypnosis. Milton H. Erickson Foundation, Inc., 3606 N. 24th Street, Phoenix, Ariz. 85016, (602) 956-6196.

> Publishes newsletters covering upcoming hypnosis workshops and seminars throughout the U.S.A. and abroad, book reviews, and "notes" about the foundation (free).

Journal Writing. Dialogue House News, 80 East 11th Street, New York, N.Y. 10003

> Mails out notices of local and national *Intensive Journal* workshops based on the work of Ira Progoff.

Rational Emotive Therapy. Institute for Rational Living, Inc., 45 E. 65th Street, New York, N.Y. 10021.

> Provides articles and books, as well as talks, seminars, and workshops "in the area of human growth and rational living."

Residential Learning Center. Esalen Institute, Big Sur, Calif. 93920.

> Offers workshops, seminars, and extended residential learning programs that focus on human potential and explore the values of human existence. Offers continuing education in many workshops such as Burnout, Holistic Health Training Program, Healing Community, Massage for Health Professionals. Catalog three times a year for $6.00. Tapes on various human potential topics available at $9.00–$16.00, as well as films of such notables as Fritz Perls, Rollo May, Carl Rogers. (Being at Esalen was one of the best experiences of my life!)

Transactional Analysis. International Transactional Association, 1772 Vallejo Street, San Francisco, Calif. 94108.

> Offers information about transactional analysis learning opportunities and clinicians throughout the United States.

MEDIA/JOURNALS

American Educational Films, 132 Lasky Drive, Beverly Hills, Calif. 90212.

> Several films on such topics as "Stress and You," "Stress, Health and You," "Relaxation Techniques," and "Learning to Cope."

Bio-Monitoring Applications Inc., 270 Madison Avenue, New York, N.Y. 10016.

> Two films especially related to education on stress management: "Life Stress Measurement and Illness Diagnosis and Treatment" written by R. H. Rake, M.D., and "Biofeedback Stress Management in Headache Pain Control."

BMA Audio Cassettes, 200 Park Avenue South, New York, N.Y. 10003, 1 (800) 221-3966.

> Extensive offering of audio cassettes on stress management and general self-help made from presentations of noted authorities. For example; "Clinical Hypnosis" by Herbert and David Spiegel; "The Power of Imagery for Personal Enrichment" by Arnold A. Lazarus; "Principles and Practice of Progressive Relaxation" by Edmund Jacobson, M.D.

Concept Media, Box 19542, Irvine, Calif. 92714.

> Several filmstrips designed for nurses and other health care professionals on stress and stress management; called the "Stress Series." Covers such topics as relaxation response, biofeedback, autogenic training, long-range life patterns, and relationship between job stress and disease.

Conscious Living Foundation, P.O. Box 513, Manhattan, Kan. 66502.

Nonprofit educational institution that offers free catalog listing books and cassettes for biofeedback stress management, relaxation, and imagery.

Learning Resources Corporation, 8517 Production Avenue, P.O. Box 26240, San Diego, Calif. 92126.

Newsletter on stress management books, workshops, and learning tools. Most of their learning tools offer experiential learning exercises for educators. Lifelong Learning Series of audiotapes made from a University of California Extension Media Center presents the principles of holistic health by leaders in the field. Examples: "Mind as Healer, Mind as Slayer" by Kenneth R. Pelletier; "Belief Systems and Cancer" by Carl and Stephanie Simonton, "Biogenic and Relaxation Exercises" by Norman Shealy.

McGraw-Hill Films, 110 15th Street, Del Mar, Calif. 92014.

Although "Managing Stress" discusses theory of stress and stress management as it relates to individuals in the business community, all the information presented is directly applicable to nursing. I often use this film in stress workshops.

Medical Self-Care: Access to Health Tools. Edited by Tom Ferguson, M.D. P.O. Box 717B Inverness, Calif. 94937.

One of the best journals on holistic self-care with a format similar to the *Whole Earth Magazine*.

Olympic Media Information, 71 West 23rd Street, New York, N.Y. 10010.

Puts out brief profiles of available hospital training and health care media information, listing the content, synopsis, evaluation, and availability. Available by subscription.

Psychology Today Cassettes, P.O. Box 278, Pratt Station, Brooklyn, N.Y. 11205. $10.95/cassette tapes. Free catalog.

Noted authorities present most essential concepts on stress management, self-help, and enhancing human potential. Offers such topics as "Rational Emotive Psychotherapy" by Albert Ellis; "Understanding and Coping with Anxiety" by Rollo May; "Deep Relaxation" by Daniel Golemen; "Assertiveness Training" by Robert Alberti and Michael Emmons.

Self-Help Report (bi-monthly), free, National Self-Help Clearing House, 184 Fifth Ave., New York, N.Y. 10010.

Newsletter reporting information on publications and articles of interest for self-help.

Trainex, P.O. Box 116, 12601 Industry St., Garden Grove, Calif. 92642.

Offers several filmstrips with cassettes on stress-related topics: "Stress, Tension and the Relaxation Response" and "Stresses."

Index